CW00501995

Black Skin, White Coats

NEW AFRICAN HISTORIES SERIES

SERIES EDITORS: JEAN ALLMAN AND ALLEN ISAACMAN

Books in this series are published with support from the Ohio University National Resource Center for African Studies.

David William Cohen and E. S. Atieno Odhiambo, *The Risks of Knowledge: Investigations into the Death of the Hon. Minister John Robert Ouko in Kenya, 1990*

Belinda Bozzoli, *Theatres of Struggle and the End of Apartheid*

Gary Kynoch, *We Are Fighting the World: A History of Marashea Gangs in South Africa, 1947–1999*

Stephanie Newell, *The Forger's Tale: The Search for Odeziaku*

Jacob A. Tropp, *Natures of Colonial Change: Environmental Relations in the Making of the Transkei*

Jan Bender Shetler, *Imagining Serengeti: A History of Landscape Memory in Tanzania from Earliest Times to the Present*

Cheikh Anta Babou, *Fighting the Greater Jihad: Amadu Bamba and the Founding of the Muridiyya in Senegal, 1853–1913*

Marc Epprecht, *Heterosexual Africa? The History of an Idea from the Age of Exploration to the Age of AIDS*

Marissa J. Moorman, *Intonations: A Social History of Music and Nation in Luanda, Angola, from 1945 to Recent Times*

Karen E. Flint, *Healing Traditions: African Medicine, Cultural Exchange, and Competition in South Africa, 1820–1948*

Derek R. Peterson and Giacomo Macola, editors, *Recasting the Past: History Writing and Political Work in Modern Africa*

Moses Ochonu, *Colonial Meltdown: Northern Nigeria in the Great Depression*

Emily Burrill, Richard Roberts, and Elizabeth Thornberry, editors, *Domestic Violence and the Law in Colonial and Postcolonial Africa*

Daniel R. Magaziner, *The Law and the Prophets: Black Consciousness in South Africa, 1968–1977*

Emily Lynn Osborn, *Our New Husbands Are Here: Households, Gender, and Politics in a West African State from the Slave Trade to Colonial Rule*

Robert Trent Vinson, *The Americans Are Coming! Dreams of African American Liberation in Segregationist South Africa*

James R. Brennan, *Taifa: Making Nation and Race in Urban Tanzania*

Benjamin N. Lawrance and Richard L. Roberts, editors, *Trafficking in Slavery's Wake: Law and the Experience of Women and Children*

David M. Gordon, *Invisible Agents: Spirits in a Central African History*

Allen Isaacman and Barbara Isaacman, *Dams, Displacement, and the Delusion of Development: Cahora Bassa and Its Legacies in Mozambique, 1965–2007*

Stephanie Newell, *The Power to Name: A History of Anonymity in Colonial West Africa*

Gibril R. Cole, *The Krio of West Africa: Islam, Culture, Creolization, and Colonialism in the Nineteenth Century*

Matthew M. Heaton, *Black Skin, White Coats: Nigerian Psychiatrists, Decolonization, and the Globalization of Psychiatry*

Black Skin, White Coats

Nigerian Psychiatrists, Decolonization, and the Globalization of Psychiatry

Matthew M. Heaton

OHIO UNIVERSITY PRESS ∽ ATHENS

Ohio University Press, Athens, Ohio 45701
ohioswallow.com
© 2013 by Ohio University Press
All rights reserved

To obtain permission to quote, reprint, or otherwise reproduce or distribute material from Ohio University Press publications, please contact our rights and permissions department at (740) 593-1154 or (740) 593-4536 (fax).

Printed in the United States of America
Ohio University Press books are printed on acid-free paper.∞ ™

20 19 18 17 16 15 14 13 5 4 3 2 1

Library of Congress Cataloging-in-Publication Data

Heaton, Matthew M., author.
Black skin, white coats : Nigerian psychiatrists, decolonization, and the globalization of psychiatry / Matthew M. Heaton.
pages cm. — (New African histories)
ISBN 978-0-8214-2070-6 (pb : alk. paper) — ISBN 978-0-8214-4473-3 (electronic)
1. Psychiatry—Nigeria–History. 2. Cultural psychiatry—Nigeria. 3. Mentally ill—Care—Nigeria—History. 4. Mental illness—Treatment—Nigeria–History. 5. Nigeria—Colonial influence—Health aspects—History. I. Title. II. Series: New African histories series.
RC438.H43 2013
362.209669—dc23 2013027515

For
Ann

Contents

Acknowledgments

I owe an enormous debt of gratitude to so many people who made the completion of this project possible. This book grew out of a dissertation written for the Department of History at the University of Texas at Austin. I am grateful for the financial support of the Department of History and the John L. Warfield Center for African and African American Studies at UT, which facilitated research trips to Nigeria and the United Kingdom in 2004 and 2005. I am also very thankful to Toyin Falola, under whose mentorship this research began and through whose friendship and advice it has continued to develop these many years. The support and advice of many others has also shaped this work. I would particularly like to thank Barbara Harlow, A. G. Hopkins, Bruce Hunt, and Juliet E. K. Walker for their formative influence, which has been greater than they all know.

This research would also not have been possible without the assistance of friends in Nigeria whose kindness and generosity sustained me and facilitated my work. Saheed Aderinto and family hosted me in Ibadan for many months in 2004 and 2005 and introduced me to the national archives there. I would also like to thank Demola Babalola and family for their generous hospitality in Lagos and Ilé-Ifẹ̀. In Kaduna, I owe Hauwa Yusuf and family more than I can ever repay for the kindness they showed me. I also want to offer my heartfelt appreciation to Olayemi Akinwumi for his generous gifts of time and help. My thanks also go out to the staff at the branches of the Nigerian National Archives, particularly "Mr. Mike" in Ibadan and Ibrahim Abdu in Kaduna. Dr. Timothy Adebowale at Aro Neuropsychiatric Hospital provided me with important insights for which I am very grateful.

I also conducted research for this project at the National Archives of the United Kingdom, Public Records Office, Kew; and the archives of the World Health Organization. I would like to thank the staffs of these organizations for their assistance, particularly Marie Villemin-Partow and Thomas Allen at the WHO.

What began as a very narrowly defined dissertation on the repatriation of Nigerian "lunatics" during Nigeria's colonial era developed into a much broader-based book on the decolonization of psychiatry in Nigeria and beyond. This transformation has occurred mostly through engagement with a variety of scholarly influences since I joined the Department of History at Virginia Tech in 2008. I would like to thank Virginia Tech for a generous start-up package that allowed me to conduct further fieldwork in Nigeria in 2009 as well as to attend several academic conferences that have shaped my thinking. A semester of junior faculty leave allowed me time to complete the first draft of the manuscript, and a Dean's Faculty Fellowship from the College of Liberal Arts and Human Sciences bought me time to complete revisions. Research assistants Scott Brennan, Amanda Clark, Charles Sanders, and Marc Egan helped to compile and organize materials. My colleagues at Virginia Tech have been immensely supportive. In particular, I would like to thank Mark Barrow, Tom Ewing, Heather Gumbert, Bernice Hausman, Dennis Hidalgo, Kathleen Jones, Marian Mollin, P. S. Polanah, Helen Schneider, Robert Stephens, and Dan Thorp for their advice, friendship, and support over the years.

This work also benefited greatly from my experience in 2011 as a fellow of the National History Center's Seminar on Decolonization, sponsored by the John W. Kluge Center of the Library of Congress and the Mellon Foundation. The research I conducted through this seminar helped shape my thinking on this project, and the comments and the advice of the seminarians were very valuable. I would particularly like to thank the organizers, John Darwin, Philippa Levine, Wm. Roger Louis, Jason Parker, Sudhir Pillarisetti, and Miriam Hauss Cunningham, for their assistance and advice.

Many people have read all or part of this project at various stages or otherwise provided commentary that has helped shape the end result. I greatly appreciate the time, energy, and expertise of Brett Bennett, Tyler Fleming, Joseph M. Hodge, Christian Jennings, Sloan Mahone, Jonathan H. Sadowsky, Brett Shadle, and Joel Tishken. Rachel Cooper, Ivan Crozier, and Roland Littlewood provided valuable insights on brain-fag syndrome at the Concepts of Health and Disease, Workshop on Culture-Bound Syndromes, held at the University of Lancaster in 2009. I also thank the anonymous readers of the manuscript as well as series editors Jean Allman and Allen Isaacman for their advice. My gratitude also goes out to Gillian Berkowitz at Ohio University Press for her steadfast assistance in bringing this book finally to press.

Finally, I thank family and friends who have helped see me through the long, sometimes dark process of completing this project. You are too many to mention, but you know who you are. To my wife and best friend, Ann: I can't tell you how grateful I am for your love, wisdom, patience, and perseverance.

Introduction

Colonizing, Decolonizing, and Globalizing the History of Psychiatry

In African psychiatry one can follow the early inception, metamorphosis, ripening and diffusion of the world psychiatry of today.

—Dr. Tigani El-Mahi, First Pan-African Psychiatric Conference, Abeokuta, Nigeria, 12 November 1961

On 12 November 1961, Thomas Adeoye Lambo convened the First Pan-African Psychiatric Conference in his hometown of Abeokuta, Nigeria. Lambo was the first indigenous Nigerian to become a Western-trained psychiatrist, and in 1954 he had become the first superintendent of Aro Mental Hospital, the first fully functioning mental hospital in Nigeria. In his foreword to the conference proceedings, Lambo recounted the goals of his historic conference. He noted the "amazing changes in the social, cultural and political life of Africa" in the previous decade. He described the "growth of factories, cities and towns, rise of business corporations, of trade unions, of new government concerns and projects, and problems in human relations" consequent to these changes.[1] He wondered how these political, economic, and environmental changes had affected the minds of individual human beings. Indeed, how had these changes affected the ways psychiatrists thought about the nature of mental illness in human beings?

Lambo's conference was held just a year after Nigeria became a sovereign state, independent from British colonial rule, and just four years after Ghana became the first country in sub-Saharan Africa to do so. It occurred just one year before the end of the bloody war of liberation in Algeria, where Frantz Fanon was chronicling the psychological impact of European power on colonial subjects. The conference was held at a time when most of the African continent had undertaken or was currently involved in an active process of decolonization. In sum, it was a time of reordering the geopolitical spectrum that had been based on the notion of white superiority for at least the previous three-quarters of a century. In other words, it was a time for defining a new normal. And when a new normal is defined, a new abnormal must be defined with it. The conference therefore took place at a time when bedrock notions about the relationship between race, culture, and mental illness were changing. They were changing because of the work of transcultural psychiatrists like Lambo, and they were being transformed through events like the First Pan-African Psychiatric Conference.

At the conference, ninety-two participants from twenty-two different countries in Africa, Europe, and North America presented cutting-edge research on mental illness and its treatment in African patients. Many major figures in transcultural psychiatry were present. They included Alexander H. Leighton of Cornell University; Sir Aubrey Lewis of the University of London; the founder of the World Federation for Mental Health, John R. Rees; and the French psychiatrist Henri Collomb, whose cross-cultural work at the Fann psychiatric hospital in Dakar spawned the Fann school of ethnopsychiatry. Ernest Gruenberg of the Millbank Foundation in the United States and E. E. Krapf of the World Health Organization, whose collaborations on psychiatric epidemiology were just beginning, presented papers. Also present was the famed (and defamed) ethnopsychiatrist J. C. Carothers, whose racialized ethnopsychiatry was becoming rapidly outdated; in attendance as well were the first three indigenous Africans to earn medical specialties in psychiatry: E. F. B. Forster, a Gambian who practiced in Ghana; Tigani El-Mahi of Sudan; and Lambo himself.

The purpose of the conference, according to its key organizers, was to advance the study of mental illness and its treatment in African countries. The emphasis in doing so was on uncovering the universal similarities of human psyches across cultural boundaries, through cooperative research endeavors and the development of networks of knowledge transfer and dissemination. In his opening remarks to the conference, Alexander H. Leighton emphasized the "unity of mankind" and declared the purpose of the conference to be the consideration "of certain universal human problems," remarking that success in this endeavor depended on "learning from experience wherever it has been had, on the exchange of information, and on the sharing of techniques."[2] Aubrey Lewis reiterated this point in his comments, stating unambiguously that "the basic principles of psychiatry seem to me of universal application, and we have no grounds for supposing that there are fundamental psychological differences between people of different ethnic groups."[3] And Lambo lamented that "there has never been a time when so many ideas and methods were employed in different parts of the world in the service of mental health as are today. They are working concomitantly, but unfortunately, too independently of each other."[4] For the key players of this conference, progress in psychiatric science would come through the organization of local, regional, and national research projects into a highly integrated global network and through the synthesis of research findings into a universal theory of human psychology based on the ideas of racial and cultural equality. The pursuance of these ideas had come to be known in the 1950s as transcultural psychiatry.[5]

The globally conscious agenda of the conference attracted a variety of international supporters. International nongovernmental and corporate sponsors included the Rockefeller Foundation and Pfizer Products. Her Royal Highness Princess Marina, a major patron of the National Association for Mental Health in the United Kingdom, sent her best wishes. A. H. Taba, the director of the World Health Organization in the eastern Mediterranean, also sent supporting words along with a gift for Lambo and Aro Hospital: a tapestry featuring Imhotep, an Egyptian official from the twenty-seventh century BCE, considered by many to be the first physician in human history and considered by politically conscious Africans as an example of the antiquity of African civilization and the essential contributions of Africans to world civilization itself. The gift was a reminder that the "Pan-African" in the conference title stood for more than a definition of scope: it was a political message referencing the power and dignity of African peoples and cultures, the need to unite to overcome oppression, and the importance of the process of self-definition, all of which, it will be seen, were as salient in the realm of psychiatric knowledge production as they were in other areas.

The political implications of an internationally recognized scientific conference trumpeting notions of racial equality and the "unity of mankind" were not lost on Nigerian politicians either. The federal government of Nigeria and the western regional government were sponsors of the event. Over the course of the five-day conference, participants met with several powerful political figures in Nigeria, including the alake of Abeokuta, the governor of the Western Region of Nigeria, the federal minister of health, and the prime minister of Nigeria himself, Sir Alhaji Tafawa Balewa. For these politicians, the conference, and its location in Abeokuta, the site of Aro Mental Hospital and the groundbreaking work of Dr. Lambo, served a strong symbolic purpose. Aro and Lambo illustrated the value attained by indigenous leadership. The conference legitimized anticolonial sentiment, decolonization processes, and by extension the First Republic government itself. The emphasis of the conference and Lambo's work in general on the "unity of mankind" underscored sentiments about racial and cultural equality in the context of anticolonial nationalism that still resonated in postindependence Nigeria. Lambo's international connections and the importance of his work beyond the borders of Nigeria represented the potential of Africa's "sleeping giant," feeding into notions held in the early sixties that Nigeria was poised to become a leading figure not only in African but in world affairs.

While participants were engaged in scientific discourses emphasizing human unity, Lambo made sure that they were also provided with extracurricular experiences that deliberately juxtaposed the richness of indigenous Nigerian cultures with Nigeria's transition into a postcolonial modernity. A tour of the alake's palace was balanced with a tour of the House of Assembly of the Western Region. A trip to the Lagos Museum was followed by a performance by egúngún dancers. Conference participants visited the University College, Ibadan, where Alexander Brown, a professor of medicine, showed them "the many attractive, modern and functional buildings" of the university as well as an "interesting collection of Nigerian Arts and Crafts." This was followed by a luncheon, "which included many Nigerian dishes."[6] The conference was clearly a site not only of scientific exchange but also of cultural and political expression. And T. Adeoye Lambo, the man at its center, had designed it this way.

This book examines the transformations in psychiatric theory and practice that accompanied the decolonization of European empires in Africa in the mid-twentieth century, taking Nigeria as a case study. The complex intertwining of scientific, political, and cultural agendas apparent in the execution of the First Pan-African Psychiatric Conference is a microcosm of the issues explored more broadly in this book. At a basic level, I make three overarching arguments in the chapters that follow. First, the transformations in psychiatric theory and practice to which psychiatrists in Nigeria contributed were inherently linked to the sociopolitical and historical contexts of their times and places. This is by no means a new argument: it has been the bedrock principle of the social history of medicine, including the history of psychiatry. The definitions, theories, and professional culture of psychiatry change over time as a result of scientific findings that both influence and are influenced by the worlds within which scientists live and work, as well as by the dreams, aspirations, and values of those scientists. In the context of this book, Nigerian psychiatrists' political and professional agendas meshed in ways that led them to repudiate racist conceptions of the inferiority of African psyches that had developed in the context of European colonial rule and to replace them with a theory of the universal similarities of human psychological processes that transcended perceived boundaries between races and cultures. These agendas were established in the context of a graduated decolonization both in Nigeria and globally, in which the structural and ideological relationships of a world dominated by European colonialism were themselves being reformed.

The second argument is that in transforming colonial psychiatric institutions and theories, Nigerian psychiatrists were intimately engaged in a contrived but nonetheless preoccupying negotiation about what postcolonial "modernity" should look like, not only in Nigeria but in the world at large. They did not simply buy into the idea that Western ideas could be universally applied to bring about the development of the emerging Third World, but they did believe that the frameworks professional psychiatry had created in Western historical and cultural contexts could be adapted and redefined to incorporate non-Western realities in ways that could then claim to be universal. Third, in the context of decolonization and independence, psychiatric discourse both in Nigeria and globally took on an intensely cross-cultural, transnational, and international character that cannot be separated from local, regional, and national developments. The Nigerian psychiatrists discussed in this monograph did not exist in a racial or cultural bubble. They worked with African psychiatrists from other countries, with white transcultural psychiatrists from Europe and North America, and were broadly aware of developments in transcultural psychiatry coming out of Asia. The transnational and international connections are as much a part of the story of the decolonization of psychiatry in Nigeria as the decolonization of psychiatry in Nigeria is to the broader history of psychiatry as a medical discipline. To keep the two separate, as has often been the custom to date, means oversimplifying narratives in ways that too often reinforce the stark boundaries between "colonizer/colonized, Western/non-Western, and domination/resistance" that Frederick Cooper has urged us to avoid.[7]

The story I am telling here could be reproduced in a variety of different contexts, if perhaps unevenly. Transcultural psychiatrists working throughout the world in the twentieth century were combating many of the same established notions of racial difference and psychological inferiority. Many other African and Asian countries were engaged in the decolonization of psychiatric institutions in the mid-twentieth century. All of these groups were contributing to the emergence of global networks of transcultural psychiatry simultaneously with those working in Nigeria. Comparative studies are needed, but Nigeria is a particularly good place on which to focus this examination for three specific reasons. First, while I am arguing here that Nigerians' contributions to a global psychiatry are a representation of the ways that non-Western persons and agendas have helped transform conceptions of psychological universals, Nigeria's case is special in some ways and cannot be extrapolated to all decolonizing spaces or non-Western environments. Nigerian psychiatrists like Lambo, Tolani Asuni, and a few others, and later a second generation influenced by them, became active organizers of international networks of knowledge production, dissemination, and application from the late 1950s. The revolutionary research and treatment methods that Lambo pioneered at Aro Mental Hospital became internationally renowned, and were used as models to be replicated and adapted in other parts of the world (see chapter 2). Aro Mental Hospital also became an important space for the collection of data about mental illness in Nigerian populations, providing resources and personnel for important cross-cultural research projects. Lambo himself had a second career in global health, rising to become deputy director-general of the World Health Organization in the 1970s.

Second, Nigeria's psychiatric infrastructure developed much more quickly and extensively than in most African countries. By the 1970s it was one of the few countries in Africa that could train psychiatrists locally. Most African countries could not or did not invest in psychiatry in the way that Nigeria did, although even Nigeria's investment has proved to be inadequate over the long term. For these reasons, developments in Nigeria serve as a particularly strong focal point from which to provide analysis of the tensions between modernization and Western hegemony, scientific universalism and cultural contingencies. Analysis of the Nigerian context helps to conceptualize historical dynamics in professional psychiatry in other postcolonial contexts without presuming that the same agendas, results, or conclusions necessarily were obtained everywhere.

Finally, although I am making a case for the historical interconnectedness of global and local dynamics in the theory and practice of psychiatry, focusing on developments in Nigeria allows for the elaboration of the local component. To examine the expansion of a global discourse on universal psychiatry that used Western terminologies and definitions as its basis from the top down would reinscribe notions of Western hegemony and of a unidirectional power flow. I want to emphasize quite the opposite: that political, social, and cultural dynamics in the context of decolonization and independence in a non-Western space transmitted outward to transform psychiatric knowledge production processes in ways that have significantly influenced what cross-cultural psychiatrists think and do today. Making this argument requires an in-depth examination of the way those political, social, and cultural factors at the local and national levels worked their way into global discussions about the nature of mental illness in diverse cultures.

POSTCOLONIAL HISTORIES OF PSYCHIATRY AND HISTORIES OF POSTCOLONIAL PSYCHIATRY

In examining the complex interactions of political, ideological, social, and scientific factors that impinged upon the transformation of psychiatry in the context of decolonization and national independence in Nigeria, this book contributes to and expands upon several emerging conceptual trajectories in the social history of medicine in Africa, most notably in the blurring of the boundaries of what constitutes colonial medicine and the decentering of the explicitly nationalist narrative of postcolonial medical history. Histories of colonial medicine in Africa since the 1980s have engaged heavily in a postcolonial critique of the ways in which European colonial governments used constructed medical knowledge to justify their intrusion in humanitarian terms and to enforce social controls that promoted white, European agendas at the expense of black, African bodies.[8] Far from seeing the imposition of Western biomedicine in African societies as an unquestioned benefit of the colonial experience, historians have shown how European colonizers presented African cultures as responsible for the heavy disease burdens that their communities experienced, for example, how supposedly "primitive" understandings of personal and public hygiene resulted in the spread of epidemic diseases.[9] Under such circumstances, colonial governments often felt justified in disrupting long-standing African political, economic, and cultural practices, both to protect themselves from contamination by Africans and on the assumption that ultimately European social engineering would be for the good of Africans' own health. Such histories often take a positivist stance, emphasizing the extent to which the actions of colonial governments were, in fact, based on shoddy scientific and medical knowledge that frequently did more harm than good in terms of understanding local conditions and providing for better health outcomes. Thus, colonial policies often failed to achieve desired results while simultaneously alienating colonial subjects from the regimes that claimed to govern in their best interests.[10] Beyond this, however, social histories of colonial medicine in Africa also emphasize a broader connection between medicalization and pathologization that has been explored in a wide variety of colonial contexts.[11]

Histories of psychiatry have also illustrated the ideological component in colonial constructions of African minds. Beginning with Megan Vaughan's 1983 examination of the Zomba Lunatic Asylum in British Nyasaland (now

Malawi),[12] historians have provided a variety of detailed accounts of the ways that European definitions of madness in colonized populations were intimately bound up with "othering" processes, in which the African mind was constructed as both opposite of and inferior to the average European psyche. In constructing this duality, with its strong racial component, the "normal" colonial subject became psychologically pathological from the colonizer's perspective. This analysis has been seconded in a small, highly coherent literature on colonial psychiatry and, in particular, the colonial lunatic asylum. Leland V. Bell, Jock McCulloch, Lynette A. Jackson, Harriet J. Deacon, and Julie Parle, among others, have consistently shown colonial asylums to be vehicles of explicit social control rather than institutions of healing throughout colonial Africa.[13] Of particular importance for this study is Jonathan H. Sadowsky's analysis of colonial lunatic asylums in southwestern Nigeria, which he describes as chronically underfunded, understaffed, and overcrowded, partly for economic and partly for ideological reasons, a sentiment that this book largely echoes in chapter 1.[14] These historical analyses have intellectual roots in Michel Foucault's articulation of the dialectic between "madness" and "reason," which reveals the innate relationship between social constructions of insanity and the social control mechanisms of the state, as well as in Frantz Fanon's radical critique of colonialism as not only constructing colonial subjects as pathological but also creating pathological colonial subjects through the physical, social, and psychological violence of the everyday colonial experience.[15]

However, histories of psychiatry in Africa have also significantly critiqued Foucault's overdetermined causalities and Fanon's Manichaean tendencies, illustrating the contingencies and limitations of colonial medical knowledge about African bodies and minds as well as the gray area between colonizer/colonized and traditional/modern dichotomies. Western biomedical science has never had a monopoly on the dialogue about the causes and treatments of physical illnesses in colonized spaces. In terms of psychiatry, Western theories of the definitions, causes, and treatments for mental illness in colonial contexts were marginally influential at best, linked explicitly to alien power structures but not particularly salient in terms of colonial subjects' perspectives or lived experiences. In all colonial African territories, the vast majority of the population had little or no interaction at all with colonial psychiatric structures, which existed mostly only in urban areas and only for the sequestration of particularly violent "lunatics." Even those with an intimate relationship to colonial psychiatric diagnosis did not necessarily buy into the supposed superiority of European knowledge about the nature of mental illness. Richard C. Keller, for example, has shown how North

African patients contested colonial psychiatrists' explanations of the nature of madness because they did not conform to prevailing cultural etiologies.[16] The diagnosed also frequently had something to say about their conditions. Sadowsky's analysis of colonial asylums in Nigeria mentioned above examined the patterns of resistance imbedded in the content of Nigerian "lunatics'" supposed psychoses.[17] Similarly, Jean Comaroff and John L. Comaroff have analyzed the speech and actions of South African "lunatics" as political expression at the individual level.[18] Although colonial regimes were authoritarian in nature, they overwhelmingly failed to establish hegemony over the domain of madness, which remains contested in the postcolonial world.

Much historical and anthropological work has also illustrated the extent to which similar contests for hegemony have characterized the dynamics of biomedicine and psychiatry in the West as well as in colonized spaces.[19] The capacity of biomedicine and psychiatry to objectify, label, and marginalize certain groups has not been isolated to European colonial environments, nor has resistance to them.[20] The antipsychiatry movement in Western countries from the 1960s argued, for example, that mental illness was a myth, and, drawing from Foucault, a social construct designed to marginalize people whose conception of reality was too unsettling for the majority.[21] And of course, even in Western countries, where biomedicine has widespread political and cultural clout, medical pluralism is still extant, with alternative, folk, and Eastern medicines and healing techniques accounting for significant shares of the medical marketplace. The recognition that such contestation pervades environments without explicitly colonial governments has begged the question of what, exactly, is colonial about colonial medicine.[22] Some have argued that Western medical science should be seen as essentially colonial everywhere in its emphasis on the universality of a particular cultural construction of disease and illness that does not and has not historically represented the beliefs of all people, even within the West.[23] Such an analysis has implications for how historians should interpret the decolonization and postindependence contexts in which the pervasive shade of a globalizing Western hegemony is often presented as distinct from and overpowering of "traditional" non-Western cultures.

Other historians have shown the extent to which the development of "modern" biomedicine in the twentieth century is inextricably bound to the historical context of European colonialism within which it developed. Just as Western understandings of disease and hygiene became a "tool of empire," facilitating the conquering of the African interior,[24] so, too, did the colonies provide spaces within which scientific and medical knowledge was produced and interpolated, shaping very basic understandings about the natural world and the relationship between man and environment.[25] Similar dynamics applied to the sciences of the mind: psychoanalysis has famously relied on anthropological accounts of colonized peoples for its explanations of the "primitive" impulses of the human unconscious, even as it has been historically criticized for representing a narrow, central European bourgeois construction of the self.[26] Keller has shown how French North African colonies offered an arena for the pursuance of invasive research agendas that were not possible in metropolitan France in the 1920s and 1930s.[27] Chapter 3 of this volume illustrates the ways research conducted on the nature of mental illness in Africans followed Nigerian immigrants to the United Kingdom in the 1950s.

The inseparability of colonial spaces and ideologies of empire from the development of "modern" psychiatry in both the colonial and the postcolonial eras is being reflected in a broadening of the lens through which we view the history of psychiatry. Temporally, historians and other postcolonial critics have traced the legacies of colonial psychiatry and the psychology of colonialism into the postcolonial era. In the Indian context, for example, Ashis Nandy and Sudhir Kakar have taken a psychoanalytic perspective on colonial and postcolonial subjectivity that criticizes the psychological violence of colonialism but also recognizes the extent to which the colonial experience inevitably shapes the way that postcolonial subjectivities are formed and articulated.[28] Studies of Francophone postcolonial ethnopsychiatry have also raised the complex problems of defining the relationship of culture to psychological disorder in the context of shifting sociocultural paradigms of health, heightened immigration and its attendant tensions, and anxieties about the effects of globalization. Alice Bullard, for example, has examined French psychiatrist Henri Collomb's efforts in the 1950s–1970s to develop a transcultural psychiatry in Senegal that was highly dependent upon local cultural explanations for the definition and treatment of mental disorders, only to be replaced in the 1970s by Senegalese psychiatrists who were much less accommodating of culturally discreet etiologies for mental illness that cited witchcraft or other spiritual phenomena as causative factors.[29] The intellectual trajectories of colonizer/colonized that one might intuit are inverted in this case, raising serious questions about how to characterize any cultural or spatial determinants in the postcolonial history of psychiatry. Didier Fassin has similarly illustrated the extent to which French ethnopsychiatrists' efforts in France since the 1960s to address the mental health needs of African immigrants in terms of "indigenous" cultural beliefs have, through their privileging of a cultural relativity based in postcolonial geographies, created scenarios in which immigrants are objectified on the basis of cultures of origin and as such denied consideration of transnational subjectivities that might better reflect their unique conditions.[30] In such cases, efforts to embrace postcolonial cultural relativity have their own capacity to colonize the minds and bodies of marginalized individuals. The result is that, as Sloan Mahone and Megan Vaughan have indicated, "there is no clear break between the colonial and post-colonial histories of psychiatry."[31] Relationships between power, culture, and individual subjectivity remain contested and unresolved, and the legacies of colonial relationships linger, even as political and ideological structures transform.

The blurring of temporal and cultural boundaries evident in these postcolonial critiques of psychiatry has also demanded a spatial reorientation in the history of psychiatry. Political decolonization brought about a marshaling of colonial health infrastructure to meet the developmental needs of the emerging nation-state, but, as Warwick P. Anderson has warned, historians should resist the temptation to compartmentalize postcolonial medical history into self-contained nationalist narratives.[32] This means breaking away from broader streams of scholarship that romanticize the rise of anticolonial nationalist movements and the emergence of independent nation-states in Africa because they were able to articulate the failures of the colonial state and delegitimize it as a political model going forward.[33] Transnational and comparative perspectives in medical history and anthropology in Africa are disrupting the modernization paradigm, allowing for a reformulation of center-periphery transmission models and an engagement with complex flows of ideas and practices that transcend nation-state normativity.[34] In some ways reflecting the supple relationship between the global and the local seen in globalization discourses, new perspectives on the history of psychiatry are also illustrating the ways that international networks have situationally reinforced or destabilized national constructs, and the ways that universalist perspectives have affected notions of cultural particularism and vice versa. As the chapters in Warwick P. Anderson, Deborah Jenson, and Richard C. Keller's edited volume, *Unconscious Dominions*, have shown, for example, the psychoanalytic construction of a universal self has had significant global impact, but in diverse ways depending on the local context in which it has been employed. Psychoanalytic conceptions of the self have had the capacity to be both oppressive and liberating, reinforcing imperial hierarchies through the pathologization of resistance to authority or subverting them in an anticolonial critique of the social pathology of colonialism and the cultural ignorance of Western-derived models for understanding non-Western psychologies.[35] As this book will show, the tensions and dynamics that exist between local and global, universal and culturally particular, can also be seen in other psychiatric developments of the twentieth century, including social psychiatry, psychiatric epidemiology, and psychopharmacology.

Even as this book focuses on the Nigerian context, the debates and engagements of Nigerian psychiatrists were never strictly national in orientation or intention. Whereas Fanon and others suggested that liberation of the colonized mind should come through oppositional violence and rejection of medicalized discourse in an explicitly nationalist context, the Nigerian psychiatrists examined here saw that liberation as coming through incorporation with and transformation of the medicalized discourse both nationally and internationally. For Lambo, Asuni, and many others, medicalization of the mind allowed for a *depathologization* to occur in that it had the capacity to bring Africans—racial "others" and former colonial subjects—into a universal medical framework that treated them as psychological equals on a global scale. In developing such a paradigm, these transcultural psychiatrists were contributing to international processes in the 1950s and 1960s, within which the knowledge-power relationship in psychiatric discourse changed to express changing social and political priorities at local, national, and international levels in complex and often ambivalent ways. The emergence of the independent nation-state was important to Nigerian psychiatrists, and they worked within its structures and for its development, but they also recognized that effectively doing so required international engagement and a globalization of locally produced knowledge.

The Nigerian and other transcultural psychiatrists examined in this book therefore straddle a complex line between being both producers of knowledge about medical and health systems and themselves subjects for the study of medical and health systems. The perspectives and methods of medical anthropology can therefore be useful for articulating not only the ideas of Nigerian psychiatrists but also the subjective experiences of the psychiatrists as they negotiated the various health systems that they inhabited. While typically concerned with contemporary processes, medical anthropology recognizes the historical influences on health beliefs and behaviors and provides insights useful for historical interpretation of the transformations of health systems. On the one hand, the psychiatrists discussed here were engaged in health knowledge production processes very similar to what Byron J. Good has called the "empiricist" school of medical anthropology, which takes biological and naturalistic understandings of disease entities grounded in Western scientific discourses as empirically "true" and then adjudges the relative rationality or irrationality of non-Western health systems based on how closely they can be explained in terms of the Western norm.[36] However, Nigerian psychiatrists were making decisions to co-opt indigenous patients into a universal model of mental illness and its treatment only partly out of a hegemonic acceptance of the scientific-rationalist basis of human health. They were also attempting to situate themselves within a field that was increasingly global in reach and to articulate the mental health needs of their patients in ways that could resonate in a world in which social change, mobility, and geopolitical interconnectivity were themselves increasingly normative. In this way, the decision-making processes of Nigerian and other transcultural psychiatrists can themselves be related to streams in medical anthropological literature represented by Arthur M. Kleinman, John M. Janzen, and others that has emphasized the negotiations of therapeutic communities in medically plural societies on their own cultural terms.[37] Emerging studies by Mary-Jo DelVecchio Good, Sandra T. Hyde, Sarah Pinto, João Biehl, and others see those negotiations as significantly influenced by the pervasiveness of disorder in postcolonial contexts: subjectivity in medical and psychiatric contexts is increasingly seen not in terms of bounded cultural constructs, but in terms of the complex blurring and layering of categories that represent the dynamics of globalization and an unstable and shifting amalgam of postcolonial modernities.[38] While anthropological case studies tend to focus on consumers of health care, in this case we can see Nigerian psychiatrists grappling with how to characterize the symbols and language of the health care they provided to patients.

Medical anthropologists who focus on the complexities of postcolonial subjectivity largely developed their critiques out of the omissions, elisions, and denials of the universalistic constructs that transcultural psychiatrists of the 1950s and 1960s espoused, but, interestingly, these critiques can also be useful in contextualizing the worldviews that motivated the very knowledge frameworks they deconstruct. In keeping with notions of the political intimacies of culture and subjectivity, it is important to note that Nigerian psychiatrists' scientific ethos was not determined strictly by the naturalistic observation of experiments, but on a clear recognition of the influence of the political on the psychological universes of their patients, and on the politics of their own psychiatric research and practice. The transcultural psychiatry of the 1950s and 1960s tended to reinforce the politics of anticolonial and civil rights activism in much the same way that colonial psychiatry had previously buttressed ideologies of racialized oppression. At the same time, however, it retained significant colonial legacies in its emergence from a psychiatric scientific trajectory with historical roots in the knowledge production processes of Western imperialist states. Nigerian psychiatrists were intimately aware of the conflicts and paradoxes imbedded in their discipline, and their work largely consisted of attempting to reconcile them. In so doing, they contributed to the establishment of a new kind of knowledge-power relationship that valued cross-cultural interaction, emphasis on universals, and the notion of the "unity of mankind" espoused by contributors to the First Pan-African Psychiatric Conference.

The transition from colonial to transcultural psychiatry examined in the following chapters therefore contributes to new trajectories in the postcolonial history of psychiatry and the history of postcolonial psychiatry in its emphasis on the blurring of the colonizer/colonized dichotomy, its negotiation of the national with the global and universal, its recognition of the legacies of colonial structures in postcolonial psychiatry, and its insistence on seeing the tensions of hybridity as residing not only in postcolonial subjectivities but also in the structures and paradigms within which postcolonial subjects operate and to which they contribute. In so doing, the chapters that follow interrogate the "precise ways in which power is deployed and the ways in which power is engaged, contested, deflected, and appropriated" in the context of decolonizing political and scientific realms.[39] They eschew any notion of a bipolar (no pun intended) world in which Western-derived values, ideas, categories, and worldviews are a single set of monolithic, universal concepts distinct from and overpowering fractious, particularistic non-Western ones. Quite the contrary, they reveal how Nigerian psychiatrists practicing since the 1950s were aware of the precariousness of their position somewhere between colonizer and colonized, between representing the relevance of "traditional" indigenous cultures and the values of a scientific rationalist "modernity." However, it argues that Nigerian psychiatrists did not see what they were doing as bridging these divides so much as attempting to unify them. The following chapters therefore underscore transcultural psychiatrists' ambivalence about whether cultural boundaries were "real" or not, and about how they should be characterized for the purposes of effective psychiatric practice. Nigerian psychiatrists' research and clinical practice reflected an uneasy effort to undermine difference where possible, to reconcile differences where they could not be undermined, and to accept differences when they could not be reconciled. In so doing, they blurred cultural, national, and professional boundaries in ways that reflected a broader transition from colonial to postcolonial "modernity."

"TRADITIONAL" THERAPY AND "MODERN" PSYCHIATRY

Examining Nigerian psychiatrists' conceptions of how to "modernize" psychiatric care in decolonizing and postcolonial contexts contributes to historical and anthropological literatures on therapeutics as well as to understandings of professionalization in African medicine. Colonial lunatic asylums mostly did not offer much in the way of therapeutic treatment for psychiatric patients, leaving little for historians of such places to discuss beyond the overt incarceration and medicalization of African subjects. Certainly the lack of psychotherapeutic care in colonial asylums was one of the main problems Nigerian psychiatrists faced when they took over old psychiatric institutions and developed many new ones after 1954. The development of therapeutic regimens for use on Nigerian patients became a site of profound negotiation between the need to provide care that was culturally appropriate on the one hand and the need to meet the medical and ethical standards of the Western medical tradition on the other. Nigerian psychiatrists' professional identity therefore rested on a fulcrum between prevailing notions of the differences between "traditional" healing and "modern" medicine. Nigerian psychiatrists thus became one of a variety of cultural brokers, intermediaries, and gatekeepers who negotiated and blurred the boundaries between indigenous/colonized and Western/colonial knowledge bases and power structures.

"Traditional" and "modern" are, of course, contingent terms. Historical scholarship in the last four decades has significantly eroded boundaries between them, as it has so many other binary constructions. The notion that "modernity" consisted of a universal set of relationships between political, economic, cultural, and scientific processes that the "West" had achieved and to which the rest of the world aspired no longer holds water. The failures of modernization theory and the rise of postmodern and postcolonial critiques of Western civilization have effectively illustrated the extent to which "modernity" is more of a contested terrain than a universally accepted and implementable package.[40] Dipesh Chakrabarty has asked us to "provincialize" Europe in thinking about political modernity,[41] and Cooper has urged historians to look more closely at the ways that modernity has been contested rather than accept its continued use as a nebulous entity with an agency of its own.[42]

Modernity has always been situational. In order for something to be "modern," it must be contrasted with something that is not. In the colonial African context, that which was European represented the "modern" and stood in direct contrast with everything that had existed in African societies prior to European intrusion. Africans, as nonmodern, were deemed primitive. They were bound by "tradition," the supposedly ancient and unchanging beliefs of their ancestors. Tradition was seen as a hearkening to a premodern past that most Africans still inhabited in the present, but which European civilization had at least partially outgrown. Colonial rule brought the prospect of "modernization" to Africans, but the transition was seen to be precarious, and in need of management to mitigate its negative consequences while maximizing its benefits. However, just as "modernity" is now seen as contested space, so, too, is "tradition." Africanist historians from the 1950s debunked myths that African societies had been static prior to European intervention, even though in so doing they created narratives of the African past that conformed very much to European conceptions about the progressive march toward "modernity."[43] Later, Eric J. Hobsbawm and Terence Ranger's seminal volume, *The Invention of Tradition*, illustrated the ways that "traditions" were not, in fact, vestiges of an ancient past but rather prone to change over time, often even constructed in recent times to serve contemporary political and cultural agendas in both European and African settings.[44]

The erosion of the boundary between a universalizing Western modernity and the culturally bound traditions of "premodern" peoples in Africa and elsewhere has opened space for the examination of the ways these categories themselves have been contested, negotiated, adapted, and adopted by diverse actors. The study of therapeutic systems in Africa has been a particularly fruitful arena for this kind of analysis. Historical and anthropological studies of African therapeutic systems have recognized the historically dynamic and pluralistic nature that healing processes have exhibited over time. Although rooted in the social structures and cultural beliefs of their communities, African therapeutic systems have also been able to adapt, change, and incorporate new knowledge and ideas, both influenced by and influencing broader social patterns.[45] For most African communities, Western biomedicine is merely a recent, and not necessarily superior, addition to the cornucopia of healing options that patients have at their disposal at any given time. Western medicine has been adapted into "traditional" healing systems even in places where prevailing political structures sought to prevent incorporation.[46] The general consensus in the field is that all healing systems, including Western biomedicine, are the products of historical and cultural contexts. They all have a social basis—they change over time with the societies in which they operate, and they reflect and reinforce the values of their societies. They interact with one another and can be explained in terms of one another in ways that make stark distinctions between "traditional" and "modern" irrelevant at best, misleading at worst.

This does not mean, however, that cultural distinctions between therapeutic systems are simply imaginary, irrelevant, or easily overcome. Efforts to integrate therapeutic systems have been particularly complicated in a post-Enlightenment world that considers only knowledge produced by scientific-rationalist methods to be true. For those who buy into the idea that only that which is measurable and observable is real, all other systems of knowledge are relegated to the realm of belief. They are characterized as serendipitously lacking insight when their methods are compatible with biomedical standards, and dangerously superstitious when they are not. Nowhere has the negotiation between Western biomedicine and indigenous therapeutic systems been more culturally relevant than in the realm of psychiatry, a discipline that is overtly conscious of its cultural interdependence. Defining appropriate therapy for African patients became a site of negotiation between "traditional" and "modern" for the psychiatrists discussed in this book. The stark, racialized divide between traditional African and modern European that colonial ideology imposed on African environments in the first half of the twentieth century was both politically and professionally precarious to address. Cross-cultural psychiatrists, even those of Nigerian origin, often presented traditional beliefs in things like witchcraft as evidence of "primitive" mentality linked on an evolutionary scale to more sophisticated, modern beliefs in secular science. Nevertheless, cross-cultural psychiatrists recognized that traditional beliefs, as constituent elements of the cultures from which they come, were central to the construction of illness in any given society and therefore had real power to affect the presentation, prognosis, and treatment of mental illnesses in ways that were not necessarily already accounted for in Western psychotherapies that defined mental illness and its treatment in terms of Euro-American cultural norms. This idea was the basis of the development of transcultural psychiatry as a subdiscipline in the years after the Second World War.[47]

However, a key argument made here is that the negotiation was not about choosing between "African" and "European" or between "traditional" and "modern" therapies. It was a struggle on the part of individual psychiatrists in the context of rapidly changing sociopolitical circumstances to define their profession as transcending these categories. Nigerian psychiatrists, indeed all cross-cultural psychiatrists, sought to decouple the "modern" from the "Western." They saw certain practices within Western psychiatry as culturally determined and by no means appropriate to present as universal. They saw many elements of traditional therapeutic systems as representative of sound psychotherapy and integratable within a universalizing psychiatric framework. In making these decisions, Nigerian psychiatrists became part of the body of intermediaries who, Karen E. Flint argues, "helped Africans to make sense of Western medical practices and practitioners."[48] However, they were more than this because they also helped medical practitioners around the globe make sense of Africans, the cultural beliefs they held, and, subsequently, the kinds of therapy that could and could not be expected to help them cope with mental illnesses. Nigerian psychiatrists were therefore intermediaries seeking to make modern Western psychiatry and traditional belief systems comprehensible to each other, ideally transforming them into one and the same thing in ways that would require compromise from each but ultimately improve the therapeutic capabilities of mental health practitioners. However, at the same time transcultural psychiatrists sought to establish themselves as gatekeepers, the only ones with the combination of cultural sensitivity, medical knowledge, and professional ethics to negotiate the appropriate integration of these belief systems into a coherent, universal whole.

The negotiation between "tradition" and "modernity" that Nigerian psychiatrists engaged in was part of the larger process of the professionalization of psychiatry in Nigeria. Professionalization is not just an internal process, however. It has an external, political dimension that has been well recognized in literature on the medical professions in Africa. Typically, medical professionals have been presented as active critics of the colonial ideologies that tried to enforce a stark division between traditional African and modern European. Going back to the early days of European colonial domination in the continent in the late nineteenth century, Africans with Western medical training were examples of the assimilability of colonial subjects into Western educational and professional models. However, racist policies and practices generally prevented African doctors from attaining the same respect or recompense that their European colleagues enjoyed. Doctors therefore frequently became vocal critics of colonial regimes that refused to recognize them as equals, indeed, that continued to maintain them in subservient positions regardless of education or experience.[49] Although they had a variety of political stances regarding the intrinsic value of the colonial state itself, African doctors undermined the hierarchies that formed the basis of colonial social and cultural politics. A large part of this undermining meant promoting the value and dignity of the traditional African cultures from which they hailed, even as they sought to be taken seriously as examples of modern medical professionals.

In so doing, African doctors were firmly entrenched in the ranks of the African elite who engaged in an identity politics of cultural hybridity and began working for an overt transformation of the colonial state from a racially hierarchical structure to one that incorporated Africans on more equal terms. African elites constructed many different political identities and thought about anticolonial activism in a variety of organizational structures. Pan-Africanists pushed for the preservation of African traditions as a means of forging a diasporic racial community. Ethnic nationalists argued for the historical integrity of specific cultural units, despite the fact that many of their "traditions" had been created in the context of colonial rule. But the model that ultimately prevailed in most cases, certainly in Nigeria, was that of the multiethnic, culturally plural nation-state based on that of the Western European nation-state, however inorganic such a construction was to African political trajectories.[50]

Decolonization and the emergence of the independent nation-state model provided African doctors trained in the Western tradition the opportunity to rise to the top of their professions and to work much more cooperatively with state power structures to achieve their aims than had been possible under colonial rule. Finally it seemed possible to be simultaneously "African" and "modern" in an official sense. And African doctors were keen to modernize medicine, to reverse colonial-era policies that had left medical infrastructure underdeveloped. As Murray Last and G. L. Chavunduka noted, "The process of professionalism became part of decolonization; it coincided with the Africanization of staff and curriculum; it was to prove, proudly, that the new independent states were not content with second best, with having only 'sub-standard' para-medicals as their doctors."[51] Decolonization of medical services was therefore connected with the emergence of the independent nation-state and with the processes of modernization and development upon which independent nation-states embarked.

Decolonization and independence did not mark a clean break with all Western ideological constructs, just the strands that claimed Africans incapable of reproducing European "modernity" in their current stage of development. In Nigeria and other independent African countries, political and professional elites bought into the project of transforming their underdeveloped colonies into "modern" nation-states. At the time, becoming an equal in global affairs meant buying into a grocery cart of universalizing ideologies like capitalism, socialism, democracy, and industrialization in their contemporary, Western-derived forms. The general consensus of the 1950s and 1960s was that there *were* universal principles that could be followed to achieve this transformation.[52] Modernization theory argued that if African countries simply followed the patterns of European political economies, they would become modern, developed countries over time. Modernization placed particular emphasis on the role of science and technology in the development process, and on the role of social scientists to study social change and provide blueprints for the mitigation of social problems that might arise in the transformation from "traditional" to "modern." The nation-state stood at the center of development processes: it was considered both the engine and the driver behind modernization. Although modernization theory proved a mirage, giving way to dependency theory by the 1970s, the idea that scientific universals existed that could be articulated in terms of Western experience and applied to African circumstances to achieve particular results was a powerful one in the contexts of decolonization and early independence for many African countries, Nigeria included.

When Nigerian psychiatrists pushed for the replacement of racist theories about the inferiority of the "primitive" African mind with a model based on the inherent "unity of mankind," they were making not only a scientific but also a political statement linked to underlying notions of the illegitimacy of colonial ideologies that underlay the anticolonial nationalisms of the decolonization era, whatever their boundaries of inclusiveness. However, at the same time, Nigerian psychiatrists were engaged in a political process that was invested in modernization and the legitimization of the specific political construction of the nation-state in the postindependence context. Lambo frequently spoke about the need to understand psychosocial phenomena in order to improve the mental health of the Nigerian workforce and, by extension, aid the economic development of the country. Politically and professionally, Nigerian psychiatrists engaged in a balancing act over how much external influence was appropriate and how much indigenous beliefs and therapies needed to be incorporated to manage the modernization transition. They had to negotiate a number of extant political and cultural boundaries. Knowledge that Nigerian psychiatrists produced at the local level fed developmentalist agendas at the national level that were themselves bound up with the same kind of universalizing ideologies that fueled the international efforts of transcultural psychiatry. The incorporation of Nigerians into networks of transcultural psychiatry contributed to the legitimization of the Nigerian nation-state internationally and gave Nigerian psychiatrists access to newly produced psychiatric knowledge that they could then apply to research and treatment on individuals at the local level. In this way, Nigerian psychiatrists were pushing the psychiatric profession to become more modern by accounting more for the effects of traditional beliefs and practices in different cultural settings. In so doing, they were integrating scientific with political agendas locally, nationally, and globally.

DIFFUSION, NETWORKS, AND THE GLOBALIZATION OF PSYCHIATRIC SCIENCE

While Nigerian psychiatrists' efforts to reformulate psychiatric theory and practice were firmly entrenched in the political and social contexts of decolonization in their country, they were also linked to broader international networks of psychiatric science that had been developing over the course of the twentieth century. Recognition of the impact that non-Western psychiatrists had on the globalization of psychiatry as a universalizing medical system is therefore important not only for understanding the history of psychiatry in African countries like Nigeria but also for understanding the dynamics of psychiatry in the world at large in the postcolonial era. This examination of Nigerian psychiatrists is therefore an effort to move the focus of scholars away from an outdated reliance on the development and spread of "Western" psychiatry and toward a theorization of a "global" psychiatry that recognizes a greater diversity of actors within psychiatric science and the complexity of flows of people, knowledge, and information that has characterized the discipline particularly since the 1950s.

Scientific networks have earned significant attention from historians. George Basalla's initial theory of the spread of "Western" science as a diffusion of scientific thinking from Europe and the United States to the rest of the world, where it would inevitably displace indigenous knowledge and take on particular "national" forms, has been effectively debunked by a body of literature that has shown the very significant roles that non-Westerners have played in the development of general scientific thinking as well as specific scientific discoveries.[53] David W. Chambers and Richard Gillespie, for example, have argued that the diffusionist approach is overdetermined, as negotiations of Western science with indigenous knowledge systems differ across space because of local political, economic, and cultural dynamics, although they see "Western" science as something very distinct from "indigenous knowledge."[54] Kapil Raj, among others, has argued convincingly for the historical inseparability of Western science from non-Western knowledge systems, however.[55]

Scientific knowledge diffusion has thus been shown to be by no means a one-way street. Not only did European scientists spread their knowledge out into the world with particular fervor from the sixteenth century, but reverse flows of scientific knowledge from colonial environments to Europe greatly influenced scientific thinking even within its metropolitan "home." Richard Grove's groundbreaking *Green Imperialism* illustrated how indigenous notions of conservationism were integral to the development of environmentalism as a Western concept through the interactions of the colonial encounter, while Richard H. Drayton has pointed out the ways that the scientific knowledge procured from indigenous lands became a moral justifier of British imperial expansion. Such a perspective invokes Daniel R. Headrick's argument that imperial conquests and colonial terrains provided testing grounds for technological advancements that have become synonymous with Western power since the mid-nineteenth century.[56] Even more recently, historians have begun emphasizing the extent to which flows of scientific knowledge in European empires often bypassed the metropole altogether and circulated between colonial environments in complex networks of interaction.[57] As Joseph M. Hodge has shown, as European empires decolonized, these scientific networks became less "imperial" and more "international" in scope.[58]

Although the role of Africans in these networks continues to be somewhat marginalized, the Nigerian psychiatrists discussed in this book were instrumental in the establishment and maintenance of networks of knowledge production and dissemination. Nigerian psychiatrists engaged actively and often in leadership roles in comparative, cross-cultural studies on psychiatric disorder. Nigerian psychiatrists also disseminated their findings on the basic equality of human psychology through a variety of international engagement efforts. They published in highly respected international journals in their field, even creating one for a short time. They organized and participated in international symposia on global psychiatry. They wrote working papers for international organizations like the World Health Organization. The knowledge that transcultural psychiatrists produced became important not only for practicing psychiatry in non-Western environments but also increasingly for practicing in immigrant communities in the West (see chapter 3). Nigerian psychiatrists therefore worked to make governments aware of the policy implications of new research findings on the psychological impact of socioeconomic changes like education, urbanization, and migration that were bringing Nigeria into ever-closer integration and interdependence with other parts of the world in the second half of the twentieth century.

The political context is also relevant in discussing the international networks to which Nigerian psychiatrists contributed. International engagement was necessary to combat the racist conceptions that the Western psychiatric tradition harbored in the 1950s. Proving that Yoruba, Nigerians, or Africans, depending on the chosen unit of analysis, were part of a psychological "unity of mankind" required the application of universal criteria to comparative studies. The political message of Nigerian psychiatrists therefore needed international, cross-cultural partners to be effective. In this way, the politics of psychiatry served as a microcosm of the broader anticolonial, antiracist struggle that blacks and sympathetic nonblacks were engaged in across the world in the mid-twentieth century.[59] As Chakrabarty has put it, anticolonial thinkers, of which we could include our Nigerian psychiatrists, "often devoted a great deal of time to the question of whether or how a global conversation of humanity could genuinely acknowledge cultural diversity without distributing such diversity over a hierarchical scale of civilization—that is to say, an urge toward cross-cultural dialogue without the baggage of imperialism."[60] A broad variety of activist groups, both governmental and nongovernmental, cooperated across cultural, national, and racial divides based on the idea that to be truly eradicated, imperialism and racism had to be combated globally. Through foreign policy approaches like nonalignment and Pan-African solidarity, newly independent nation-states like Nigeria sought to strengthen their national identity through international engagement.[61] Just as it would be a simplification to say that decolonization was a process that each African country undertook in isolation, it would be erroneous to present decolonization of psychiatric institutions and practices as a geographically bounded process.

The insertion of African agents into international scientific networks like those of transcultural psychiatry provides yet another way to look at the contingent nature of modernity. Nigerian psychiatrists adopted signs and symbols of a culturally bounded Western psychiatric tradition as universal norms partly out of belief in the basic tenets of their field, but also partly to have a language and set of methods that could be used to make comparisons relatable to each other.[62] In so doing, they reinscribed notions of the basic "truth" of Western models, but in adopting these signs and symbols, Nigerian psychiatrists changed the meanings of the terms embedded in them to account for local circumstances and to achieve nationalist and developmentalist aims. It is therefore impossible, or at least highly inaccurate, to conflate "modern" psychiatry with "Western" psychiatry in the postcolonial context. The core practices and principles of psychiatry have been adopted by non-Westerners and adapted through networks of scientific knowledge production and diffusion such that they are no longer, if indeed they ever were, the preserve of a "Western" civilization, however nebulous its boundaries.

METHODOLOGY AND ORGANIZATION

Since the arguments of this book are centered on Nigerian psychiatrists' efforts to transform discourses on mental illness and its treatment within global psychiatric circles, the source material used to write it is largely that which was widely disseminated. Published materials that reached a relatively large audience and that represent the scientific thinking of a broad body of professionally active Nigerian psychiatrists are therefore liberally consulted. Journal articles, conference proceedings, government reports, and other policy documents are all analyzed here as having both medical and political messages regarding how best to conceptualize human mental health. In several chapters, documents from colonial psychiatrists and the colonial government of Nigeria are used to illustrate the entrenched ideas about African mental illness that characterized the field when Nigerian psychiatrists like T. Adeoye Lambo and Tolani Asuni entered the profession: they formed the mainstream discourse with which transcultural psychiatrists had to engage and against which they provided counterdiscourse. The practicalities of how these changing ideas affected actual patient care are discussed in the following chapters only insofar as Nigerian psychiatrists presented their ideas as leading to improvements in care over what had obtained previously. It is well beyond my expertise and, indeed, beyond the scope of this book to make any value judgments about what mental illness "really" is or, by extension, how one "really" goes about healing it. It is merely my intention to show that ideas about how to define and treat mental illness changed significantly in the twentieth century, and they changed because of confluences of political, social, and scientific processes, at the crux of which stood several prominent Nigerian psychiatrists and their professional networks.

Chapter 1 examines the establishment of psychiatric institutions in Nigeria and the networks of psychiatric knowledge production and dissemination to which Nigeria became connected over the course of the colonial era. It shows how the ideological underpinnings of psychiatric theory and practice in colonial Nigeria were inextricably connected to the ideological basis of state power: both defined colonial subjects in Nigeria as inherently different from Europeans and psychologically threatened by European "civilization." These ideas were still very salient and operational in Nigeria as of the mid-1950s and were still mainstream thought in the burgeoning international networks of scientific knowledge dissemination to which Nigeria was connected. Chapter 2 explores the decolonization of these psychiatric institutions and networks. The main figure in this story is Thomas Adeoye Lambo, who took over Aro Mental Hospital in 1954. Lambo revolutionized clinical practice in Nigeria, providing both Western-derived treatments such as pharmaceutical care and electroshock therapy for the first time. However, it was his development of a community-care model based on indigenous social structures and cultural beliefs called the Aro Village Scheme that really brought Lambo into international acclaim. Lambo's work was very much inspired by notions of anticolonial nationalism and a desire to contribute to the development of an independent Nigerian nation. His research agenda explicitly denounced the racist theories of colonial-era psychiatry and sought to replace them with an egalitarian model of universal human psychological dysfunction. Lambo used the tools and language of the Euro-American psychiatric tradition to make these arguments, but in so doing was able to communicate his ideas to other transcultural psychiatrists and to contribute to changing the basic assumptions and definitions that psychiatric language had previously connoted.

But one of the key arguments of this book is that not all flows of scientific knowledge and resources flowed from the West to Nigeria. Nigerian psychiatrists were also engaging with the rest of the world, as were Nigerians more generally. Chapter 3 examines the problems posed to transcultural psychiatry by migration, specifically the migration of Nigerians to the United Kingdom since the 1950s. The chapter examines the ways that psychiatric authorities viewed Nigerian migrants who developed psychiatric troubles while abroad. While many psychiatric authorities in the UK believed that such people should be repatriated to "familiar surroundings" in language clearly influenced by colonial psychiatric notions of culture clash, Nigerian psychiatrists tended to argue that the much more viable long-term solution to the problem would be for the governments of the United Kingdom and Nigeria to promote cross-cultural understanding and to provide resources to aid Nigerian migrants with their acclimatization processes while abroad. Rejecting notions of difference and separation, such arguments presaged developments in cross-cultural psychiatry in later decades, when concerns about meeting the mental health needs of large migrant communities, many of them of African or Caribbean origin, became inescapable in many European and American cities.

The ways networks of knowledge production and dissemination were used to emphasize the universality of psychiatric disease entities is the focus of chapter 4. Through an explicitly cross-cultural research agenda, Nigerian psychiatrists, again Lambo chief among them, argued that both schizophrenia and depression were present and relatively prevalent in rural, non-Westernized Nigerian populations. This argument overturned previously held ideas that depression was extremely rare in Africans and that the greatest threat to the development of full-blown schizophrenia in Africans was the inability to cope with the sociocultural changes brought about by the intrusion of complex, individualistic European civilization into the simplistic, communal cultures of most Africans. The chapter concludes with a section illustrating the extent to which Nigerian psychiatrists in the 1970s and 1980s had become so invested in the universalist notions of transcultural psychiatry that they vehemently fought against the suggestion that a specifically "culture-bound syndrome" known as brain-fag syndrome existed in Nigeria. The disavowal of brain-fag syndrome, like the idea that schizophrenia was caused by culture conflict or that African cultures were incapable of producing depression, was inherently bound up in a cultural politics that rejected notions of African psychological difference.

If major mental illnesses like depression and schizophrenia could be identified as universal but with significant cultural variations in presentation, then it stood to reason that therapy might also be constructed as universal in nature but culturally variable in practice. Chapter 5 explores the existential quandary of Nigerian psychiatrists as they sought to find a place for themselves in a medically pluralistic landscape to which they were a recent and culturally alien addition. How different was the psychotherapy that Western-trained psychiatrists practiced from that provided by "traditional" healers? Could Western-trained psychiatrists work within traditional belief systems, or with traditional healers? What could they learn from one another? Could psychiatric principles coming from a Western cultural trajectory be effectively integrated into traditional belief systems to form a holistic universal therapy? No clear consensus emerged on these questions, but in all cases, Nigerian psychiatrists posited themselves as the possessors of the "real" knowledge that would ultimately serve a Nigerian population destined for a postcolonial modernity, and as the only ones with both the scientific and the cultural expertise to negotiate the integration of traditional beliefs and practices into that modernity.

The ambivalence over the importation of Western methods of treating psychiatric disorder carries over into a discussion of drug therapies in chapter 6. The invention of antipsychotics, anxiolytics, and antidepressants that significantly reduced the severity of the key symptoms associated with major mental illnesses also helped to foster the reemergence of biological notions of the nature of the human mind. While on the one hand Nigerian psychiatrists embraced the psychopharmacological revolution because it contributed to the notion of universal psychological similarity, on the other they saw the influx of psychoactive substances as socially and culturally dangerous. Although Nigerian psychiatrists used psychopharmaceuticals freely, they tended to see them in much the same terms as they saw other psychoactive substances like alcohol, marijuana, and methamphetamines: as foreign imports that people needed to cope with a changing sociocultural landscape that was much more psychologically precarious than that which had come before. Heavy regulation of these substances was needed, and once again psychiatrists saw themselves as natural gatekeepers between indigenous Nigerians and the foreign substances that helped them cope with the perils of modernization.

The book concludes with some remarks on the confluence of fissures in the alliance between international, national, and scientific interests in the field of transcultural psychiatry since the late 1970s. The universalist framework advanced by Lambo, Asuni, and countless other Nigerian psychiatrists and transcultural psychiatrists around the world was, as I have argued, just one way to make sense of an extraordinarily complex and often contradictory agglomeration of data and interpretations of that data. It was a particularly attractive model partly because new scientific methods and researches supported it, but, more importantly I think, also because the sociopolitical context within which those new scientific methods and researches were undertaken had changed to the point that it could support no other construct. However, by the late 1970s, this was no longer the case. Cross-cultural psychiatrists and medical anthropologists began to question whether the universalist theory had, in fact, gone too far. They began to assail the idea that Western-based terminologies and definitions that were themselves culturally determined could account for the ways diverse cultures understood something as culturally imbedded as mental illness. Similarly, in Nigeria, the idea that psychiatry and the modernizing state were on the same page slowly eroded. After the civil war of 1967–70, the increasing disillusionment with government structures throughout the 1970s and, ultimately, the crash of the Nigerian economy in the 1980s, a new generation of psychiatrists in Nigeria was as likely to implicate the state as a cause of psychological distress in the citizenry as to promote it as a partner for the development of good mental health and the overall strengthening of Nigerian society.

Throughout this book, terms like "mental illness," "psychiatric disorder," "psychological distress," and the various diagnostic entities used to represent them (e.g., schizophrenia, depression, brain fag, ọdẹ orí, witchcraft), are liberally used. However, their use is intended to represent only their functions as explanatory categories, not their material "reality." The conversation about these issues is not over: the basic questions about the relationship between nature and nurture, individual and society, and cultural particularism and humanistic universalism remain as salient in psychiatric discourse today as they were a hundred years ago. While all societies have found ways to define particular types of abnormal behavior as indicative of an illness of the mind, they do so differently and contingently, in ways that are apt to change over time. What J. C. Carothers considered depression to be and what T. Adeoye Lambo considered it to be were different. What an indigenous Yoruba babaláwo called wèrè did not connote the same notions of cause, presentation, treatment, or prognosis as what Western-trained psychiatrists called "psychosis," "neurosis," or any *DSM* subcategorization therein. Indeed, one of the main arguments of this book is that the belief that all the different forms of mental illness human beings conceive and experience could be calibrated into a single, coherent framework was itself historically contingent, the product of a confluence of political, cultural, social, and scientific changes that accompanied the shift from a colonial to a postcolonial world order. The Nigerian psychiatrists discussed here represent only one group through which to examine the interconnections between local, national, international, transnational, and global forces that have characterized psychiatric discourse since the 1950s. The opportunities for comparison and synthesis are numerous.

1 Colonial Institutions and Networks of Ethnopsychiatry

African mentality—East, West and South—is, for certain reasons, more uniform than that of literate cultures, such as that of Europe.

—J. C. Carothers, 1953

The position of lunatics in prisons is considerably worse than it would be if they were left to wander the streets.

—C. E. Marlow, Acting Secretary of Health, Nigeria, 1957

WHILE THIS BOOK IS NOT CENTRALLY CONCERNED with colonial psychiatry, it is important to provide some early background on psychiatry in colonial Nigeria in order to establish the professional context that Nigerian psychiatrists encountered in their efforts to transform psychiatric institutions from the 1950s. This chapter makes three arguments about the nature of psychiatric theory and practice in colonial Nigeria that will continue to resonate through the remainder of the book. First, the ways that psychiatric institutions developed in colonial Nigeria were intimately bound up with the philosophy and ideology of European power. The British colonial government throughout most of the colonial period sought to minimize public service expenditures both as an economical measure and because it had little desire to actively transform indigenous communities through heavy-handed policy initiatives. As such, colonial mental asylums were purely institutions of social control designed to house only the most dangerous and criminal "lunatics." They were strictly custodial in nature, providing little to no psychiatric medical treatment. And because the colonial government was not willing to make psychiatric service allocation an administrative priority, colonial asylums remained chronically underfunded, understaffed, and overcrowded throughout the colonial period. The state of psychiatry in colonial Nigeria was therefore a perpetual embarrassment to the colonial government and a source of alienation for Nigerian subjects who had no reason to consider psychiatry a legitimate healing system prior to T. Adeoye Lambo's intervention at Aro Hospital beginning in 1954.

Second, the minimalist approach to psychiatric service provision was at least partly justified by a body of knowledge called "ethnopsychiatry" that sought to understand the psychological functioning of non-Western peoples, particularly in comparison to what were considered to be European "norms." Ethnopsychiatric studies in Africa were generally conducted in colonial settings and, as such, inherited many of the racially hierarchical assumptions that formed the basis of social relations in colonial environments. Ethnopsychiatry became a remarkably consistent body of knowledge that functioned on the assumption that European and African psyches were inherently different and, as such, that the rapid transformation of African societies along European lines was likely to do much more harm than good in the short term. In these psychological constructions, African psyches, lumped together on the basis of racial affinity, were imperiled by the social and cultural transformations of colonial rule, which they were considered psychologically ill-equipped to negotiate. Mental illness in Nigeria, as in other parts of the continent, was primarily seen as a problem for colonial subjects who deviated from constructions of "normal" African psychology. In the colonial context, the most easily recognizable deviation from the African "norm" was the "detribalized" African whose "traditional" worldview was being assailed by the attempt to assimilate European "civilization." The psychologically disturbed and the "detribalized" came to be indistinguishable in many colonial settings, linked by virtue of being "insufficiently 'Other,'" as Megan Vaughan has put it.[1]

Third, and most important for the overall focus of this book, constructions of and policy approaches to mental illness in colonial Nigeria were the product of both local and international forces. The colonial government of Nigeria thrice brought in international experts to examine its psychiatric infrastructure and provide advice on how to improve it. While these experts suggested the extension of European-styled psychiatric facilities, they also reinforced notions of racial difference and the concern that culture clash between the races was likely to result in more, not less, mental illness among African populations. These experts were part of an international community of psychiatrists who were reaching similar conclusions. Local attitudes toward mental illness among colonial officials in Nigeria were conveniently reinforced by scientific knowledge that was international, more or less unanimous in its assumptions, and therefore unequivocal in its application. The broader body of knowledge about the nature of the African psyche contributed to the entrenchment of a basket of binary oppositions: between white and black, between European and African, between "civilization" and "primitivity," and between "modern" and "traditional" at the level of international science. This coherent body of ethnopsychiatric literature on the nature of the "African mind" had clearly established the terms, language, and debates in professional psychiatry in relation to Africa by the 1950s.

INDIRECT RULE AND COLONIAL ASYLUMS

The history of colonial mental health services in Nigeria is for the most part one of neglect and inertia. The first large-scale asylums for the confinement of the insane opened in 1906 in Yaba, a suburb of Lagos in the southwest; and Calabar, in the southeast. Although chronically overcrowded and underfunded, these two remained the only centrally run asylums in Nigeria until the opening at Lantoro in 1946 of a third asylum, which was designed specifically as a place to send mentally disturbed soldiers returning from overseas deployments in World War II. Prior to the opening of Aro Mental Hospital in Abeokuta in 1954, mental institutions were strictly custodial in nature, designed to protect the general population from violent offenders whom the courts deemed too dangerous to be placed in the general prison population or to be remanded to the custody of relatives. The asylum system in Nigeria offered no curative or therapeutic treatment for its "patients"; indeed, other than the brief tenure of Matthew Cameron Blair in the early 1920s, Nigeria did not boast a single qualified European-trained psychiatrist until the arrival of Dr. Donald Cameron in 1949.[2] Even the most violent and dangerous "lunatics," to use the parlance of the times, could not be housed in the two overcrowded government-run asylums, and instead were placed in segregated sections of local prisons or in native administration asylums, most of which lacked trained medical staff qualified to look after the needs of the mentally ill. Conditions in asylums were often dilapidated, unsanitary, and cruel, with inconsolable inmates sometimes chained to walls or rings anchored in the ground. Those mentally disturbed individuals who were neither dangerous nor criminal tended to remain in the care of friends, relatives, and communities to be treated by indigenous medical practitioners as deemed appropriate by their caretakers.[3]

The overcrowded, unsanitary asylum system that could not claim to offer curative care to any of its patients was a continual embarrassment to the colonial government. The general opinion among government officials throughout the colonial period was that the existing conditions in Nigeria's asylums were unacceptable, but at no point was a suitable plan of reform implemented. This was to a great extent because the issue of mental health policy was intricately tied to one of the key debates regarding the philosophy of the colonial project in Nigeria, namely whether the emphasis of the colonial regime should be on providing stability to the subject population or on undertaking grand projects of social transformation. In other words, should colonial rule be based more on the philosophy and practice of indirect rule or on the idea of modernization? "Indirect rule" implied a general desire for the preservation of indigenous political structures and cultural traditions. "Modernization" implied the deliberate erosion of traditional ways and their replacement with European models. This dialectic is, of course, overly simplistic. The history of colonial Nigeria is redolent with stories of individuals, institutions, and policies that sought to negotiate some middle ground between these ideological positions. However, in the case of mental health policy, colonial administrations tended to favor a reliance on the indirect rule approach, with the result that the embarrassment of the existing asylum system was determined to be less damaging than the economic and social costs associated with expanding facilities and services to meet approximated need.

The conflict between "indirect rule" and "modernization" and efforts to reconcile them date back to the onset of British colonial occupation in the second half of the nineteenth century. British colonial rule spread in fits and spurts over the course of roughly forty years, beginning with the annexation of Lagos in 1861 and culminating with the defeat of the Sultan of Sokoto in 1903 and the incorporation of his remaining territories into the Northern Protectorate under the governorship of Lord Frederick Lugard. Colonial administrations that developed throughout Nigeria all relied on some variation of indirect rule, whereby British colonial officers ruled through indigenous authorities, whether they were Yoruba obas,[4] Fulani emirs,[5] or the infamous "warrant chiefs" of southeastern Nigeria.[6] However, colonial officials in different parts of Nigeria had different agendas regarding the levels of economic and social transformation that should accompany British colonialism. Particularly in the early years of British rule, many colonial officials in the southern territories of Nigeria believed in the construction and expansion of European-styled institutions and infrastructure. For example, Lagos quickly became a locus for the creation of British-inspired institutions. By 1898, the colonial government in Lagos had established a medical department, which employed eleven European and three African doctors; a police service; and a public works department charged with the maintenance of public buildings and roads and the extension of electric lighting, telegraphs, piers, and public transport.[7] Progressive-minded British colonial administrators in the south heavily promoted the extension of European education, among other things.[8] From 1906, the Yaba and Calabar asylums served partly as a symbol of the colonial government's power to intern the mentally ill, but also as a symbol of the nascent commitment of British colonial rule in the south to a colonial policy bent on the "modernization" of public institutions.

In the northern territories, however, indirect rule conformed to a different set of circumstances and took on an ideological mission very different from what had developed in the south. Lugard believed that the rapid and widespread extension of European ideas and institutions was likely to serve as a destabilizing force for colonial subjects, particularly in the north, where the overwhelmingly Muslim population had very little precolonial experience with Europeans. Lugard explained the form of indirect rule he developed in the north in terms of a "Dual Mandate" to run the colonies to the economic benefit of Britain, while at the same time promoting a tempered notion of progress toward Europeanization for colonial subjects. However, unlike the colonial administrators in the south, Lugard believed that the purpose of colonial rule was theoretically to alter only those customs, traditions, and institutions that the British deemed harmful to Nigerian progress, leaving existing cultures intact to the greatest degree possible. Unlike what was occurring in the south, the development of social services under Lugard's indirect rule was to be undertaken only by local native administrations, not the colonial government, at their own expense and more or less on their own terms. Lugard believed that for the British colonial government to embark on such activities was a direct violation of the Dual Mandate, in that it constituted unnecessary colonial expenditure and purposelessly brought about the erosion of traditional social structures.[9] In 1914, Lugard oversaw the amalgamation of northern and southern Nigeria into a single administrative unit. As the first governor-general of a unified Nigeria, Lugard decided that his form of indirect rule should be extended throughout Nigeria. As a result, the development of colonially funded education services and health-care systems ceased to be an administrative priority.

The entrenchment of an indirect rule philosophy based on the concept of budgetary parsimony and justified in terms of cultural unobtrusiveness had a strong effect on the development of psychiatric services in Nigeria. Some officials, particularly those associated with the Department of Medical and Sanitary Services (DMSS), repeatedly argued in the interventionist spirit that the colonial government had a responsibility to expand its facilities to meet the needs of Nigerians deemed mentally ill. However, colonial officials dedicated to the philosophy of Lugardian indirect rule believed that mental health was a cultural issue and, as such, should be left to the care of indigenous communities. Such cultural arguments were generally secondary and used circumstantially to justify the primary consideration: cost.

Mental hospitals of the European style were expensive to build, maintain, and staff. They required a lot of land, access to large amounts of water, and had to be prepared to maintain patients for possibly many years at a time. European-styled mental health services were far beyond the budgetary means of the colonial government for most of the colonial period.

An examination of the specific debates surrounding the building of additional government-run asylums in Nigeria clearly illustrates the extent to which the philosophical undercurrents of indirect rule were influencing decisions to keep psychiatric facilities underdeveloped. By the mid-1920s, officials in the Department of Medical and Sanitary Services had begun to push for the erection of a new mental hospital in Abeokuta to reduce the number of "lunatics" who had to be housed in local jails.[10] As of January 1926, the Yaba asylum was at 200 percent capacity, housing 48 patients in space designed to accommodate 24.[11] The DMSS proposed that given such conditions, there was a need to develop a new lunatic asylum and to appoint an official, qualified alienist to oversee it.[12]

While the DMSS pushed for the expansion of mental health facilities in both size and scope, other officials saw such proposals as beyond the responsibilities of the colonial government. Rather than expand facilities at the expense of the colonial government itself, many officials saw the establishment of native administration asylums as the ideal solution to accommodate mental patients. In fact, in the Northern Provinces, native administration asylums were the most common institution for the confinement of the mentally ill. By 1925, native administration asylums had been established in Bauchi, Bida, Maiduguri, Ilorin, Kano, Katsina, Keffi, Kontagora, Makurdi, Ibi, Sokoto, Yola, and Zaria.[13] In 1926, the acting secretary of the Northern Provinces justified the use of native administration asylums in true indirect rule style, arguing to the director of Medical and Sanitary Services in Lagos that there was no "urgent need for Government intervention in such parts of Nigeria where native laws and customs exist as opposed to administration on European lines."[14] Such comments reflect the constant struggle of colonial officials to reconcile the fact that the existing asylum system was inadequate with the belief that direct intervention to improve the system would be both costly and culturally intrusive.

Seeking practical solutions to the debate between the DMSS and the secretariat described above, the Colonial Office commissioned an independent third party to report on the forms of mental illness in Nigeria and make recommendations for future care of the mentally ill. In 1928, Bruce Home toured twenty-five regions of Nigeria and compiled data from questionnaires sent to colonial residents and medical officers. Home's conclusions came down strictly on the side of the DMSS. He declared Nigeria's asylums woefully inadequate for the treatment of mental patients. He noted that asylum facilities were overcrowded, unsanitary, and at times inhumane, particularly in the use of chains to restrain the more restive patients. He compared the government-run asylums at Yaba and Calabar to prisons in their focus on containment rather than treatment, and urged the government to remodel Nigeria's asylum system based on the design and methods of European mental hospitals. In addition to offering more therapeutic and curative treatment for mental patients, Home also urged the government to expand the size of its existing facilities to be able to accommodate at least four thousand patients on the intuition that demand for mental health services among the Nigerian population was likely to rise over time.[15]

Based partly on Home's recommendations, the colonial government approved plans in 1928 to build a new government-run mental asylum in the Southern Provinces in order to relieve overcrowding in existing institutions and increase space for future admissions.[16] Dr. Home himself accompanied a government entourage to the alake of Abeokuta, roughly sixty miles inland from Lagos, to request a lease of 150 acres upon which to build the new asylum. According to the acting resident of Abeokuta Province, the alake and his council "needed no pressing whatever to grant the lease."[17] With the site selected, final building plans had only to be finalized.

The intended size and scope of the new asylum continued to be a sticking point for some colonial officials, who could not get behind the need for a heavy expenditure on a government-run mental asylum. Home suggested that the new asylum should have at least five hundred beds, enough presumably to handle not only the violent and criminal lunatics but also a sizable number of "harmless" lunatics. The acting chief secretary to the government, however, made it clear that although a new asylum was to be built, it would not be as large as medical authorities envisioned, both on account of cost and because top administrative officials did not want to encourage the relatives of mentally ill persons "to transfer their burden to the Government."[18] Some authorities suggested that the new asylum should originally contain only fifty beds, with space available to expand facilities over time.[19]

A compromise was reached in 1930 by which the asylum would be built piecemeal in three separate units. Unit A would accommodate 230 males; Unit B 58 males; and Unit C 188 females, bringing the ultimate total accommodation of the new asylum to 476 patients, very near Home's suggested total of 500. However, the building would be a long-term process. In fact, the total estimated cost for building the three units of the Abeokuta asylum was set at just over £40,000. However, in 1930–31, the first year of construction, the asylum was budgeted only £7,000, not enough even to build Unit B, the smallest of the three units.[20]

One of the main reasons that the colonial government was even willing to undertake such a large project was because an opportunity arose from 1929 in the form of the Colonial Development Fund (CDF), through which the colonial government could apply for imperial grants and loans from Britain to fund agricultural, industrial, and social service programs in the colonies.[21] However, as the economic crisis in Britain and the colonies deepened in the early 1930s, most of the public health projects financed through the CDF were abandoned.[22] The mental hospital at Abeokuta quickly became one of these abandoned public health projects. Before construction could even begin, the lieutenant governor of the Southern Provinces ordered that all work on the new mental hospital at Abeokuta should cease, owing to "financial pressure."[23] Funding for the asylum was not killed, but was rather perpetually deferred to future budgets. No mental health facility would be constructed in Abeokuta for nearly twenty-five years.

In response to continued criticism of the policy of housing "lunatics" in prisons in the years after the Home report and the failed attempt at building a new asylum in Abeokuta,[24] the colonial government commissioned Dr. R. Cunyngham Brown, a one-time deputy commissioner of lunacy for Scotland,[25] to conduct another independent study of mental health policy in Nigeria in 1936. Brown canvassed Nigeria from June to September 1936, visiting mental asylums, prison asylums, and even indigenous medical practitioners. Ultimately, however, Brown found that mental health services had changed very little in terms of material conditions or treatment options in the time since Home's tour eight years earlier. As a result, the critiques and recommendations offered in Brown's report were largely similar to those provided by Home. In his report, Brown criticized the overcrowding of Nigeria's asylums generally and the government-run asylums in the south specifically.[26] He also repudiated the use of prisons to house lunatics and lamented the paucity of staff and lack of curative or therapeutic treatment.[27] Although Brown did not expect the conditions in Nigeria's asylums to compare favorably with those in Europe, he noted that overall they fell below the standards that should be expected of even colonial circumstances.

Brown's recommendations focused on the issue of accommodation, arguing for the building of new facilities, such as the moribund project at Abeokuta. Although Nigerian asylums cumulatively housed roughly five hundred lunatics at the time of Brown's visit, he noted that the number of Nigerians needing mental health care was likely to increase in the future, with the result that any new asylums built should be "at least three or four times in extent that which would be adequate for the numbers to be accommodated at the time of purchase." Brown also recommended the demolition of the existing asylum at Lokoja in the Northern Provinces and the erection of a new asylum capable of housing a thousand patients.[28]

Brown, however, made clear that most mentally ill patients should continue to be treated outside official psychiatric institutions. In a move that pleased even the most stalwart proponents of indirect rule, Brown suggested that the emphasis of mental health policy should be on supporting the treatment of patients in their home communities. He argued for the establishment of a domiciliary care system in which officially sanctioned mental health professionals would have the power to select and approve the local guardians of lunatics, followed by regular if infrequent inspection of the care of patients in their homes. Brown argued that such a system made sense for a country like Nigeria, where "the family care of the insane, thanks to the widely diffused and deeply rooted family system of West Africa, already exists." Although Brown believed home care in Nigeria was "greatly in need of visitation, medical guidance and aid," he argued that such a system need not be particularly disruptive to local customs and institutions. "In the administrative and medical services with the cooperation of chiefs of wards and headmen of villages," argued Brown, "the structure of such organization and means of aid are already furnished." Furthermore, he continued, domiciliary care would actually save the colonial government money by freeing up space in Nigeria's asylums, thereby reducing both the expenditure on construction of new asylums and the recurrent expenditure on maintenance of a large number of patients. Brown's idea of domiciliary care seemed to be based on the understanding that the colonial government was likely to balk at any suggestion that sought solutions only in the form of great capital expenditure.[29]

Colonial officials, both within the Department of Medical and Sanitary Services and in other branches of government, lauded Brown's recommendations for domiciliary care. The acting chief commissioner of the Northern Provinces noted that Brown's report correctly recognized that "existing institutions for the care of lunatics are unsatisfactory," but also had the foresight to realize that "it is essential to frame any proposals for the amelioration of existing conditions with the strictest regard for economy." Brown's domiciliary care proposal provided an invaluable alternative by showing "that the organization for the care of lunatics which has come into being almost fortuitously can be utilized as the basis for a more highly-developed scheme." However, the acting commissioner did have one caveat to Brown's recommendations. Whereas Brown suggested that home care should be monitored to ensure that the mentally ill were receiving humane and proper care, the acting commissioner disavowed this kind of cultural encroachment, arguing that "anything in the nature of registration should be avoided," and that "these people should be encouraged to declare their charges to Village Heads and to avail themselves of the facilities provided at district dispensaries." This would presumably reduce expenditure even more by eliminating the need for a bureaucratic process or the hiring of medical staff to conduct home visits.[30]

In essence, the forms and processes of domiciliary care would continue exactly as they had prior to Brown's report. The director of Medical and Sanitary Services agreed that domiciliary care would be a viable compromise.[31] Nevertheless, he pointed out that domiciliary care did little to improve conditions prevailing in Nigeria's asylums, where "detention and not treatment" of dangerous and criminal lunatics would continue to be the emphasis for the foreseeable future.[32] Colonial officials therefore cherry-picked from Brown's report those recommendations that justified the status quo, while dismissing as too ambitious those that required a significant outlay of new effort and expenditure.

Conditions in Nigerian asylums were largely unchanged in 1955, when the colonial government commissioned yet another report on the psychiatric services of Nigeria. Conducted by J. C. Carothers, the most famous ethnopsychiatrist with experience in Africa, this survey came in the context of the decolonization of Nigeria. Carothers's mission was therefore not only to report on the nature and functioning of psychiatric services in Nigeria, but also to offer suggestions on how mental health services should be administered in an independent Nigeria. Carothers toured Nigeria between September and November of 1955. With Aro Mental Hospital open for business but not yet accepting inpatients at this time, the institutional structure and conditions within Nigerian asylums did not differ much from those reported by Brown nineteen years earlier. In the case of the Yaba asylum, Carothers noted that Brown's assessment continued to apply, "except that it is now more crowded and much more dilapidated."[33]

Overall, Carothers lamented, "It is sad to reflect that, if Dr. Brown's excellent advice could have been followed at that time, there might have been no need for the present commission of enquiry."[34] As such, Carothers's recommendations in many ways mirrored those of Brown, whose own recommendations had looked very much like those of Home before him. Whereas Brown had suggested the building of an asylum with accommodation for a thousand patients, Carothers expanded upon this, arguing that there should be one psychiatric bed per ten thousand of gross population. Thus Nigeria, "with a population of 33 million, should provide a minimum psychiatric accommodation of 3,300 beds."[35] This was far in excess of the roughly 1,150 beds that existed in Nigeria at the time of Carothers's visit, and about half of those were in prison asylums, which Carothers believed should be abolished entirely. However, like Brown, Carothers also believed that the vast majority of mental patients could continue to be cared for in their home communities by family, friends, and indigenous medical practitioners.

Carothers also pushed for the development of regional parity in the extension of psychiatric services. Under the constitutional reforms of 1946, 1951, and 1954, Nigeria became a federated state, split into three regions—North, West, and East—with a Federal Territory at Lagos. Under the 1954 constitutional revisions, medical services, including psychiatric confinement and care, became the purview of the regional governments. It was therefore important to Carothers that each regional government have available the necessary resources to handle the mental health needs of the region. As of 1954, they did not. Due to issues of overcrowding, many mental patients had to be transferred to asylums in regions other than their home region, with the result that at the time of Carothers's survey, "not less than one in five, and probably one in four," of all detained lunatics were "accommodated in Regions other than their own."[36] Such a situation became problematic in a federated Nigeria because once regional governments took control of the psychiatric services, they were no longer required to provide accommodation to lunatics from other regions. The problem was further exacerbated by the fact that Aro Mental Hospital was located within the Western Region and once fully operational was likely to benefit only the Western Region, not Nigeria as a whole. It was therefore imperative that each region expand its psychiatric services to be able to meet its specific needs.[37]

The issue of the cost of implementing Carothers's recommendations once again plagued colonial officials after the release of the report. In a particularly intemperate memo to the acting secretary of the Southern Provinces, the acting secretary to the government at Lagos proclaimed: "We discussed the cost of a Lunatic Asylum and you have mentioned figures from £750,000 downwards. I should say that there is not the faintest hope of getting any sum of this order. . . . It constantly mystifies me that the medical mind in particular can never see any half way house in matters of this nature, and I flatly refuse to believe that £100,000 could not build reasonable accommodation for 1,000 lunatics."[38] According to the secretary, "To think in terms of £750,000 for 300 lunatics is merely baying for the moon and can only perpetuate the present situation which I gather is plainly disgusting."[39] The disparity between Carothers's recommendations and what the colonial government was willing to do was so stark that some colonial officials even suggested scuttling the publication of the report so as to keep its findings secret.[40] In such a climate, it is not surprising that Carothers's recommendations largely went the way of Home's and Brown's for the remainder of the period of British colonial control.

BROWN, CAROTHERS, AND PSYCHOLOGICAL RACISM

The colonial government's desire to keep expenditures on psychiatric services minimal was clearly based on a basic premise of indirect rule that cultural matters were best left to "traditional" institutions. While this idea was economically efficient, it was also ideologically connected to racist notions of African incapacity to adjust to social transformations along European lines. As increasing numbers of Africans moved from rural to urban environments, adopted and adapted European religious and cultural norms, and, in so doing, demanded more active and participatory forms of government, traditional and presumably historically static social structures were significantly undermined in ways that threatened the stability of both indigenous societies and individual psyches.[41] Ideas about the innate psychological difference of colonial subjects were apparent in the reports that Brown and Carothers supplied to the colonial government. As such, these reports tended to reinforce notions central to the philosophy of indirect rule that Africans were likely to suffer from too rapid social change. Therefore, even as the Brown and Carothers reports called for a much wider extension of modern European-styled institutions to service the needs of Nigeria's mentally ill population more effectively, they nevertheless revealed the extent to which their basic conceptions about African psychology had been influenced by prevailing notions of racial difference that characterized colonial ideology.

Both Brown and Carothers argued that in a large, multiethnic country like Nigeria, recognition of the differences in culture across space was of paramount importance to the understanding and treatment of mental illness. Ultimately, however, both fell back on a tendency to lump all Africans together as a more or less homogeneous cultural unit and to define that unit primarily in contradistinction to Europeans. For example, Brown argued that cultural difference within Nigeria should be a concern to mental health officials because "the presumed causes of mental disorder . . . vary from tribe to tribe in consonance with locally current mythology and belief," and it was therefore important for psychiatric experts to know the cultures within which they were treating. Brown had no such specific cultural understanding himself, however, having spent only a few months on a whirlwind tour of Nigeria. As a result, he quickly fell into familiar patterns of cross-cultural generalization, noting that Nigerian beliefs in the causes of mental illness were "fairly general," with "the most commonly entertained" being "first, possession by evil spirits (especially in the cases of acute and chronic mania), and second, 'ill-wishing' by evil-minded persons (especially in delusional forms of insanity)." Brown attributed the predominance of supernatural etiology to Nigerians' stage of "racial development," suggesting that at one point Europeans believed such things, but, as a race, had evolved beyond this point. Brown clearly viewed Nigerians as culturally similar to each other and to other Africans primarily in terms of their negative deviation from what he considered to be European psychological norms.[42]

Of course, Brown was an outsider with no previous experience in Nigeria and did not claim to have any specific understanding of cultural differences within Nigeria other than that they certainly existed. But he also illustrated in his report the extent to which racialized definitions of human mentality impinged upon his judgment. For example, he was quick to point out "the wide dissimilarities in mentality, including in this term intellectual, emotional and ethical qualities, which in the average distinguish the West African from the European." Brown refused to comment on the ongoing debate about the causes of these differences, and explicitly stated that the recognition of racial difference was "no question of good and bad, or of superior and inferior, but only one of difference," a fairly liberal idea for its time. Nevertheless, it is clear that at a basic level he defined culture in terms of race. "The fact remains," argued Brown, "that the emotional or affective processes, which are at once the source of feeling, habit and custom and the mainspring of conduct, are so deeply implanted in every individual and race that they are peculiarly insusceptible of alteration by external conditions with which they are not in essential agreement, and persist beneath the surface, in powerful operation, generation after generation." Perhaps most telling, a close reading of Brown's report reveals that he makes several references to the "African" and a few to "Mohammedans," but not a single reference to any of Nigeria's hundreds of ethnically or linguistically discreet groups.[43]

Interestingly, although Brown defined Africans as a more or less homogeneous group based on their presumed shared differences from Europeans, he placed little to no belief in the psychological effects of sociocultural change.[44] The Carothers report from 1955, on the other hand, tended to define Nigerian cultures primarily in terms of degrees of "detribalization." Carothers, like Brown before him, argued that Nigerian cultures were significantly different across space and that cultural differences did likely result in differences in the psychological makeup of people. For this reason,

Carothers believed that there was a strong need in Nigeria to reorganize the asylum system on regional lines because, in his opinion, Nigerian cultures varied significantly from region to region (but apparently not within regions). As a result, he argued, "the incidence of insanity and even the forms that mental derangement takes may be expected to vary somewhat on this basis and the psychiatric needs are thus also likely to vary on these [regional] lines."[45] The delineation of regional boundaries was itself ultimately a political process heavily influenced by colonial occupation and only very loosely reflecting substantive cultural divisions within Nigeria, but for Carothers these boundaries had real cultural and psychological implications.

For Carothers, the primary marker of cultural difference between the regions was the relative extent to which British values and cultural norms had infiltrated the lifestyles of indigenous societies. Of the Eastern Region, Carothers declared, "The people by and large are ambitious and adventurous and have availed themselves in high degree of the European type of education, and often travel or go to work outside their Region. In these circumstances conflicts between the old ways and the new must often be acute and take a corresponding toll in mental health and happiness."[46] Comparatively, Carothers described the people of the Western Region as:

> hav[ing] developed, independently of recent European influence, a way of life to which they are firmly attached and which includes a considerable degree of urbanization. In these circumstances it would seem, firstly, that European ways make less appeal to them than to peoples of the Eastern Region and secondly, that they can absorb these ways more easily and less conflictually than can many African groups. In these circumstances an increase of mental breakdown due to the impingement of the new ways on the old is likely to be less dramatic.[47]

In extreme distinction from the Eastern and Western Regions, which were both located in southern Nigeria near the coasts and which therefore had the greatest amount of historical contact with Europeans, Carothers defined the predominantly Muslim Northern Region as "on the whole . . . and especially by comparison with the peoples of the southern Regions . . . hav[ing] in common a considerable complacency in regard to their traditional ways of life and little inclination for their change. In all those circumstances it is not to be expected that demands for psychiatric care and treatment are likely to increase very rapidly unless they are powerfully encouraged to do so."[48]

So far as Carothers was concerned, the cultural differences within Nigeria existed primarily at the regional level, and these cultural differences were based primarily on the relative exposure of the peoples in these regions to British culture, education, and social institutions. Those with high exposure to British ways, the significantly "detribalized," were assumed to be in greater danger of developing a mental imbalance because of cultural conflict, and therefore Carothers suggested that mental health infrastructure needed to be boosted in the Eastern and Western Regions that made up southern Nigeria, where there was a greater concentration of such "detribalized" Nigerians. In the north, where British influence was less significant, Carothers argued that there was less need for an expansion of mental health infrastructure and services.

Ultimately, both Brown's and Carothers's reports very much adhered to the basic assumption that Africans, as a race, were culturally similar because of the ways they differed from European cultures. As such, their analysis focused on the extent to which "modern" European-styled mental health services should be provided at a basic level, but not at the expense of African cultures and institutions. While their recommendations for expansion of European-styled mental institutions largely fell on deaf ears, their comments on cultural matters conformed broadly to colonial administrators' fears of the destabilizing effect that the active transformation of "traditional" cultures and institutions would have on African societies. In other words, they reinforced the social assumptions of indirect rule in Nigeria even as they called for a change in its practice through the expansion of psychiatric facilities.

COLONIAL NIGERIA AND NETWORKS OF ETHNOPSYCHIATRY

The racialization of psychological functioning was not an isolated dynamic within colonial Nigeria. The assumptions and debates about the nature of the "African mind" that the Brown and Carothers reports presented were commonplace in scholarship about the psychology of Africans and the effects of colonialism on African psychology. Jock McCulloch has argued that because the political and ideological frameworks of European—particularly British—colonialism were similar across the continent, the key concepts in ethnopsychiatry tended to be remarkably similar across space, despite the fact that ethnopsychiatrists tended to work in isolation.[49] This may be true; however, it is also important to note that by the 1950s, ethnopsychiatric literature defining the "African mind" as different from that of the white man and threatened by European civilization had become the basis of scientific knowledge about psychology in Africans at an international level. Ethnopsychiatrists published not only in regional journals like the *East African Medical Journal*, but also increasingly in much more international fora like the *British Medical Journal* and the *Journal of Mental Science*. Although McCulloch argues that ethnopsychiatry never became a mainstream methodology of the broader disciplines of either anthropology or psychiatry, it must be recognized for our purposes that ethnopsychiatric literature did account for most of the firsthand scholarship on the nature of African psychology by the 1950s. While I am not arguing that the specific reports produced in Nigeria were particularly influential in the development of ethnopsychiatry as an international body of knowledge, I am suggesting that the theory and practice of psychiatry in colonial Nigeria was part of a widely held, broadly based and, by the 1950s, somewhat integrated set of beliefs about the relationship between culture, psychology, and race that had established the debates and discourses that transcultural psychiatry took up and transformed.

J. C. Carothers had not been randomly chosen to survey Nigeria's psychiatric infrastructure in 1955. Indeed, Carothers was probably the most internationally renowned ehtnopsychiatrist with clinical experience in Africa at the time. He had spent more than twelve years, from 1938 to 1951, as the head of the Mathari Asylum in Nairobi, Kenya, and during that time had published many scientific papers concerning the psychology of the "African mind" as he had experienced it. By the time he conducted his survey in Nigeria, his stature as a vanguard ethnopsychiatrist was such that the World Health Organization (WHO) had commissioned him to write a monograph for international dissemination on the current status of scientific thinking about African psychology. In 1953, the WHO had published Carothers's *The African Mind in Health and Disease* to serve as the synthesis of mainstream scientific knowledge about African psychology. It was on the basis of these credentials that the Nigerian government approached him to survey its psychiatric institutions in 1955.

Carothers's WHO monograph therefore serves as a good starting point for examining the views on the nature of the African psychology that served as the basis for his analysis of Nigeria and the recommendations that he made to the Nigerian government. Carothers's monograph represents to a great extent a consensus of ethnopsychiatric opinion on the nature of the "African mind" presented and analyzed by the leader of the field in the waning years of the colonial epoch. In addition to Carothers's own perspective, *The African Mind in Health and Disease* cites dozens of works by other colonial psychiatrists with experience in Africa over the course of the first half of the twentieth century. As such, it is the example par excellence of how ethnopsychiatrists conceived of the "African mind" and of the extent to which these ideas formed a coherent, interrelated body of knowledge by this time.

In this book, Carothers defined the "African mind," as it had been determined by European philosophers and scientists, to consist of the following traits:

> conventional, highly dependent on physical and emotional stimulation; lacking in spontaneity, foresight, tenacity, judgment, and humility, inapt for sound abstraction and for logic, given to phantasy and fabrication, and, in general, unstable, impulsive, unreliable, irresponsible, and living in the present without reflection or ambition, or regard for the rights of people outside his own circle. To counteract these ruderies, he has also been described as cheerful, stoical, self-confident, sociable, loyal, emotionally intuitive, and eloquent, and as bearing grudges and having an excellent memory, a large vocabulary, and an aptitude for music and dance.[50]

It is important to note that this definition applied for all black Africans, regardless of religious or cultural background. Although Carothers recognized some distinction between African societies, primarily between Christian/Muslim and indigenous religious practitioners and between the "tribal" and the "detribalized," he also believed that those distinctions masked a set of core traits that all Africans possessed. According to Carothers, "Although many, if not most, Africans today diverge in some degree from the model as defined, the ancient cultural modes are a far more vital force than these remarks imply."[51] The conception that African cultures and societies were largely similar, at least when compared to European cultures and societies, was, according to Carothers, "indeed the chief justification for the writing of this monograph."[52] Carothers based this definition of the "African mind" on the idea that Africans, as a race, were largely similar in terms of mentality, character traits, and social and cultural organization, particularly vis-à-vis Europeans. African groups or individuals who did not conform to this definition were considered deviations from the norm, not evidence of normlessness.

Carothers was working well within the established practices of other European ethnopsychiatrists with experience in Africa. As Geoffrey C. Tooth put it in his study of mental illness in the Gold Coast as late as 1950, "There is . . . no doubt that races and individuals differ widely in their natural endowment, in the use that they make of these two components of mentation [feeling and thinking] and in their ability to switch from one to the other."[53] European colonial psychiatrists, working from an assumed position of racial difference based on European superiority, did not question *whether* Europeans and Africans had distinct psychologies. The main goal of most ethnopsychiatrists was to determine *why* Africans developed such negative character traits. A psychological racial binary therefore became the starting point for scientific research, not a theory to be questioned in its own right.

Notions that biological differences separated African from European mentality were no longer in vogue by the 1950s.[54] Replacing them was a social evolutionist discourse that cited African culture as the culprit of African backwardness. According to the cultural causation models, which were heavily influenced by psychoanalytic theories of childhood development, African intellectual development stagnated at a relatively early age—curiosity was stifled because the universe was explained only in supernatural terms; social development ceased because an adolescent was considered an adult and could interact as a social equal with his elders. Any deviation from communal practices was considered antisocial, and as a result innovation was deemed suspicious and individual accomplishment without honor. There was no incentive for intellectual development in the individual, and as a result, group development also stagnated.[55] Some Europeans argued that loose sexual mores were the cause of arrested development of adolescent Africans.[56] Because Africans were lumped together as a single demographic unit based on race, ethnopsychiatrists also tended to talk about African culture as a uniform thing, undifferentiated across space.[57] Carothers's generalizations were therefore meant to apply broadly to African societies across the continent.

The communally oriented, extroverted, unambitious, superstitious, unintelligent African, lacking introspective insight and living only in the present and without a care for the future, became for ethnopsychiatrists the "normal" African. Mental illnesses in Africans were characterized by some deviation from this norm. However, most ethnopsychiatrists believed that rates of mental illness were very low among Africans living in their "natural" environments, where socialization occurred in the ways described above.[58] The same forces that caused the African mind to be so underdeveloped and inferior compared to the European were also responsible for this low level of mental illness in African societies. European ethnopsychiatrists presumed that levels of stress were low in African societies because the communal lifestyle expected very little of the individual, while the cosmology of so many African societies prevented the existential curiosities that drove Europeans into despair and torpor.[59] Ethnopsychiatrists believed that in such a secure social environment, levels of mental illness were likely to be much lower than in the fast-paced, individualistic "modern" world.

Conceptions of mental illness prevalence based primarily on ideas of racial difference seemed to be supported by statistical analysis. As of 1939, the rate of institutionalization for mental derangement in England and Wales stood at 4 per 1,000 of the total population. In contrast, colonial statistics indicated that institutionalization rates in African colonies were much lower. Tooth estimated the rate of institutionalization in the Gold Coast to be 0.3 per 1,000 in 1950.[60] In Nyasaland (Malawi), Horace Shelley and W. H. Watson estimated the rate to be 0.06 per 1,000 as of 1936.[61] Carothers estimated an institutionalization rate of 0.1 per 1,000 in Kenya in 1953,[62] and, according to the commissioner for mental hygiene, the rate was 1.2 per 1,000 in South Africa in 1950.[63] Such numbers led to the general belief that incidence of mental illness was much lower among African populations than among European populations, even though there were widely recognized problems with the data.[64]

The general assumption among colonial psychiatrists was that the "traditional" lifestyle of "primitive," rural Africans provided stability for the intellectually stunted "African mind." But in the context of European colonial rule, this lifestyle was in flux, as African cultures came into ever-closer contact with Europeans. The general tenor was that African societies represented an earlier, static stage of human social evolution and that, in time, African societies could evolve along the lines that Europeans had. However, "modernization" along European lines had consequences. In the short term, ethnopsychiatrists feared that social change could be dangerous to Africans not equipped to cope with what they assumed were the more sophisticated, modern, and civilized cosmologies and social institutions that Europeans brought with them. As P. Gallais and L. Planques, working in French Algeria, declared, Western civilization "swamped these countries [African colonies]" with "a veritable tide of political, social, and religious ideas, entirely new, . . . submerging the natives under an ocean of concepts for which nothing had prepared them, and in which they were incapable of discriminating good from bad. Already the frequency of mental states among uprooted natives (soldiers, sailors, dockers), with their frequent frenzies, bears witness to the influence on their mentation of a conditioning quite different from that of the environment to which they were adapted."[65] European specialists called the social process whereby Africans were forced to adapt to European ways of life "detribalization," and most of them considered it the greatest single threat to the stability of the "African mind."

European ethnopsychiatrists concocted a broad array of psychological consequences attendant to "detribalization." They argued that detribalization brought psychological distress because it required so much change on the part of Africans. Exposure to European education brought literacy, which exposed Africans (assuming they were from previously nonliterate societies) to ideas and customs that would cause them to disconnect from and question their traditional worldviews. If enough literacy were achieved, it could lead to better-paying, more individualistic and urban employment, which would take Africans farther from their "traditional" homes, exposing them to loneliness, isolation, and alienation in ways they were unprepared to handle.[66] The better pay and the need to live in cities, often far from the traditional extended family, put a great deal of pressure on detribalized Africans to succeed. The literate, detribalized African was expected to maintain his traditional responsibilities in addition to his modern ones, and even to distribute his largesse back to his community of origin. Detribalized Africans were therefore faced with a dilemma of whether or not to cut ties with their traditional past in order to effectively adapt and live a modern existence. The stress of this circumstance, according to ethnopsychiatrists, could easily lead to mental unbalance.[67]

The possibility that mental illnesses in Africans might be caused by detribalization remained a prevalent theory throughout the colonial period and into the postindependence era despite the inconclusiveness of data on the subject. In his WHO monograph from 1953, Carothers pointed to studies that showed Africans who lived away from their rural homes showed a higher institutionalization rate than Africans who did not migrate to cities, as well as studies suggesting that mental breakdowns among rural Africans tended to be less severe than detribalized urbanites. However, Carothers made clear that these studies failed to provide "sufficient evidence to justify any firm conclusions, one way or another," because their conclusions could all be explained away by faulty methodology or unknown variables. Nevertheless, he appeared to believe that the psychopathological effects of detribalization were simply facts awaiting scientific proof. He declared that even among detribalized Africans, the rates of incidence were significantly lower than in American and European populations, concluding that "if one relates this finding to the high rate for Negroes in America, there do seem to be grounds for thinking that psychotic incidence in Africans is related to deculturation."[68] Indeed, his recommendation that the growth of the psychiatric service sector in Nigeria should be targeted to communities with the highest exposure to European civilization is an indication of the extent to which he had internalized the detribalization theory of psychiatric disorder.

The work of ethnopsychiatrists on the nature of the "African mind" meshed particularly well with the gradualist notions of social and cultural transformation that characterized the indirect rule philosophy of colonial administration in Nigeria and other parts of Africa. Not only was rapid modernization seen as politically destabilizing to African societies, it was also presumably psychologically destabilizing to individual Africans. Since Africans tended to be considered psychologically similar as a race, interpretations of psychological makeup in a particular African community could easily be applied to other African territories. Therefore, it is not surprising that Nigerian officials reached out to ethnopsychiatrists like J. C. Carothers who had no particular expertise on Nigeria to provide feedback on how to improve treatment of the disordered African minds in their territory. The approach that the colonial government of Nigeria took toward the development of psychiatric services was therefore linked to a broader set of processes that had established a widely applicable theory of the nature of African psychology. Ethnopsychiatrists working in Nigeria and a variety of other African environments had developed a coherent set of key terms and debates that defined African psychology diametrically against European psychology. Though generally regarded as unproven theories, the key terms and debates of ethnopsychiatry had become internationally synthesized through scientific networks by the 1950s and framed the scholarly discourse on mental illness in Africans at the time that Nigerian psychiatrists came on the scene.

CONCLUSION

By the mid-1950s, despite frequent declarations by officials and visiting specialists that Nigerian mental asylums were unsanitary, overcrowded, and unsuitable for confinement of the mentally ill, conditions remained largely what they had been in the 1920s. In 1954, the medical officer for the Yaba asylum reported that 255 lunatics were being confined in space allotted for just 180.[69] By 1957, the prison asylums in the Eastern Region, at Calabar, Enugu, and Port Harcourt, housed 400 lunatics in space designed for 333.[70] Material conditions within the asylums had not improved either. In 1955, the superintendent of prisons noted that the accommodations for lunatics in prisons in Port Harcourt remained "as deplorable as ever. I saw several violent lunatics shivering naked in dark damp cells chained like animals to a ring in the floor; others also naked, wandered aimlessly around a barbed wire enclosure. Since the more violent destroy any clothing or bedboards issued to them they are obliged to sleep naked on damp cement."[71] These circumstances were partly the consequences of an indirect rule philosophy that stressed economy and nonintrusion into cultural matters. This philosophy was greatly reinforced by scientific knowledge constructed by ethnopsychiatric experts in colonial environments across the continent that stressed the essentially similar psychology of Africans as a race and its incommensurability with that of Europeans, even while it preached for extension of medical and custodial services for the mentally ill in Nigeria. This knowledge was produced and disseminated internationally and therefore, through its application to Nigerian circumstances, linked governmental justifications for the ways it exerted power over the mentally ill to an international scientific discourse that both legitimized government inaction and reinforced racialized conceptions of humanity. In the 1950s, a new generation of psychiatrists would engage this body of knowledge to decolonize both the Nigerian psychiatric institutions that had so poorly served the population and the international networks of psychiatric science that had so denigrated its character.

2 Decolonizing Psychiatric Institutions and Networks

When I was there, I know all the politicians, I was able to participate in getting them better when they were ill. So psychiatry had a tremendous life, boost, and at the same time I was able to push it.

—T. Adeoye Lambo, 1977

Psychiatric thought and practice in Nigeria underwent a revolution in the 1950s and 1960s. This chapter focuses on the two specific developments during this period that contributed most to the transformation of psychiatry in Nigeria. The first was the emergence of Nigeria's first native-born but Western-trained psychiatrist, Thomas Adeoye Lambo. From his first day on the job in 1954, Lambo actively sought to decolonize both the custodial asylum system in Nigeria and the racialized ethnopsychiatric knowledge that had constructed Africans as mentally and culturally inferior to Europeans. The second was the establishment of Aro Mental Hospital near Abeokuta, the first European-type institution in Nigeria designed to provide therapeutic treatment for psychiatric disorders. It was at Aro that Lambo and others pioneered efforts at transcultural psychiatric treatment and research that contributed to the deracialization of psychiatric knowledge not only in Nigeria but globally. The scientific and medical contributions of Lambo, coupled with the creation of a full-fledged mental hospital at Aro, set the foundation for the development and expansion of the psychiatric profession in Nigeria from the 1950s.

Just as ethnopsychiatry had been both a contributor to and a product of colonial political ideology, so, too, was the transition to transcultural psychiatry a reflection of the changing political and economic context of the postwar period. Major increases in development planning funds at this time led to expansions in infrastructure, education, and health care throughout Nigeria, while the political gains of anticolonial nationalist movements moved the country gradually toward self-rule and independence. The work of Nigerian psychiatrists like Lambo reflected these changes. Lambo asserted through his research and clinical practice the ignorance, incompetence, and arrogance of colonial attitudes toward mental illness in Nigerians. As a counterargument, he began to produce research arguing for the basic universal similarity of human psychology, irrespective of race, religion, ethnicity, or geography. In so doing, Lambo contributed to anticolonial nationalist discourses by debunking notions of hierarchical racial difference while simultaneously illustrating the value of indigenous leadership for effective application of "modern" science and social service provision in African settings. At the same time, Lambo's accomplishments were both illustrative of and a contribution to changing attitudes about the processes of "development" and "modernization" in an impending postcolonial world order.

The decolonization of psychiatric theory and practice in Nigeria reflected national political and social circumstances. But the Nigerian context was intimately connected to developments in psychiatry internationally. Lambo recognized that challenging racialized notions of the "African mind" required an engagement with international networks of scientific knowledge production and dissemination in order to produce the kind of comparative data necessary to reformulate psychiatric conceptions of the boundaries of cultural units and their relationship to one another. He therefore positioned Aro Mental Hospital and the University of Ibadan, where he had become a faculty member by the early 1960s, as nodes for international research in transcultural psychiatry. The projects that Lambo participated in produced new knowledge about the nature and prevalence of mental illness in Nigerian populations using Western scientific methods and actively compared findings with studies done elsewhere in the world. Lambo published in national, regional, and international journals, many of which had previously been instruments for the dissemination of colonial psychiatric knowledge. He engaged actively in the international scientific community, organizing international conferences and serving on international bodies. In so doing, Lambo blurred the line between nationalism and internationalism, between "Western" science and "indigenous" knowledge, and between cultural particularism and global universalism in ways that would characterize Nigerian psychiatry and transcultural psychiatry more broadly for the next several decades.

NATIONALISM, DECOLONIZATION, AND THE "MODERNIZATION" OF PSYCHIATRIC SERVICES

At the conclusion of World War II in 1945, the colonial government of Nigeria began the long, slow, negotiated process of decolonization that would end with official independence on October 1, 1960. Decolonization contained both political and economic components, both of which were important for developments in psychiatry. Politically, by the end of World War II, nationalist politicians in Nigeria were coalescing into official political parties pushing for the independence of Nigeria from British colonial rule. Working within increasingly regionalized ethnic bases, nationalist politicians and their supporters put pressure on the colonial government for gradual constitutional reforms that granted ever more power to indigenous leadership. Three constitutions were produced, in 1946, 1951, and 1954, respectively, which established the framework for the emergence of a delicately balanced sovereign federation in 1960. Despite the subnational cleavages that existed between politicians, the road to independence, however tenuous, was paved with rhetoric that painted colonial rule as failing to bring the "civilization" and progress that it had promised. For nationalist politicians, whatever their other differences, the best chance for a better future would come through independence and indigenous rule, which they believed would provide more effective and responsible governance than racist and alien British colonialism had.[1]

Partly as a response to increasing political pressures from anticolonial nationalist politicians, the colonial government also embarked on massive development-planning schemes that were supposed to bring about the deliberate "modernization" of Nigeria in ways that would have been unconscionable in the prewar context. A ten-year development plan was instituted in 1945 that provided millions in infrastructure and agricultural improvements, as well as major expansions in social services. As part of the ten-year plan, £7.7 million was allocated for education and £10.4 million for medical and health services.[2] New schools were needed to train Nigerians to take on skilled positions in a modernizing economy, while the medical and health funds were earmarked for building new hospitals, controlling endemic diseases like leprosy and malaria, and conducting research in tropical medicine. The total availability of Western education increased dramatically after 1945. In 1947, there were roughly 100 secondary schools in all of Nigeria; by 1960 more than 700 were in operation in the Western Region alone.[3] In 1948, Nigeria opened University College, Ibadan, as its first degree-granting institution. Growth of hospitals was equally dramatic. From 116 in 1945, the total number of hospitals in Nigeria grew to more than 300 by 1960, the bulk of the increase coming from the establishment of new government-run hospitals.[4] The expansion of education and medical facilities meant that the number of practicing doctors—both Nigerian and expatriate—also rose in the postwar era, from roughly 150 total in 1945 to more than 1,000 by 1960.[5] As part of this expansion of medical infrastructure, after nearly twenty years of inaction, the colonial government finally approved £350,000 for the construction of Nigeria's first mental hospital in 1945.[6]

In the context of an actively developmentalist policy, the dilapidated and coercive psychiatric infrastructure was a particularly damaging blight on the colonial government's record. By the 1940s, colonial mental asylums had become easy targets for anyone who wished to point out the incompetence of alien rule. In 1945, the *West African Pilot*, one of the largest independent Nigerian newspapers, run by Nnamdi Azikiwe, a prominent nationalist politician who became the first president of independent Nigeria in 1960, ran a story excoriating the Yaba asylum. The article drew on many of the well-known issues of overcrowding and poor sanitation, using vivid imagery to illustrate the horrendous conditions in the asylums. Among other things, the *Pilot* accused Yaba employees of using the same buckets to draw water that were used for latrines, leaving some rooms vacant while crowding patients into others, and leaving nurses and inmates in the sun to the point of fainting.[7] Although most Nigerians had little direct interaction with colonial Nigeria's psychiatric infrastructure, such stories certainly publicized the ways that colonial medical policy appeared to be more oppressive and damaging than beneficent and healing.

Those who were so unfortunate to have friends or loved ones locked away in colonial asylums showed a great deal of disappointment and anger over their treatment there. Nigerians with family members in asylum custody regularly petitioned for their release.[8] For example, Moses Ogede revealed his frustrations in a letter requesting the release of his wife from the Yaba asylum in Lagos in 1951. "Don't you know that if a person dies," wrote Ogede, "there must be some people to take him to the grave? I am on my knee begging for permission to take my wife from the hospital for the worriness [*sic*] of her parents are becoming greater day in and day out. I cannot endure any further. I am fed up with her position there. I therefore want his honour to give me a note to the doctor in order to discharge her at once."[9] Many people wanted their loved ones released in order to take them to traditional medical practitioners in whom they had greater faith than the custodial asylum.[10]

While such requests might have fallen on deaf ears before the 1940s, the colonial government recognized that some reform and expansion of the psychiatric infrastructure was clearly needed in the context of increasingly powerful and organized anticolonial sentiment. Efforts by the colonial government to expand Nigeria's asylum system and move toward providing actual therapeutic care actually began in the mid-1940s, roughly ten years before T. Adeoye Lambo began practicing psychiatry at Aro. In 1944 the colonial government took over a native administration prison at Lantoro, near Abeokuta, and converted it into a hospital for psychologically disturbed soldiers returning from active duty in Burma.[11] In 1948, Aro, just a few miles from Lantoro, was chosen as the site for the new mental hospital, and construction was set to begin. Progress was slow and still well below required capacity, prompting the overwhelmingly negative assessment of colonial psychiatric facilities found in J. C. Carothers's 1955 survey discussed in chapter 1. The hospital at Aro was not high on the priority list of development projects, and the facility was not in a position to admit inpatients by the time Lambo arrived in 1954.

The late 1940s also saw the posting of a full-time psychiatrist in Nigeria for the first time in twenty-five years.[12] In 1949, Dr. Donald Cameron, a British psychiatrist, arrived to oversee the operation of Lantoro and the nascent construction of nearby Aro Mental Hospital. While the arrival of a full-time in-residence psychiatrist might have seemed like an opportunity for the improvement of mental health services, Cameron's tenure in Nigeria was tumultuous and, ultimately, fairly unproductive. While waiting for construction of Aro to be completed, Cameron put his professional expertise toward centralizing control over Nigeria's much-maligned asylums. Cameron ruffled feathers by claiming that "few of the Medical Officers have any idea how to 'run' an Asylum,"[13] and issued directives demanding that all institutions that housed "lunatics" submit annual reports to him on the demographic and diagnostic makeup of their charges.[14] Recognizing the onerous nature of this process, Cameron suggested that a panel of medical officials be established in each region and that these panelists should all come to Abeokuta for "a month's course of instruction."[15] Perhaps unsurprisingly, colonial medical officers across Nigeria resented any implication that they might do better by their patients and refused to comply with Cameron's demands. The director of Medical Services for the Northern Region simply refused to provide the data in 1952, arguing that such an effort would be futile owing to the fact that the north had no central asylums like Yaba or Calabar, and, as such, "no [medical] superintendent is whole time, nor does he administer it [the asylum] from an office in the institution."[16] He concluded on behalf of all medical officers in his region, "Any information gained, owing to its paucity and doubtful accuracy, would not be worth the work involved."[17] To the request that northern medical officers travel to Abeokuta for training, the director of Medical Services stated that they simply did not have the time, and suggested that if Cameron wanted to instruct them, he should "go on tour himself" so as to advise them "on their home ground."[18] Cameron received a similar response from the Eastern Region.[19] Once again, administrative inertia was stymieing any effective modernization of psychiatric practice.

Cameron agreed to tour the asylums in the north, but soon grew frustrated by his observations. After visiting asylums in Zaria and Kano, he produced a report declaring that the native-administration lunatic asylums were "not putting first things first."[20] He excoriated the asylums on the grounds that patients there "get no treatment for their illness; apparently they get no examination to search for possible causes of their illness."[21] He refused to tour any more northern asylums until he had some proof that action was being taken, noting that circumstances in other northern asylums were "not likely to be different."[22] As a result, little came of Cameron's efforts to reform Nigeria's asylum system even minimally. Shortly before Lambo arrived at Aro, Cameron left Abeokuta to become the medical superintendent of the Yaba asylum. He left Nigeria "very disgruntled" shortly thereafter.[23]

Cameron's efforts illustrated the extent to which widespread, systematic reform of the psychiatric infrastructure of Nigeria was unlikely to occur in the short-term. Despite a modest growth of funding for psychiatric services, staff constraints and general inertia on the part of government officials meant that meaningful reforms would have to come not so much through policy reform as through practical changes to the conduct of psychiatric care by vested individuals. Furthermore, in order for the practice of psychiatry in Nigeria to decolonize and modernize, it had to be significantly distanced from the colonial asylum system both for purposes of administration and for purposes of gaining popular support. This was exactly the approach that Lambo took on arrival at the still-incomplete Aro Mental Hospital grounds in 1954.

DECOLONIZING PSYCHIATRIC INSTITUTIONS: T. ADEOYE LAMBO AND ARO MENTAL HOSPITAL

Lambo was born in Abeokuta, in southwest Nigeria, in 1923. Educated in local mission schools, he traveled to the United Kingdom to undertake his medical training at the University of Birmingham.[24] Upon returning to Nigeria in 1951, he was briefly stationed at the Yaba asylum. The experience, along with the encouragement of Dr. Samuel Manuwa, who would become Nigeria's first indigenous director of Medical Services and, later, president of the World Federation for Mental Health,[25] convinced him to make psychiatry his specialty. He then went back to the UK for further study at the Maudsley Hospital in London. The Maudsley was famous in psychiatric circles for its innovative approach. It shunned the notion of psychiatric hospital as custodial asylum, and instead focused heavily on treating voluntary psychoneurotic patients on an outpatient basis, a characteristic that greatly influenced Lambo's approach toward clinical practice.[26] When he returned to Nigeria to take over at Aro, Lambo immediately began to do things very differently than previous expat experts. Rather than work within the colonial-era construct that Western-styled psychiatric care was too expensive and culturally intrusive to work on African populations, which so many colonial officials had argued before him, Lambo went about actively trying to integrate "modern" psychiatry with local cultural modalities. Indeed, Lambo's conviction about the importance of cultural sensitivity in psychiatric practice was so strong that he declared not Sigmund Freud or Emil Kraepelin, but the anthropologist Margaret Mead as the intellectual model for his pursuits.[27] In emphasizing the importance of culture not only in presentation but also in the treatment of mental illness, Lambo sought to transform psychiatry from a profession associated with ineffectuality and incarceration to one that Nigerians could associate with progress, national development, and, most importantly, positive therapeutic results.

The construction site for Aro Mental Hospital was located just a couple of miles outside Lambo's hometown of Abeokuta, making Lambo particularly well-suited for the task of developing strong relationships between the hospital and the surrounding communities. Rather than wait for the construction of the hospital to be completed, Lambo immediately began developing ways to provide psychiatric care outside the confines of the hospital walls. The result was the Aro Village Scheme, through which Lambo began to offer outpatient therapy in 1954. Based loosely on the famous community-care schemes organized in Gheel, Belgium, in the nineteenth century, and, more recently, of Tigani El-Mahi in Sudan, the latter of which Lambo had toured personally,[28] the Aro Village Scheme provided a holistic, community-based therapeutic experience. Lambo made arrangements with local chiefs and elders for his patients to live in four villages surrounding Aro Hospital. Patients arrived with a family member—usually a mother, aunt, or sister—who would keep watch over the patient during his or her stay.

Patients attended the hospital during the day for regularly scheduled treatments, which sometimes included such "modern," up-to-date psychotherapeutic methods as electroconvulsive therapy, insulin coma therapy, and, by the late 1950s, psychopharmaceutical treatment, then returned to the village at night, where they rented out rooms in the homes of villagers. Patients and villagers engaged in community projects and activities together, including church services, films, plays, dances, and eventually in agricultural activities, which were meant to help patients develop qualities of sociability and responsibility that they would need for effective social reintegration when they returned home.[29]

No doctor resided in the Aro villages, but there was a twenty-four-hour psychiatric nurse service established for day-to-day administrative matters and to handle any crisis situation that might occur. Urgent cases were immediately reported to the resident doctor in the hospital. Nonurgent matters were communicated to the doctor during his daily rounds of the village. Some drug therapy was given in the village, particularly in the form of sedatives, and some occupational therapy activities were organized in the village as well. Such activities were kept minimal, however, so as not to make the village feel like an extension of the hospital, as it was believed this would detract from the overall benefit patients received from community therapy in a "normal" environment.[30]

Patients residing in the Aro Village complex were admitted on a voluntary basis and could stay and receive treatment for as long as they liked. In practice, however, most stayed for less than three months. Factors determining length of stay were numerous. Some patients improved dramatically and went home. Others did not improve as much as hoped, and family members decided to leave to seek alternative treatment. Still others left involuntarily, being unable to afford to stay longer paying rent in the village while not working at home.[31] Regardless, Lambo was able to declare that African patients treated within a culturally familiar community environment showed lower levels of chronicity and higher levels of permanent recovery than those treated in mental hospitals in Europe or the United States, and at a lower cost than prolonged inpatient care.[32]

Aro Village catered specifically to the needs of nondangerous psychotic and neurotic patients. Seriously disturbed, uncontrollable, or criminal patients were not accommodated at Aro Hospital. Rather they were sent to Lantoro, which remained a closed unit affiliated with Aro Hospital. As of 1967, Lantoro housed about three hundred patients.[33] Even at Lantoro, however, patients received care and treatment unlike anything seen in colonial-era asylums. Asuni noted that patients in the closed ward were treated very humanely. They spent most of their time out in the open, interacting with one another. In fact, the gates to the asylum were not locked and some of the patients were allowed to leave the grounds on their own accord. Such an approach was deemed to be both therapeutic and socially beneficial, as it reduced "the feeling of incarceration" along the same lines as the village scheme, if to a lesser degree, and helped to combat the stigma Lantoro carried with the general population due to its history as a prison and colonial-style lunatic asylum.[34]

While the hospital and the patients clearly benefited from association with the local villages, the villagers of Aro also had much to gain from their association with the hospital. Not only did the rents of patients and their relatives provide a steady source of income for villagers, but the hospital also became involved in the development planning of the village. Landlords could borrow money from the hospital to expand their operations and take in more patients.[35] The hospital helped to bring piped water, pit latrines, and mosquito eradication equipment to the village in the late 1950s.[36] Aro Hospital staff also provided medical treatment to villagers and their families.[37]

With the village scheme up and running, Aro Hospital itself continued to grow. It began admitting inpatients in 1957. Although originally designed to house two hundred inpatients with plans to increase to five hundred beds over time, by the late 1960s, only about a hundred beds were in use at any given time, owing to staff constraints and a desire to maintain a focus on outpatient therapy. Despite the small number of inpatients served, by the late 1960s, Aro boasted "two admission wards, two infirmaries, three general treatment wards, and two disturbed wards," as well as a "staff dining room, kitchen block, laundry, treatment block, student hostel, occupational therapy, main dining hall, administrative block, operating theater, gatekeeper's lodge and gate, and a number of both senior and junior residential buildings."[38]

Aro Hospital also became a major medical training center. The hospital opened its own Psychiatric Nurses School in 1956 and quickly became the center of psychiatric nursing in the country, receiving nursing students from other Nigerian institutions, including the University of Ibadan, for rotations in the hospital and village by the mid-1960s.[39] In 1979, Aro Neuropsychiatric Hospital, as it was by then known, became an official World Health Organization Collaborating Centre for Research and Training; and in 1983, the hospital added a Drug Addiction Research and Treatment Centre providing round-the-clock service for substance abusers, the first facility of its kind in Nigeria.[40] It also established a department of psychology and began to provide postgraduate psychiatric training in conjunction with the West African

College of Psychiatrists and a postgraduate program in clinical psychology in conjunction with the University of Ibadan.[41]

In 1963, Lambo left Aro Hospital to take up the position as the chair of the newly formed Department of Psychiatry at the University of Ibadan. He took the Aro Village Scheme with him. From this point, the "Community Mental Health Center" housed in the main village of Abule Aro became the "Field Research Unit" of the university department, and formal connections between the village and Aro Hospital were severed.[42] Daily rounds from nearby Aro Hospital were replaced with weekly rounds from the much more distant University Hospital, Ibadan, some forty miles away.[43] Tolani Asuni, who had done his medical training in Dublin and arrived as an attendant physician at Aro in 1957, became the new director of Aro Mental Hospital, a position he would hold until 1976. Asuni developed two new village schemes at Olomore and Idi-Ori, continuing Aro Hospital's dedication to the outpatient community care model.[44]

Lambo's efforts to expand psychiatric service provision and tailor it to Nigerian needs and expectations should be seen not only in the context of a medical desire to provide effective care to individual patients, but also as a contribution to the development and modernization processes that Nigeria was undergoing alongside its political decolonization. Lambo, like ethnopsychiatrists before him, believed that psychological maladjustment was on the increase in many African countries, including Nigeria, in the 1950s and 1960s. Although Lambo did not attribute this rise in maladjustment to any unique shortcomings of the "African mind," as we will see below, he argued that the high levels of social disruption brought about by the widespread and rapid political, economic, and social change affecting Nigerian society in the context of decolonization, development, and modernization schemes would be psychologically disruptive to human beings from any racial or cultural background. "It is easier to see new buildings and new roads as evidence of progress," declared Lambo, "but unfortunately delinquency, prostitution, drug addiction and other social disasters accompanying 'progress' are often tucked away from full view."[45] As rural-urban migration dislocated families and communities, and as values and lifestyles fluctuated to adjust to new possibilities and changing circumstances, Lambo believed that psychiatry had an important role to play in ushering Nigerians through this tumultuous time. He urged that the research agenda in the social sciences should be "to investigate more scientific ways of preserving, activating, and mobilizing . . . human resources for the balanced survival of our peoples and their optimal functioning in the new world."[46]

Lambo did not think it was sufficient, however, for psychiatrists and social workers to shoulder the burden of the psychosocial fallout of Nigeria's development processes. He saw psychiatry as having a preventive medical component through its research and knowledge-gathering processes. If effective knowledge about the psychological effects of change on specific cultures could be produced, that information could then be transmitted to political leadership, which could in turn direct governmental policy toward an optimal balance between socioeconomic change and the public health needs of the population. In this way, he believed that "psychiatry . . . could contribute to national and individual productivity,"[47] noting, for example, that schizophrenia tended to afflict young adults in the prime of their productive years. Finding a way to prevent psychotic breaks and to treat them effectively when they occurred had the potential to save Nigeria a great deal of cost in terms of long-term care, as well as prevent the wastage of manpower upon which development of the country relied. Lambo was himself active in integrating his psychiatric practice with the social and economic development of Nigeria. For example, at Aro Village Lambo helped to organize occupational therapy programs focused on farming. Patients receiving psychiatric care also therefore learned skills that would allow them to contribute productively to the survival of the village and to be productive members of society.[48] In a speech to some of the young men engaged in these farming projects, Lambo urged his patients to "make a good success of what you are doing" so as to "contribute to the economic and social life of Nigeria."[49] For Lambo, the psychological health of individual Nigerians was inextricably linked with the development of the country as a whole.

DECOLONIZING PSYCHIATRIC NETWORKS: LAMBO AND TRANSCULTURAL PSYCHIATRY

The development of outpatient care and the orientation toward therapy and treatment rather than inpatient incarceration helped to reduce the stigma associated with Western psychiatric care in Nigeria, although most Nigerians continued to see traditional healers as an option of first resort. In 1965 Aro Hospital staff had treated a total of 2,000 outpatients.[50] This number had grown to 86,253 in the two-year period from January 1984 to December 1985.[51] Lambo's original mission to make psychiatric care relevant and available to Nigerians had improved dramatically over what had obtained previously, even though the vast majority of Nigerians still had no access to Aro. The decolonization of psychiatric institutions within Nigeria was only part of Lambo's grand vision for Nigerian psychiatry, however. For Lambo, the decolonization of psychiatry needed to be undertaken not only at the level of patient care, but also at the level of scientific research on the nature of the "African mind" that had so reinforced colonial governments' attitudes toward psychiatric care of African subjects.

When Lambo took up his post at Aro he began to confront the racist generalizations of ethnopsychiatry. In early published works, Lambo declared that existing research on mental disorder among Africans was "extremely inadequate," because too often "the clinical conclusions were founded on the treacherous sands of unscientific methodology."[52] He lambasted colonial psychiatrists for declaring their work to be scientifically objective when, in fact, Lambo believed, "at their worst they have been but glorified pseudo-scientific novels or anecdotes with a subtle racial bias; at their best, they are abridged encyclopedias of misleading information and ingenious systems of working hypotheses, useful for the guidance of research, but containing so many obvious gaps and inconsistencies, giving rise to so many unanswerable questions, that they can no longer be seriously presented as valid observations of scientific merit."[53] These unscientific conclusions about African mentality had led to a situation in which the advancement of the field was hampered not so much by ignorance, but "by knowing so much that is not strictly true."[54] Lambo took the greatest offense to Carothers's equation of the "African mind" with simplicity and fantasy. Referencing a paper in which Carothers had declared that African mentality corresponded generally to that of the lobotomized European, Lambo called such exaggerations "a good example of one of those attempts by some authors who, confronted with the baffling problems of the incomprehensible, adopt the popular procedure of making sweeping generalizations behind a veritable smoke-screen of technical terms, involved abstractions and semantic confusion."[55] Lambo's research sought to ameliorate some of the most heinous injustices that he observed in ethnopsychiatry.

Convinced that colonial psychiatrists' belief in the low prevalence of psychiatric illness among "primitive" African peoples was based on predetermined assumptions that conflated race and culture among Africans into a homogeneous, undifferentiated unit, Lambo went about examining the effect of culture on the form and presentation of mental illnesses. Lambo fought against the racialized conceptualizations of culture that had characterized colonial psychiatry. "There is no such thing as 'African culture' and therefore 'African mentality,'" argued Lambo. As far as Lambo was concerned, race should be eliminated as a demographic category for determining cultural difference. "Culture, strictly speaking," argued Lambo, "implies environment but in its totality. The racial concept is based on the assumption that genetically determined mental differences do exist between different races but the fact should be stressed that, in the light of our present knowledge, while the range and levels of innate mental capacities between races have not been proved to exceed those that are usually encountered in individuals of the same race, there is no evidence to support the view that psychological differences between groups are racially determined."[56] By focusing specifically on differences between cultures within Africa and similarities between African cultures and other world cultures, Lambo opened the door for a more nuanced brand of psychological research.

Lambo published many articles detailing the ways that culture affected the form and content of psychiatric disorders, particularly among the Yoruba ethnic group of which he was a member. In so doing, Lambo embarked on revolutionary research that tended to emphasize the similarities of psychological disorder across races and cultures rather than the differences. Arguing for the basic similarities of human psychology did not mean, however, that cultural understanding was not important for the effective practice of psychiatry. Quite the contrary, Lambo consistently argued that colonial ethnopsychiatrists had reached such erroneous conclusions about the nature of the "African mind" mainly because of their poor understanding of the ways that psychological disorders manifested in different cultures. For example, he argued that schizophrenia was far more common among rural Africans than had previously been believed and that depression was more common among both rural and urban Africans than ethnopsychiarists considered possible. Lambo believed individuals expressed symptoms of these diseases differently in different cultures because the signs and symbols that social groups used to identify sickness were to a great extent culturally determined. The symptom complexes that Europeans had used to identify schizophrenia and depression were calibrated to European cultures; African cultures, according to Lambo, expressed these universal diseases differently (see chapter 4).

If cultural factors were important in recognizing and diagnosing mental illnesses, it stood to reason that they would also be instrumental in treating them. In order to better understand local conceptions of mental illness, Lambo worked closely with traditional medical practitioners, even incorporating them into the Aro Village Scheme. Although he knew that this practice was "indefensible by western standards," Lambo was unwilling to believe that traditional medical practitioners did not provide real therapeutic care, and chalked up objections to his incorporation of them at Aro to "a form of arrogance of the 19th and 20th century Europe."[57] The incorporation of indigenous medical practitioners served two purposes for Lambo. In the first place, they helped the European-trained psychiatric staff understand the cultural factors that might be affecting the presentation of mental illness, therefore allowing for more complete and effective diagnoses. Secondarily, they also allowed for patients to be treated within cultural frameworks with which they were familiar and comfortable, thereby engendering trust in the therapeutic process and improving the likelihood of eventual recovery (see chapter 5).

Indeed, the Aro Village Scheme was itself part of a process of exploring the universal similarity of human psychology. Lambo did not see the idea of community therapy as something particularly attuned to Yoruba, Nigerian, or even African cultures. The specific employment of a rural village was designed to appeal to cultural specificities of Nigerians, but Lambo believed that the community therapy model would work in all human cultures if effectively adapted to the appropriate cultural markers. Speaking about the concept of community therapy to the United Nations, Lambo pontificated:

> There is no reason why an adapted form could not really take place in every society. . . . All human beings are the same, you know. We all want to be liked . . . we want to be loved. And these are the basic ingredients to positive mental health. . . . There is no reason why in New York City on Manhattan any form of community mental health which may have some affinity towards the social structure . . . could not be formulated and be carried out. There is no reason why in other African countries what we do in Nigeria could not be adopted to fit in with their either political or social-economic ideology and so on. . . . If we look at the basic ingredients, the basic philosophy of it, it's applicable everywhere among all societies where we use the word "human beings."[58]

The need to have psychotherapeutic regimes tailored to specific cultural milieus was therefore itself a universal human psychological characteristic as far as Lambo was concerned. Others appeared to agree. By the early 1960s, the Aro Village Scheme had garnered significant international attention. In 1960, the United Nations filmed a documentary in Nigeria lauding the accomplishments of Lambo and his staff called *The Healers of Aro*.[59] Adaptations of the Aro Village Scheme were attempted in several additional locations in Africa from the 1960s, including other parts of Nigeria, Senegal, and Tanzania.[60]

The idea that psychiatry needed to become more centrally concerned with cultural issues and with cross-cultural comparisons that took account of similarities as well as differences was part of a broader international movement in psychiatric science in the 1950s that came to be known as transcultural psychiatry. In the Euro-American history of psychiatry, the emergence of transcultural psychiatry is linked to the psychological turmoil of the Second World War. As Jatinder Bains has said, "Psychiatrists and social scientists believed that their insights into how culture/environment interacts with personality and mental illness could be utilized to solve major problems, in essence the problems caused by World War II, such as migration, rapid sociocultural change and tensions between nations."[61] After the war, John R. Rees founded the World Federation for Mental Health, which encouraged comparative studies; and in 1956 the departments of psychiatry and anthropology at McGill University in Montreal, under the leadership of Erik D. Wittkower, founded a newsletter titled *Transcultural Research in Mental Health Problems*, which later became *Transcultural Psychiatric Research Review*, the first academic journal to emphasize transcultural psychiatric research. The field remained small and funding opportunities minimal, but by 1960 efforts to organize and conduct transcultural psychiatric research had been undertaken in North and South America, the Caribbean, Europe, Africa, and Asia.[62] Transcultural psychiatry was divided from the very beginning about whether the primary goal should be to adapt Euro-American psychiatric theory and practice to non-Western cultures or to explore the influence of local cultures on mental health. Ultimately, the agendas of transcultural psychiatrists differed significantly within the subdiscipline. The emphasis on international, cross-cultural, and comparative projects, however, made transcultural psychiatry a fruitful outlet for the realization of Lambo's efforts to deracialize ethnopsychiatric theories about the inferiority of "African minds."

An early classic text in transcultural psychiatry came from a direct collaboration between Aro Hospital and the program in social psychiatry at Cornell University. Published as *Psychiatric Disorder among the Yoruba*, the results of the Cornell-Aro Mental Health Research Project provided a blueprint for how to conduct effective cross-cultural comparisons of psychological function and dysfunction, and Lambo was central in its conception and completion. The spark for the project was lit in 1959, when Alexander H. Leighton, a professor in the Department of Sociology and Anthropology at Cornell, visited Lambo for a tour of his increasingly famous Village Scheme at Aro. While there, Lambo and Leighton realized a shared interest in psychiatric epidemiology and began to discuss the possibility of an intercontinental comparative study of major psychiatric disorder between West Africa and North America. By January 1961, plans had been made and a methodology defined for conducting the study. The overall goal of the study would be to interview as many people as possible in fifteen Yoruba villages and the urban center of Abeokuta—all within five miles of Aro Hospital—and, using a standardized questionnaire, determine the relative mental health of individuals within these settings by classifying them on a scale from A to D, with A being clear-cut psychiatric disorder and D being psychologically "well." The findings of the research team in Nigeria were to be compared with the results of a nearly identical 1948 survey that had been conducted in Stirling County, a rural community in Canada, to determine what basic similarities and differences existed between the two communities in terms of rates and types of psychiatric disorder as well as broad social and cultural influences on the development of psychiatric disorder in the respective communities.

The development of appropriate terms of comparison between Canadian and Yoruba conceptions of mental illness became a difficult task for the research team, as did the translation of the Stirling County survey from English into Yoruba in ways that would elicit desired understanding of the meanings of highly subjective terminologies for things like feelings and emotions. The result was that the Cornell-Aro project found it very difficult to work within the existing constructs of the first edition of the *Diagnostic and Statistical Manual of Mental Disorders* (*DSM-I*), which had been published in 1952. For example, the Cornell-Aro team veered away from creating a diagnostic category called "depression" due to widespread uncertainty within psychiatric circles about whether or how to diagnose depression in Africans. While the ethnopsychiatric literature claimed that depression was exceedingly rare in Africans, Lambo had come to believe through his clinical practice that depression merely presented in different symptom patterns among Africans than Europeans. For this reason, the Cornell-Aro team decided that "rather than predetermine the issue we would employ a general category for affective disturbance and see what patterns turned up in it."[63] A similar propensity to keep diagnostic groupings as general as possible was applied to schizophrenia, mental deficiency, and a variety of other categorizations.

The Cornell-Aro team chose to use large, umbrella categories for diagnostic purposes because they recognized that most of their psychiatrists were from Western backgrounds and did not have the cultural expertise necessary to make fine distinctions (with the possible exception of Raymond H. Prince, who had done fifteen months of clinical work in Yorubaland previously). They also recognized that Western definitions and categorizations of psychiatric disorder were likely to differ substantially from Yoruba cultural conceptions of mental illness. As part of the background data gathering, the team discussed local conceptions of mental illness with indigenous Yoruba healers. In general, the team concluded that the Yoruba recognized the same types of symptoms as evidence of psychiatric disorder that Westerners held—generally socially unacceptable behavior in the form of excessive excitability, violent temperament, or, conversely, extreme withdrawal and lethargy. For example, a Yoruba healer described to the research team a clear case of mental illness of one of his patients who "wanders around talking to himself, apparently hearing voices when no one is speaking. He has sleep difficulty. He takes other people's things and exchanges them for cigarettes and 'is rather disobedient to instructions to refrain from particular actions'" (*PDY*, 107). Regardless of what the specific diagnosis of this individual would be in Western or Yoruba terms, it is clear that at a general level both Western and Yoruba cultures considered this type of behavior as abnormal, unacceptable, and an indication of an illness of the mind. Although in Yoruba cultures psychiatric symptoms were combined into different patterns and defined as different disease entities than obtained in Western cultures, according to the group, "None stood out as being unsuited to one or more of the psychiatric symptom categories" (*PDY*, 109). This did not mean that Yoruba mental illness categories corresponded one-to-one with Western categories, but that the component parts of Yoruba categories could also be recognized as component parts of Western categories.

Convinced that enough cross-cultural similarity existed to communicate the terms of psychiatric disorder interculturally, the team moved forward with its survey. Over the course of seven weeks in early 1961, four full-time psychiatrists—Alexander H. Leighton, Dorothea C. Leighton, Charles Savage, and Raymond H. Prince—conducted interviews with hundreds of Yoruba villagers and several dozen urbanites; while two anthropologists—Jane M. Murphy and Charles C. Hughes—surveyed the communities to better understand their social and cultural makeup. Lambo and Asuni oversaw the process and contributed to interviews where possible, often double-checking Yoruba-English translations. The cultural and linguistic expertise that they brought to the proceedings as indigenous Yoruba persons was, indeed, the only absolutely essential individual contribution to the ability of the project to go forward. Overall, the team interviewed 262 Yoruba individuals from fifteen different rural villages around Aro; 64 individuals from eight sections of Abeokuta, a city of an estimated population of 80,000 in 1960; and 59 patients from Aro Hospital, not all of whom were Yoruba (*PDY*, 125). The results showed that, in general, the Yoruba experienced a somewhat lower overall incidence of psychiatric disorder than the rural Canadians of the Stirling County survey, although the Yoruba respondents tended to experience more psychiatric symptoms than the Canadians. A further difference appeared in the gender breakdowns. Whereas in the Stirling survey women had experienced a significantly higher propensity for psychiatric disorder than men, in the Yoruba sample men and women had a nearly equal propensity for psychiatric disorder, an indication that socially something was happening in Yorubaland that Stirling County was not experiencing in the same way.

The easy answer for the higher prevalence of psychiatric disorder in Yoruba males would have been "detribalization"—rapid sociocultural changes that were affecting men more directly and immediately than women as the area urbanized, modernized, and Westernized. However, the Cornell-Aro team sought to complicate this model by examining not just the intensity of "change" that was occurring in Yoruba villages, but the general levels of "integration" and "disintegration" that Yoruba villages were experiencing in relation to that change. The authors defined *disintegration* as "the breakdown or disruption of the inter-relationship" of established patterns of sociocultural interaction between people. Both integrative and disintegrative processes are constantly under way in any community; however, "at a point in time when the social network undergoes change, there is likely to be a disruption of the previous forms of interaction, and it is appropriate to say that the community is in a state of reorientation, in which a preponderance of either integrative or disintegrative processes may come to the fore. Changes that occur in such a manner as to permit substitutions and adaptations while the functioning of the system of relationships continues with effectiveness will not involve disintegration to any significant degree" (*PDY*, 177). Based on the anthropological surveys, the Cornell-Aro team was able to categorize their fifteen villages on a three-tiered scale of "integrated," "intermediate," and "disintegrated" according to the effectiveness of local government, intensity of social organization, and material conditions of the village. In so doing, the authors concluded, first, that the levels of urbanization, cultural change, and socioeconomic status were not directly proportional to the level of integration/disintegration. A rural community could be significantly disintegrated, and a poverty-stricken community could be significantly integrated. When the team correlated their findings on psychiatric disorder, they were able to determine that rates of disorder corresponded more closely to the integration/disintegration axis than to those of rural/urban or illiterate/literate. The team concluded that in the Yoruba villages, "disintegration . . . is a common but not a necessary accompaniment of cultural change and modernization. In the Yoruba villages we received the impression that prevalence of psychiatric disorder is associated with disintegration rather than with cultural change as such" (279). The Cornell-Aro team was more inclined to see psychiatric disorder as brought about by disruption in human social networks rather than as the clash of cultures within an individual psyche.

The results of the integration/disintegration analysis showed a great deal of similarity with those of Stirling County in Canada, which had also seen higher rates of psychiatric disorder in disintegrated than in integrated communities. Despite the gender differences noted earlier, this finding, in conjunction with the background data on comparability of psychiatric symptom identification across cultures, led the team to conclude that "by and large . . . the similarity in the two samples is much more impressive than the differences" (*PDY*, 274). Taking a swipe at the ethnopsychiatric literature that had defined Africans as psychologically different from Euro-Americans at an essential level, the Cornell-Aro team claimed that their findings raised "some question as to whether the emphasis on cultural difference has been overdone. Perhaps a more balanced approach is appropriate, and the 'why' of similarities now emerging is just as interesting as the 'why' of difference" (274). Lambo's interests in examining similarities rather than differences therefore meshed well with the interests of transcultural psychiatrists internationally. Lambo's interests, findings, and organizational abilities had been essential to the cooperative network of knowledge production and exchange that resulted in the production of *Psychiatric Disorder among the Yoruba*.

The insertion of Lambo and Aro Mental Hospital into international networks of transcultural psychiatry had political as well as scientific implications for a decolonizing and modernizing Nigeria. So while *Psychiatric Disorder among the Yoruba* became an important foundational text in transcultural psychiatry for its innovative and rigorous methodology, the conclusions it reached also served larger political purposes for Lambo and other cultural nationalists who were interested in promoting the basic equality of nonwhite cultures. The comparability of the prevalence of many psychiatric disorders—and their universal connection to social integration/disintegration—between Yoruba and Canadian communities suggested that large-scale comparative experiments in transcultural psychiatry might go a long way toward eradicating persistent ideas of a cultural superiority/inferiority dichotomy between Westerners and Africans. Lambo's growing international prestige was therefore connected with both the emergence of the independent, indigenously controlled Nigerian state and a larger Pan-African nationalism that promoted the intellectual and cultural contributions of Africans to the world. The connection between international science and cultural nationalism was not lost on Lambo, who deliberately connected his political and scientific agendas through such projects as the First Pan-African Psychiatric Conference held at Aro in 1961, discussed in detail in the introduction to this book. While the First Pan-African Psychiatric Conference was a means to insert cultural politics into a psychiatric framework, Lambo also engaged in the insertion of psychiatry into networks of cultural politics. For example, in 1962 Lambo contributed to the *Proceedings of the First International Congress of Africanists*, an organization whose officers included some of the most distinguished intellectuals and social activists in West Africa, such as Kenneth Onwuka Dike, Alioune Diop, Aimé Césaire, James Ojo Coleman, Michael Crowder, and Ezekiel Mpahalele, among others.[64]

Lambo's international fame led him to a second career in international public health. Within three years of leaving Aro Hospital for the University of Ibadan, he had become the dean of medicine and, in 1968, vice-chancellor of the university.[65] He resigned from the university in 1971 to become the assistant director general of the World Health Organization (WHO), with responsibility over the divisions of Mental Health, Noncommunicable Diseases, Therapeutics and Prophylactic Substances, and Health Manpower Development. From 1973 to 1988, Lambo served as deputy director general of WHO, overseeing the development and implementation of projects in not only global mental health, but global health in general. While at the WHO, Lambo worked for the integration of the biological and social components of health care, and for the active incorporation of non-Western health systems into global health structures and beliefs. As deputy director, Lambo appointed the WHO's expert committee on mental health for much of the 1970s and 1980s.[66] He was also a major force behind WHO efforts to recognize and incorporate "traditional" medicine within the larger global health paradigm.[67] For Lambo, the move to the international arena made perfect sense, considering the extent to which his culturally nationalist approach to psychiatric practice in Nigeria had always contained an intrinsic engagement with the political process and with international networks of knowledge production and dissemination.

TRANSCULTURAL PSYCHIATRY AND CULTURAL BOUNDARIES

The entire purpose of the transcultural psychiatry that Lambo and others practiced from the 1950s was to determine scientifically acceptable ways to account for the relationship between cultural factors and the development, presentation, and treatment of mental illnesses. Lambo's personal identity was itself transcultural in the sense that he was a Yoruba man who had attained the highest levels of Western European education. This transcultural identity placed Lambo in an ideal position to negotiate the decolonization of Nigerian psychiatry as a symbol of an indigenous but modernizing Nigerian nation. In this way, Lambo fit the mold of many of the nationalist political activists who negotiated political independence for Nigeria and most other sub-Saharan African countries.[68] Such highly educated elites like Lambo were themselves proof of the basic flaws in the racialized hierarchies that had characterized colonial societies in Africa and the ethnopsychiatry that had emerged within them. That nonwhite psychiatrists like Lambo would be both interested in and good at debunking racist theories of human psychology is perhaps not particularly surprising. However, while Lambo and other transcultural psychiatrists like those of the Cornell-Aro project were relatively convinced that cultural beliefs and worldviews did not themselves *cause* mental illnesses to be more or less prevalent in a given society, they did believe that cultural factors influenced the ways that individuals experienced and expressed their psychological turmoil. Culture still mattered. However, the accepted boundaries (race) that had been used to differentiate cultures for the purposes of psychiatric research in Africa were being significantly disrupted by the 1950s. Reconstructing the relationship between individual, culture, race, and species in psychological terms was a daunting and unclear process for Lambo—indeed for all transcultural psychiatrists—and one that he never fully reconciled over the course of his career.

In early works, Lambo was as likely to use accepted terms and definitions of ethnopsychiatry as he was to contest them. Although Lambo argued that there was no such thing as a uniform African culture, he also tended to lump African cultures together when it served the interests of his counterdiscourse. For example, in a 1955 article very early in his career, Lambo had no problem essentializing African cultures when comparing them to other "civilizations" throughout time, arguing that "African cultural institutions . . . may lack the beauty of the Greek, the durability of the Chinese, the profound mysticism of the Hindu, and the effective knowledge of scientific facts and control over natural forces acquired in the West."[69] In a discussion of the Yoruba of southwestern Nigeria, Lambo declared, "There is no evidence . . . to support the view that Yoruba cultural institutions are significantly different from those of the other African tribes. A review of the literature on this subject reveals the fact that there are important points of similarity. Insofar as his personality structure is influenced by the cultural pattern, a rural (non-literate) Yoruba, for practical purposes, is a fair representative of the primitive African."[70] Lambo's reference to the "literature" in the above quote is also something of a contradiction. Presumably this is the same literature that Lambo had previously disregarded as racist and unscientific. His use of "primitive" to describe Africans who had little to no cultural interaction with Europeans is also clearly a holdover from ethnopsychiatry that implied an evolutionist understanding of culture. This was a term that Lambo used not infrequently.

However, by the mid-1960s, Lambo was less willing to make these kinds of generalizations. For example, in a 1965 article he refused to suggest that any of the data produced in *Psychiatric Disorder among the Yoruba* had any direct applicability outside southwestern Nigeria, urging researchers to be "extremely cautious in using this data because [the] study is confined to a fairly homogenous section of the population."[71] He wrote in 1972 that the "great diversity of tribes and cultures, in the face of rapid social and cultural changes, makes any attempt at isolation of the characteristic features of Nigerians particularly difficult," and doubted as a result that his comments about child psychology in Nigerians could be "generalized to other African groups."[72] He became adamant that his use of the term "African" be seen as applying "in a purely generic fashion with the knowledge that there is no such thing as 'African culture' or an 'African mind.'"[73]

Similarly, early in his career, Lambo had been instrumental in redefining the parameters of psychiatric diagnoses to make them more universally applicable to the ways that his patients expressed their psychological disorders. Lambo tended to speak of mental illness in non-Western cultures predominantly in terms of the mainstream psychiatric discourse of the time. For example, when determining the universal similarity of psychiatric disorder between the Yoruba and other cultures, Lambo discussed Yoruba mental illnesses as culturally specific variants of schizophrenia. Schizophrenia then was the "real" disorder that Lambo suggested could be discerned by peeling the cultural onion. He was similarly convinced that Africans experienced the disease known in psychiatric terms as "depression" far more commonly than ethnopsychiatrists had previously believed. However, Lambo believed that the symptoms of depression were culturally determined, and that African cultures therefore expressed depression differently than Euro-American cultures.

On a certain level, Lambo's acceptance of existing categories and terminologies seemed unavoidable. As a Western-trained psychiatrist, Lambo was invested in and beholden to the tools and concepts of the European psychiatric tradition. It was necessary for him to be able to communicate with other psychiatric professionals around the world in order for his message to have any influence or be taken seriously at all. Because of the nature of his own training and the need to integrate his work into established discourses in order to have any impact in transforming those discourses, Lambo worked within preexisting scientific language and symbols developed in a Euro-American cultural and historical tradition. However, he did this to illustrate the drawbacks of existing methods where they existed, and to prove the extent to which African psychology compared similarly to Western-defined "norms" as a means of overcoming the racialized bias that had historically characterized psychiatric interpretations of Africans.

Lambo recognized this adherence to psychiatric terminologies of Western origin as something of a clumsy fit for the explanation of mental illness in African cultures. By the 1960s, Lambo had become heavily critical of adopting Western methods and procedures for the interpretation of research and the conduct of clinical practice in non-Western settings, particularly in Africa. For example, in 1965 he declared that, ideally, social workers who intended to work in Africa should be trained in Africa, "in order to be conversant with the current social problems of Africa, and at the same time to be aware of the many potential local resources which could be used without falling back on the importation of alien ideas."[74] In a 1972 article Lambo criticized Western medicine, particularly psychiatry, as "largely concerned with disease in the civilised white man," and, by virtue of its incongruence with cultural patterns in most African settings, he believed that "its importation into Africa in its present form is ill-suited to the mental health problems of the present or the future."[75] He urged psychiatrists practicing in the developing world to "decontaminate themselves intellectually from Freudian and neo-Freudian theories" on the grounds that they represented "at their best, a spectrum of possible ideas emanating from Hellenic and Judaeo-Christian culture and tradition" and as such were not particularly useful in describing the mental processes of individuals who did not identify with that cultural tradition.[76] By the 1980s, Lambo had become deeply conflicted by the problem of terminology and found the lack of an effective common language to be one of the main drawbacks to real progress in transcultural psychiatry.[77]

Lambo also became increasingly critical of the materialist worldview that he felt undergirded so much of Western perspectives on the definition of "health" and how to achieve it. Particularly during his time at the WHO, Lambo used the visibility of his position to argue against what he saw as a neocolonial project to define health, psychological or otherwise, in non-Western environments strictly in terms of material affluence or access to the technologies that increasingly defined the "modern" existence.

In a 1979 editorial in *World Health*, the public-relations magazine of the WHO, Lambo lamented that "the claim of contemporary Western societies to possess high-powered technology and wealth, and the excessive reliance they place on these material possessions in an effort to keep in the swim, are not very conducive to the quality of life so earnestly desired by non-Western societies."[78] By the early 1980s, he had begun to identify reliance on materialist indicators as something of a rigged game, seeing the development promises of the 1960s and 1970s as increasingly chimerical. Knowledge production about health and medicine remained overwhelmingly an investment of wealthy Western countries, to the extent that "the developing countries today feel profoundly that they have been deserted, that they are isolated from knowledge, from hope."[79] Western medical science, in Lambo's view, relied heavily on technological advancement at the expense of social and preventive medicine that he believed was much more appropriate and feasible for developing non-Western countries, as well as wealthy Western ones.

All was not lost, however. While Lambo continued to argue for the basic universal equality of human cultures and of individual needs to attain mental health and treat mental illness, he believed that Euro-American scientific cultures could not continue to dominate approaches to knowledge production about the psychological and psychiatric patterns of non-Westerners. And he believed that global organizations like the WHO could be enormously powerful vehicles for the promotion of a humanistic approach to health care. Lambo believed that if African psychiatrists conducted research free from the implicit ideological fetters of Western psychiatric discourse, it would turn out that "thinkers from the Third World could offer positive challenge to the established institutions and practices in the West."[80] The terms used to communicate about mental illness in different cultures and the meanings those terms implied to people from different cultural backgrounds would continue to be an enormous obstacle. Indeed, the difficulty of reconciling the idea of universal human psychological characteristics with the specific cultural markers that affect the ways people understand and talk about "normal," "abnormal," and "insane" behaviors continues to be the primary conflict within the disciplines of cross-cultural psychiatry and medical anthropology.

In this regard, it is important to note that Lambo and other Nigerian psychiatrists were not disinterested or disconnected men of science. Lambo and his followers were products of sociopolitical circumstance and professional culture. Just as Lambo advocated for the equality and respect of African psyches vis-à-vis other human societies, he also advocated for the professional relevance of psychiatry, which implied a certain reliance on terms, methods, and principles developed in a cultural setting different from the one in which he worked. The line Lambo walked was tenuous, laced with potential hazards and contradictions that he himself recognized but, lacking perfect solutions, had to work within and around. Nevertheless, Lambo's efforts were critical in undermining much of the racist thinking that had characterized the ethnopsychiatry of the colonial era and in adapting a universalizing psychiatric practice to Nigerian cultural particularities and vice versa, both within Nigeria and at an international level.

EXPANSION OF NIGERIAN PSYCHIATRY

Lambo paved the way for the growth of the psychiatric profession in Nigeria. Although at no time has the supply of psychiatrists met the country's demand, the growth of the profession since the late 1950s has nevertheless vastly improved the availability of psychiatric care over what obtained during the colonial era. In addition to Lambo's prestigious image, Tolani Asuni also became a major and prolific fixture in the psychiatric profession, both in Nigeria and internationally in the 1960s. In 1960, Charles Oshodi became the first indigenous psychiatrist to offer his services in the Northern Region.[81] Over the next two decades, a new generation of Nigerian psychiatrists, including Ayo Binitie, Amechi Anumonye, Olufemi Morakinyo, Roger O. A. Makanjuola, R. Olukayode Jegede, Michael O. Olatawura, A. O. Odejide, John C. Ebie, and clinical psychologist Peter O. Ebigbo, among many others whose contributions will be discussed in detail in the following chapters, completed their studies, took up posts throughout the country, and began to contribute to international networks of psychiatric knowledge production and dissemination.

Initially, all Nigerian psychiatric specialists received training abroad. Even with the development of university teaching hospitals in the 1960s and 1970s, no Nigerian institution provided specialties in psychiatry until the 1980s.[82] Nigeria's medical schools and psychiatric institutions, however, did undertake the training of psychiatric nurses within the country. Nevertheless, the number of psychiatrists working in Nigeria grew steadily from the late 1950s. From three in 1955, the professional ranks grew to eight in 1968, twenty-five in 1975, fifty in 1983,[83] and roughly one hundred by 2001.[84] Facilities for the practice of psychiatry also grew. Aro Mental Hospital had started treating outpatients in 1954 and inpatients by 1957. By the mid-1960s, both Yaba asylum and the asylum at Calabar had been converted into full-fledged mental hospitals as well.[85] Aside from these mental hospitals, there were eleven other psychiatric centers in Nigeria by 1980, six of which were units of university teaching hospitals engaged in both clinical practice and scientific research.[86] The rest were mostly wards of general hospitals across the country.[87] All of these facilities had at least one psychiatrist on full-time staff.[88]

The development of the psychiatric profession remained indebted to Lambo's example. Not only were Nigerian psychiatrists engaged in patient care, but they also continued with Lambo's mission to strengthen local practice through international engagement and to grow global psychiatric knowledge through cross-cultural studies. Nigerian psychiatrists were very active in conducting, discussing, and publishing research related to the practice of psychiatry in African environments. Partly this was accomplished through creating and engaging with national and international professional organizations. In the late 1960s, Lambo and Asuni founded a national association of psychiatrists in Nigeria. By the early 1990s, membership was about fifty.[89] Nigerian psychiatrists became active members in the WHO, the World Psychiatric Association, and the World Federation of Mental Health.[90] In 1970, the Association of Psychiatrists in Africa was formed with Asuni as its president. The association coordinated several Pan-African psychiatric workshops at which psychiatrists from across Africa could meet and discuss their research.[91] Nigerian psychiatrists also published their findings frequently in major international journals housed in Great Britain, Canada, and the United States, as well as in bulletins of the World Health Organization.[92] Two major psychiatric journals were founded in Africa. The first, *Psychopathologie africaine*, published out of Dakar, began its run in 1965. In 1975, the African Psychiatric Association began publication of the *African Journal of Psychiatry*.[93] Nigerian psychiatrists contributed significantly to both journals.

It must also be noted that in order for effective cross-cultural psychiatric discourse to develop, Nigerian psychiatrists worked closely with psychiatrists from other parts of the world. Several expatriates contributed to the development of the psychiatric profession in Nigeria and to the creation of new knowledge about African psychology. Most notably, in the late 1950s, Raymond H. Prince, a Canadian from McGill University in Montreal, came to work with Lambo at Aro, where he contributed to the production of knowledge on the relationship between culture and mental illness in Yoruba patients.[94] In 1961, Alexander Boroffka, a German psychiatrist, came to Yaba asylum and aided in its transformation into a full-fledged mental hospital along the lines of Aro.[95] In this way, Nigerian psychiatrists integrated themselves, both externally and internally, into an international, cross-cultural network of collaborative research.

CONCLUSION

By the 1960s, the psychiatric profession in Nigeria had undergone a revolution small in size but enormous in political and scientific weight. With the arrival of T. Adeoye Lambo and the development of Aro Mental Hospital, mentally ill Nigerians for the first time had access to modern psychiatric therapies, although on a limited scale. Custodial asylums along the lines of those that existed during the colonial period continued to operate throughout the country, but increasingly they were at least accompanied by medical options. Traditional healers also continued to thrive. Lambo's research and clinical practice, particularly his development of the Aro Village Scheme, were centered on integrating psychiatry into Nigerian cultural frameworks and vice versa. He worked for the deracialization of psychiatric knowledge and for the decolonization of psychiatric practice in Nigeria. In so doing he became a nationalist symbol in Nigeria and an important player in the field of international public health. His approach became the foundation upon which the psychiatric profession in Nigeria grew, and his influence would be apparent in subsequent research conducted by Nigerian psychiatrists.

Lambo's career illustrates the extent to which anticolonial nationalisms and decolonization processes had the potential to influence, even transform, international scientific agendas, as well as the extent to which international scientific networks had the capacity to reinforce nationalist political positions much as they had previously reinforced imperial structures and ideologies. However, there are also major continuities between colonial and postcolonial psychiatry that are evident in Lambo's approach to the profession. Although the questions asked and knowledge produced led to different conclusions than that which had preceded it, Lambo's explication of mental illness in Nigerians, even with its cultural peculiarities, was explained wholly in terms of the Euro-American psychiatric definitions, nosologies, and diagnoses. This adherence to established terminology reflects the idea that international science needs a universal language and set of symbols in order to make knowledge relatable and comparable across space and time.[96] Lambo also utilized the networks of scientific knowledge dissemination constructed in the context of European imperial power, even as he strove to expand on them and transform the knowledge disseminated through them.

The career of T. Adeoye Lambo brings focus to the complex blending and overlapping of ideologies that pervaded the thinking of many non-Western scientists of the late colonial and early independence era. In the context of a peaceful, negotiated decolonization process in Nigeria, Lambo worked his entire career at achieving a tenuous integration of the "Western" and the “indigenous”; the “modern” and the “traditional”; the scientific, the political, and the cultural; and the national, international, and global in ways that were influential if never fully reconciled. The remaining chapters of this book explore the ways that Nigerian psychiatrists negotiated specific tensions as they sought to apply and advance the transcultural psychiatric agenda.

3 Mentally Ill Nigerian Immigrants in the United Kingdom

The International Dimensions of Decolonizing Psychiatry

THE PREVIOUS CHAPTER made the argument that T. Adeoye Lambo engaged in international networks of transcultural psychiatry as a means of undermining racialized ethnopsychiatric theories about the relationship between race, culture, and mental illness. This international engagement was central to the effective decolonization of psychiatry in Nigeria. However, in the 1950s and 1960s, Nigerians were increasingly living outside Nigeria, migrating to other parts of the world, most notably to the United Kingdom, the imperial mother country and land of educational and employment opportunity. This chapter examines the ways that psychiatric authorities thought about the causes and possible treatments for Nigerian immigrants who became psychologically disordered while in Great Britain. The question of the relationship between race, culture, and mental illness was central to psychiatric conceptions of mental illness in Nigerian migrants at the time. Some elements of ethnopsychiatric thinking clearly applied to psychiatrists practicing in the UK in the 1950s and 1960s, who often, although by no means always, argued that the best treatment for mentally ill Nigerians would be to remove them from British social surroundings, which they intrinsically could not handle, and repatriate them back home where they would be more likely to thrive in familiar surroundings. Nigerian psychiatrists T. Adeoye Lambo and Amechi Anumonye argued, however, that repatriation was a poor solution to the problem of mental illness in Nigerians. For these Nigerian psychiatrists, the cause of immigrant psychological disorder was more a problem of a lack of cross-cultural understanding that needed to be ameliorated by integration and provision of mental health services for immigrant communities in British society. Lambo and Anumonye saw little value in segregating Nigerian immigrants from British society as this approach ultimately reinforced ethnopsychiatric notions that cultural boundaries necessarily correlated with racial and geographical ones.

Two sets of sources provide the material for this chapter. Since psychological studies of black immigrants in the United Kingdom did not begin to emerge until the late 1960s, in order to understand the extent to which racialized notions of African psychology were operational in the UK in the 1950s I examine the case files of individual Nigerians who were repatriated on the grounds that it was in the best interests of their mental health. These patients came from a variety of backgrounds and suffered from a variety of diagnosed maladies, but all were deemed unlikely to recover substantially while in the UK. Patients' names have been anonymized to protect their identities. The second set of sources includes the writings of Nigerian psychiatrists from the 1950s and 1960s about the problem of mental illness in Nigerian overseas students in the UK. Nigerian psychiatrists focused on the mental health of students as opposed to other migrant groups partly because students made up the bulk of the Nigerian population in the UK, but also because the performance of students reflected upon the Nigerian government, which, in many cases, sent students abroad. These students also represented Nigeria's capacity for future modernization and progress as a strong independent country.

Transcultural psychiatry itself was founded partly out of an interest in the psychological problems of migrant individuals after the devastation of World War II. That emphasis on the relationship between immigration and mental illness then became part of a stream of transcultural psychiatry that dealt with the psychology and mental health needs of immigrant communities in Western countries after the war. In the same way that ethnopsychiatry had reinforced the racialized social order in the colonial context, so, too, did theories about black psychology have the capacity to reinforce racialized social orders in the United Kingdom in the 1950s and 1960s, a time when anti-immigrant sentiment was high. For Lambo, Anumonye, and other transcultural psychiatrists, understanding the mental health needs of immigrant communities and promoting cross-cultural interaction were simultaneously psychological tools for protecting patients and political tools taking the antiracist, culturally relativist rhetoric that characterized nationalist discourse in decolonizing territories to the shores of the motherland by arguing for a deracialization of British society and the active fostering of a multicultural Britain. In this way, this chapter argues that Nigerian psychiatrists' focus on black immigrant mental illness was an integral part of the larger agenda to link the decolonization of psychiatry in Nigeria to the development of a global transcultural psychiatric network that had both theoretical and practical influence not just within Nigeria, but also at the international level.[1]

BLACK MIGRATION AND MENTAL ILLNESS IN POSTWAR BRITAIN

In the British Empire colonial peoples were historically viewed as British subjects and, with few exceptions, had enjoyed full rights of entry and residence in the United Kingdom regardless of their race. However, few nonwhites had made use of this right prior to the 1940s.[2] Although by this time blacks had been present in Britain for more than four hundred years, their numbers had been very small. They had often lived in relatively segregated communities, and, although they faced periodic race-baiting and violence, they posed little threat to the established social order. A significant proportion of blacks in the UK at any given time prior to the 1940s were colonial seamen or students; both groups that typically intended to stay in the country only temporarily before returning home. The relationship between race and citizenship had been sublimated because, for the most part, nonwhite British subjects had stayed where they "belonged."

Black migration into Britain began to increase rapidly in the late 1940s, however. Most of the new black immigrants came from the West Indies, with smaller numbers from African colonies. In the period between 1955 and 1961, the United Kingdom saw an estimated net inward migration of 227,700 West Indians, compared to just 12,350 West Africans.[3] Whereas most West Indian immigrants came to fill working-class jobs created by a major postwar labor shortage, West African immigrants tended to come for educational purposes, intending to return home in a matter of just a few years. Regardless, due to the disparity in numbers and a shared skin color, Africans and West Indians experienced many of the same racial prejudices from a domestic British population faced for the first time with the prospect that imperial connections could turn Britain from a country of net emigration to one of net immigration. Negotiations of race and citizenship became major elements in British political and social discourse at this time, as the imperial homeland struggled to determine whether black colonial subjects and Commonwealth citizens could really be considered "British" and in what sense.

To a great extent, the British Empire had been built on a racialized ideology claiming white right to rule over dark-skinned peoples. Colonial ideology had defined Europeans and blacks as inhabiting different cultural worlds. Overlap between these worlds had been defined as dangerous, undesirable, and potentially destabilizing (see chapter 1). The influx of black immigrants into the United Kingdom brought the possibility that the clash of cultures could affect not just the empire, but also the homeland. Political and social rhetoric coalesced around the notion that the new black immigrants were decidedly *not* British in cultural terms, regardless of their colonial subject or Commonwealth citizen status. Mainstream British depictions of black colonial immigrants conformed largely to the process of racialized "othering" that had occurred in colonial contexts.[4] Politicians expressed fears that black immigrants could not effectively assimilate into British society and, as a result, would do more to destroy British character in the long term than to rebuild a British civilization decimated by years of brutal war.[5] Black immigrants were pathologized as "quarrelsome, suspicious, violent, unlikely to settle down, and in need of disipline."[6] They were often presented as unsanitary, prone to criminality, and sexually promiscuous. The political and public debate about the immigration problem in the 1950s ultimately led to calls for immigration restriction, even the repatriation of immigrants already resident in the UK. In 1962, Parliament passed the Commonwealth Immigrants Act, which for the first time severely limited the rights of current and former colonial subjects to enter and reside in the UK, and largely did so on the basis of racial background.[7]

The widespread (but by no means universal) belief that black immigrants could not effectively assimilate into British society had implications for perceptions of black psychology. If blacks in Britain were defined largely as exhibiting antisocial, "abnormal" behavior, it stood to reason that they would be seen as more likely to exhibit patterns of mental illness as well. Indeed, studies finding particularly high rates of schizophrenia among the West Indian population began to emerge in the 1960s.[8] Although the vast majority of black immigrants were from the West Indies and came to fill working-class positions,[9] the pathologization that they experienced also applied to immigrants from African countries, including Nigeria. By the early 1960s, the notion that West African students were more likely than other groups to suffer mental breakdown in the United Kingdom had become something of a truism. Margaret J. Field, for example, noted that "in England, Ghana, and Nigeria, at the present time [1960] concern is being expressed about the large number of young Africans who go to Britain for study-courses and there suffer mental breakdown."[10] In a 1960 article on a syndrome dubbed "brain fag" in Nigerian students (see chapter 4), Raymond H. Prince noted the "good deal of concern expressed in the Press, both in Nigeria and Ghana, over the high incidence of psychiatric disturbance among West African students in the United Kingdom."[11]

Studies conducted in the United Kingdom on psychiatric morbidity in student populations seemed to uphold the idea that Nigerian students were particularly vulnerable to mental breakdown while abroad. For example, in a 1960 study of mental health in overseas students at Leeds University, R. J. Still found that Nigerian students had a much higher rate of "psychological reactions"—ranging from the "severe" to the "trivial"—than other groups of students. Overall, 28.1 percent of Nigerian students had experienced psychological symptoms during their stay at university compared to 14.0 percent of overseas students as a whole and 10.7 percent of native British students.[12] Cecil B. Kidd, of the Department of Psychiatric Medicine at Edinburgh University, found in a 1965 study of psychiatric morbidity in Edinburgh University students that "prevalence of psychiatric disorders was significantly high for men who did not have a western cultural background," specifying "conspicuously high case rates" for Nigerian men.[13] Kidd's and Still's studies made no effort to explain why this discrepancy existed, but it is important to note that while these studies found psychological disorder to be statistically high among immigrants as a whole regardless of racial background, they found black Africans to be even more vulnerable than other immigrant groups.

Although these studies did not emerge until the 1960s, they had come about as a response to the perceived need to study a recognized problem that dated back many years. The connection between migration and mental illness has long been recognized. Dating back to the nineteenth century in both European countries and the United States, asylum statistics regularly showed that the foreign-born had a proportionally higher chance of developing serious mental illness than the native-born.[14] In psychiatric terms there were essentially two conceivable explanations in the 1950s and 1960s for why rates of mental illness would be higher in immigrant populations. The first explanation focuses on environmental factors. The argument is that the process of emigration and the lifestyle of living as an immigrant in a host country carry extraordinary environmental stressors that contribute to higher levels of psychological disorder. The second explanation focuses on the constitutional makeup of immigrants. The argument goes that migrants may be more predisposed to the development of mental illness than nonmigrants. This may be because individual migrants have a biological predisposition: for example, schizophrenic personalities have been characterized as by nature more itinerant, less likely to settle in any one place for a long period of time because, in essence, they find it difficult to "fit in" anywhere. Another possibility is that the group from which the immigrant originated has a higher propensity for certain types of mental illness, and therefore migrants from this group are more likely to develop those mental illnesses than their host populations.[15]

A third explanation for higher rates of psychiatric diagnosis in immigrant groups emerged in the 1980s and claimed that cross-cultural dissonance frequently results in native-born psychiatrists' diagnosing immigrants with severe mental illnesses at significantly higher rates than the native-born. This can be the result of miscommunication, lack of cross-cultural understanding regarding mental illness, and possibly latent prejudice and racism. Both the psychiatrist and the patient can contribute to these cross-cultural difficulties, but the result is that the immigrant patient is likely to be pathologized in an extreme way as a result.[16] These explanations are not mutually exclusive. All are likely in operation at all times, and complicated further by the recognition that there are different types of immigrants. Refugees fleeing civil war and expatriates relocating because they were promoted at work inhabit different psychological universes and should not be lumped together as "migrants" for scientific evaluation purposes. However, in the 1950s and 1960s, the argument that psychiatrists were prone to overdiagnose mental illness in immigrants was not an expressed concern of British doctors, although their Nigerian patients sometimes felt their diagnoses to be the result of racist objectification, as we will see below.

SEGREGATING AFRICAN MINDS: REPATRIATIONS OF THE 1950S

Examination of the files of mentally ill Nigerians in the 1950s indicates that psychiatric experts in the United Kingdom tended to believe that Nigerian immigrants who developed a mental illness while in the UK were incapable of assimilating into British society. Since they saw the problem as at least partly due to the constitutional makeup of Nigerians, the solution was frequently seen to be repatriation—the return of the immigrant to his (they were almost all males) community of origin, where his constitutional capacities were more suited to recovery and social reintegration. Of course, not every Nigerian mental patient in the UK was repatriated; however, the many cases that do exist indicate a strong belief among many psychiatric specialists at the time that a viable short-term solution to the problem of mental illness in Nigerian immigrant communities was the reinforcement of geographical and cultural barriers between the races: the segregation of "African minds" from the stressors of "modern" civilization.

Repatriation had legal implications. Committed patients, who gave up many of their individual rights, could be moved only if it could be proved that returning them home would be in their best medical interests. The British government had periodically made agreements with other sovereign states for the reciprocal repatriation of committed mental patients dating back to the mid-nineteenth century, but such policy was never adopted within the empire.[17] Throughout the British Empire, no legislation ever existed allowing for the forced repatriation of a certified "lunatic," regardless of racial, cultural, or even national origin. The general rule both in the United Kingdom and throughout the empire was that "wherever people become lunatics, there they remain,"[18] although this proved not always to be the case. Voluntary mental patients retained their own power of attorney and could not be repatriated against their will under any circumstances. As British subjects, Nigerians had full right of residency in the UK, and as a result had to formally apply for repatriation even if they were undergoing treatment for mental illness.

Psychiatric responses to mental illness among African patients in the United Kingdom were implicitly connected to ethnopsychiatric arguments that had tended to portray Africans as intellectually and culturally inferior to Europeans and consequently psychologically threatened by exposure to Western "civilization." The similarities with ethnopsychiatric theories developed in colonial contexts are probably partly to do with the general circulation of ideas about the relationship of race and culture to psychology, but also partly intuitive to psychiatrists working within a racially charged political and social climate that was moving inexorably toward strict immigration controls in the 1950s. Migrant Nigerians (indeed, all racial minorities) in the UK were physical evidence of the erosion of cultural and racial barriers over which ethnopsychiatrists in Africa had so anguished. Although ethnopsychiatrists had made no particular study of the effects of overseas migration on African psyches, their general preoccupation with the psychological consequences of "detribalization" meant that any kind of migration was likely to be more psychologically detrimental to "primitive" Africans than to other, presumably more advanced groups. Indeed, within African settings, ethnopsychiatrists frequently made connections between rural-urban migration and increasing rates of mental illness. J. C. Carothers, for example, concluded in a study on migrant Kenyans that "so long as an African remains at home he is very unlikely to be certified insane, but as soon as he leaves his home his chances of being certified are much increased."[19] If local urbanization processes threatened African psyches, certainly the presence of "primitive" Africans in "civilized" Europe would be even more dangerous to the stability of African minds.

A few specific examples will suffice to illustrate the extent to which psychiatrists in the United Kingdom identified constitutional factors as the precipitating problem for psychologically disturbed Nigerian immigrants. Take, for example, the case of U.U., who had left his home in Bende, Nigeria, in 1954 without telling his family where he was going or what he intended to do. He arrived in the UK the next year but soon applied for repatriation as a distressed British subject. At the time, officials in the office of the secretary of state for the colonies declared that U.U.'s mental health was "giving cause for concern."[20] During the ensuing months, while officials in Nigeria attempted to verify U.U.'s nationality and trace his relations, U.U. went to prison in Brixton for smashing several windows. The medical officer at Brixton prison indicated that U.U. was in a "restless, uncooperative state, and has torn his clothing." He was not, however, certified as a mental patient, and repatriation proceedings continued under the condition that he would be escorted back to Nigeria under guard.

After further examination, the medical officer of the prison determined the cause of U.U.'s disturbance:

> He tells me that he has fallen in love with a white girl of about twenty years old. He says he has never been able to talk to her, and that he does not know her name because he has been warned off her by men bigger than himself. He says that he wants no other girl but this one and yet he realises that she is unattainable. In this pent up state he has seen men of colour that he knows by sight out with girls similar to the one he covets. This raises such jealousy in himself that he relieves his tension by smashing their windows. He says he has done this three times.[21]

The medical officer concluded that "in such a man as the prisoner I do not believe that these are insane actions. In my opinion he cannot be certified as insane under the Lunacy Act, nor is he in need of medical treatment."[22] So U.U. was not insane, according to the medical officer. It would seem perfectly reasonable that sexual frustrations in the context of race prejudice and social alienation might very well cause someone to commit such a crime of passion, as it were.

However, in U.U.'s case, it became clear that the medical officer did not see this as a case primarily rooted in deep-seated British social pathologies, but rather in the inadequacy of U.U.'s overstimulated, fragile psyche. According to the medical officer, the reason U.U.'s actions could not be regarded as indications of mental illness was because "he is a Nigerian coloured man of low normal intelligence, of poor education." He went on to declare that U.U. "appears to me to come from a primitive culture," and that "this should be borne in mind when assessing his peculiar attitude and conduct."[23] U.U. was not insane: he was simply out of his element and had not been able to cope with the stress of transitioning from a "primitive" to a "modern" society. His inability to possess a "white woman," a symbol of the civilization into which he was trying to assimilate, served as a constant reminder of the outsider, indeed "primitive," status that he could not overcome in the United Kingdom. Under the circumstances, U.U. himself welcomed repatriation as a means to forget the heartache had had suffered. Nevertheless, the British psychiatrist seemed to be implicitly invoking ideas common in ethnopsychiatric literature that identified the "normal" African as pathological.

Although psychiatric authorities did not believe that U.U. suffered from any specific mental illness, they did promote repatriation for many other cases that had been diagnosed with a wide variety of very severe psychiatric disorders. When M.O., a nineteen-year-old Nigerian with schizophrenia, applied for repatriation in 1950, the hospital staff in Nottingham supported the repatriation on the unexplained grounds that "the boy is unlikely to make a full recovery until he gets home."[24] Similarly, G.N., a twenty-six-year-old patient in Bristol Mental Hospital diagnosed with "reactive depression with gross hysterical phenomena," applied for repatriation in 1952. Psychiatric authorities considered his repatriation "essential to complete recovery."[25] In 1956, the doctor of P.A., a Nigerian "said to be suffering from serious mental disability," declared that "in view of his mental condition, he would best be treated in his own country."[26] N.U., who suffered from "schizophrenia of an intense and paranoid type," applied for repatriation in 1958. Despite (or perhaps because of) his "vigorous delusions of a grandiose type, such as that Princess Margaret was his wife and that he had invented some wonderful space-travel apparatus," the consultant psychiatrist at Long Grove Hospital in Surrey informed the Colonial Office that "it would be in the best interests of the patient if he could be returned to his country of origin."[27] Medical authorities supported repatriation in all the above cases, despite the varying diagnoses and degrees of mental illness exhibited by the patients.

Patients put up for repatriation also required varying degrees of further care once they returned to Nigeria, ranging from suggested further institutionalization in Nigerian asylums to immediate release to the custody of relatives. However, Nigerian asylums were notoriously overcrowded and underresourced, and before Aro began to support inpatient care in 1957, none could claim to provide more than basic custodial care. While in some of the cases it is clear that the patient himself sought repatriation, it seems that some patients were ambivalent to repatriation at best. The medical report of one patient named B.A. indicates that at the time psychiatric authorities requested his repatriation in 1952, he refused even to write to his relatives in Lagos.[28] Nevertheless, the psychiatric authorities supported his repatriation presumably on the grounds that it would be in his best interest to be nearer them. One patient repatriated to the Yaba asylum in 1953 was slated for release as soon as possible upon return. However, once he arrived Yaba staff were unable to trace his relations because he was "absolutely inactive, docile, mute and altogether inaccessible. He has not spoken a word and therefore [has been] incapable of giving any account of himself or his relations."[29] Some patients were clearly not fit for travel. A.H. had arrived in the United Kingdom in 1953. He had left his native Nigeria, for reasons unknown, having stowed away on a British vessel. Not long after A.H. arrived in the UK, he applied for repatriation back to Nigeria, presumably as a distressed British subject. Before his repatriation could be accomplished, however, he suffered a mental breakdown and entered Long Grove Hospital, Epsom, in 1954. Authorities temporarily postponed his repatriation as a result, but on November 18, despite his unstable condition, A.H. sailed for home aboard the *Apapa*. On November 26 he jumped overboard and was lost at sea.[30] Although in A.H.'s case hindsight is twenty-twenty, it is unclear how repatriation was intended to be medically beneficial for many of these patients.

As with U.U.'s case, however, psychiatrists seemed to believe that removing severely mentally ill Nigerians from British surroundings would be inherently useful regardless of other complicating medical factors because Nigerians were implicitly better suited to exist socially in Nigeria than in the United Kingdom. Take, for example, the case of O.O., who arrived at Winwick Hospital in Warrington sometime before 1950 suffering from inactive pulmonary tuberculosis and an apparent mental disorder. According to medical reports issued at the time he applied for repatriation in 1952, O.O. "remains sullen, suspicious and excitable with impulsive outbursts. He also has ideas of reference and persecutory beliefs. He has periods in which he appears fairly rational, but at others takes no interest in his surroundings and mutters to himself. He remains untidy in his habits and requires care and supervision."[31] O.O. was himself "very keen to be repatriated," and the medical superintendent at Winwick Hospital believed that "the sure knowledge of this would probably be a factor in extending his well behaviour over a period."[32] However, O.O.'s personal desire to return to Nigeria was only part of the reason that medical authorities thought repatriation was a good idea. The medical superintendent went on to state that "because of his unreliable mental state . . . he will not be able to take care of himself *in this country*."[33] Unfortunately, O.O. died in Winwick Hospital on April 4, 1953, before he could be repatriated.[34]

J.M. received a similar prognosis from medical authorities. Suffering from what hospital authorities diagnosed as severe paranoid schizophrenia upon his admission in 1957, J.M. received a "prolonged course of physical treatment" including twenty bouts of electroconvulsive therapy, after which the physician superintendent at the hospital determined he was "as well as he is likely to be."[35] The physician superintendent supported J.M.'s repatriation to Nigeria on the grounds that "in the event of returning there, his chances of obtaining work are probably quite good," while, in the opinion of the physician superintendent, J.M. was "not likely to become self-supporting if he remains in the United Kingdom."[36] In these cases, the medical authorities stressed that British society was in some way causing their patients' mental illness or, at the very least, that their patients' mental illness prevented them from functioning in British society. They might, however, be able to take care of themselves in their own country. Therefore, leaving Britain and returning to Nigeria was the presumed best chance for these patients to improve their living conditions in the long term.

Sometimes returning Nigerians back to their country of origin did not necessarily constitute effective repatriation in the minds of psychiatric authorities in the United Kingdom because there were areas of Nigeria that might be too "modern." For example, one mental patient named M.S. wished to return to Nigeria in 1950. Despite the fact that hospital authorities could identify no next of kin who could take responsibility for him, they nevertheless supported repatriation in M.S.'s "best interests."[37] However, before M.S. returned to Nigeria, authorities in the UK wanted to know "whether he could receive suitable treatment on his return."[38] The government of Nigeria, as it had done in other cases, argued that M.S. could not receive suitable treatment if he returned to Nigeria. In a letter to the secretary of state for the colonies, the acting governor of Nigeria, A. F. F. P. Newns, declared:

> It would not be possible to put [M.S.] in Yaba Asylum unless he is certified and without medical details it is not possible to say whether he is certifiable or not. If he were brought here now and not put in the asylum, it appears he would be both destitute and helpless.
>
> While, therefore, on humanitarian grounds this Government would be willing to pay for the repatriation of [M.S.] if it is likely his

> health would benefit thereby, it seems that, if he were repatriated now, he would be in a far worse position than at Freirn Hospital in the United Kingdom.[39]

Eventually, Nigerian authorities located M.S.'s father. By this time, however, nearly a year had passed and the government of Nigeria wished to know if M.S. would still require "the same handling and treatment" that hospital authorities had suggested the previous year.[40]

The response by the physician superintendent at Freirn Hospital indicated the extent to which concerns over the psychological effects of "detribalization" played into the decision to repatriate. According to the physician superintendent, "The answer to this depends on whether his home is in a large town or in a small village in the country. In the first case he would be in need of hospital care, but it is quite possible that he might be looked after by his family in a small country district."[41] The assumption apparently made by the medical authorities at Freirn was that M.S., as a black African, must be innately of a "primitive," rural background. As such, repatriating him to an urban area in Nigeria would expose him to the same kind of stressors that he had been unable to cope with in the United Kingdom. The "modern" urban lifestyle was apparently too much for M.S., who needed, first, to be removed from such surroundings in the UK and, second, to be isolated from reminders of such surroundings once back in Nigeria.

Interestingly, M.S. did not return to Nigeria at this time. Since his father was in the major urban hub of Lagos, M.S. would have been placed in the Yaba asylum if he returned. Since the asylums in Nigeria were by all accounts inferior to those in the United Kingdom, M.S. remained at Freirn. Five years later, in November 1956, the consultant psychiatrist at Freirn reported that M.S. "has made considerable improvement in the last few weeks, and as he does not wish to go back himself at this juncture it is felt that he should be given an opportunity of further improvement and possible discharge from hospital."[42] However, always ready for the possibility that the improvement would not last, the consultant psychiatrist concluded that "in the event of his improvement proving to be transitory I will get in touch with you again concerning the possibility of his repatriation."[43] It is not clear from the documentary record that this repatriation ever occurred.

The general argument behind UK psychiatric authorities' decisions to support repatriation of Nigerian mental patients in certain cases was anchored on two assumptions: first, that their individual psychology was ill-equipped to function under British social circumstances; and, second, that availability of advanced medical services and facilities mattered little for their prognosis. Such cases were based on assumptions that, perhaps, psychiatric processes were not universal, that the background of the patient mattered, and that cross-cultural interaction often resulted in greater alienation than assimilation. However, by the 1950s, these ideas were increasingly debatable, for both political and scientific reasons. M.S.'s case above raises the important fact that, of course, not all Nigerians who manifested mental illnesses in the United Kingdom returned home as a result. Many recovered within short periods of time and reintegrated back into British society. In fact, sometimes, medical and governmental officials in Nigeria mounted cases against the repatriation of Nigerians on the grounds that patients might be better off remaining in the UK. This was particularly true of cases in which psychiatric experts believed the patients would require continued institutional care once returned to Nigeria.

Such disparities led some officials even within the colonial government of Nigeria to question the value of repatriating mental patients from overseas. In 1955, after the United States had abruptly deported several mentally ill Nigerians and placed them on a chartered flight to Kano,[44] one colonial officer in Nigeria posed the question to the acting secretary of health for Nigeria: "Why do we accept them back. . . . It would surely be better to leave them where they can be well treated and looked after, possibly even cured?"[45] The conditions of overcrowding and inadequate resources in all Nigerian asylums in the 1950s made it difficult for Nigerian authorities to believe that repatriation was necessarily a beneficial medical intervention, particularly for severely incapacitated mental patients.

Colonial government officials in Nigeria sometimes argued that, despite protestations from UK psychiatrists that repatriation was in the patients' best interests, conditions would likely be worse for patients in Nigeria. For example, in 1951, the director of Medical and Sanitary Services (DMSS) for Nigeria reluctantly agreed to the repatriation of J.O., who had traveled to the United Kingdom in 1946 as a stowaway. By 1950, he had entered Winwick Hospital suffering from schizophrenia. According to hospital records, J.O. desired to be repatriated, but was still manifesting symptoms of mental illness. He was "excitable and emotionally unstable," and was sometimes "abusive and aggressive." He had "the habit of spitting on the floor or his bedding" and could be "resistive to attention." Under the circumstances, the medical authorities at Winwick Hospital determined that there was "no immediate prospect of his recovery." J.O. "would require mental hospital treatment on repatriation."[46] The DMSS in Nigeria acquiesced, stating that J.O. could go to Lantoro Mental Hospital if he were repatriated. However, the DMSS made it clear that conditions would not be opportune for J.O.'s recovery at Lantoro, noting that "the most modern methods of treatment of these cases are not yet fully available in Nigeria and without having full details it would be impossible to say whether any effective remedial measures could be carried out here."[47] From the perspective of the Nigerian officials involved, the type of medical treatment that J.O. could receive absolutely should bear on the decision whether or not to repatriate. J.O. returned to Nigeria in 1952, but on arrival medical authorities deemed him recovered enough by Nigerian standards to be released to the custody of a cousin.[48]

In other cases, Nigerian officials argued that repatriation should not occur because the patient in question had likely become too acculturated to life in Britain to reintegrate effectively back into Nigerian society. Take the case of B.A., mentioned above, who was born in 1902 and had come to Britain in the early 1930s to study medicine at Manchester University. In 1935, he had committed a murder, for which he received a verdict of not guilty by reason of insanity. He entered Broadmoor Institution, where he lived for the next twenty-one years. Diagnosed with paraphrenia, B.A. was "violent and had auditory hallucinations." Medical authorities declared in 1956 that he "requires—and will continue to require—care and attention." Nevertheless, Broadmoor desired to repatriate B.A. in 1956, citing that "he has gradually improved," and, although he continued to have hallucinations, "he has not been violent since 1952."[49] The doctors vaguely asserted that it would be "in the best interests of the patient if he could be returned to his country of origin," but to colonial officials in Nigeria it was unclear why this would be the case. The governor-general of Nigeria, acting on advice from the DMSS, responded to the secretary of state that under the circumstances,

> the medical authorities in Lagos are of the opinion that the above named person should not be returned to Nigeria for the following reasons—
>
> (a) after over 20 years in the United Kingdom he would have no relatives or interests in Nigeria to assist in ameliorating his condition.
>
> (b) conditions at Yaba Mental Hospital are extremely overcrowded and he would find this most upsetting.
>
> (c) there are no facilities at Yaba for special diets, etc., and by now he would be completely used to English-type food.[50]

After further deliberations, the Colonial Office decided not to repatriate B.A., based on the notion that he would likely experience culture shock from returning to his country of origin.

Protestations against repatriation such as occurred in the case of B.A. revealed chinks in the armor of ethnopsychiatric conceptions of the relationship between race, culture, and mental illness. Clearly even some colonial officials recognized that the boundaries of culture were not racially defined and subsequently were willing to argue that being back home among one's racial cohorts did not necessarily constitute being back in a familiar culture. Furthermore, repatriation did not necessarily reflect the patient's best medical interests in the view of governmental and medical authorities in colonial Nigeria. However, contestations were somewhat rare and tended to come from officials in Nigeria concerned primarily about the overcrowding of Nigerian asylums.

The general concept that repatriating immigrants suffering from mental illnesses might be therapeutically beneficial is not necessarily an indication of the influence of the racialized constructions of colonial ethnopsychology on psychiatric practice in the United Kingdom. No doubt, the stress of travel and of assimilating into a new society is significant. Adding to the pressures that Nigerians faced in Britain was the race prejudice that followed them everywhere they went. Often persecuted, discriminated against, and isolated in a foreign place, it is not surprising that some Nigerians suffered mentally. Nor is it surprising that many would wish to return to the relative comfort of their homes and families or that psychiatric authorities would consider repatriation a potentially therapeutic process under the circumstances. However, I am arguing here that the ways that psychiatrists and government officials in the UK talked about the particular nature of the psychological problems that Nigerian immigrants experienced in the UK were frequently put in the familiar terms of ethnopsychiatry. References to the primitive background of Nigerian subjects, assumptions of their innate rural lifestyles, and concerns that they could not normalize their psychology in a "modern" environment because of these presumed cultural characteristics conjured up associations with the "detribalization" thesis of ethnopsychiatry that applied to black African subjects more significantly than other migrant groups. Instructively, British psychiatric authorities often suggested that, although returning to familiar home surroundings might not result in significant improvement in the patient's mental state, returning to Nigeria might allow the patient to better function in his current impaired condition, a clear indication that psychiatric authorities assumed an essential difference between British and Nigerian societies. Such characterizations reflect the general racialized hierarchies of ethnopsychiatry prior to the development of transcultural psychiatry and the decolonization of European empires in Africa from the 1950s.

TRANSCULTURAL PSYCHIATRY AND OVERSEAS STUDENTS

The frequency of repatriations occurring in the 1950s was noticeable to the rapidly decolonizing Nigerian government. So much so that in 1957, the government of Nigeria's Western Region approached T. Adeoye Lambo about conducting a study on the mental health problems of Nigerian students in the United Kingdom as a means of trying to reduce what appeared to be a growing problem. From the perspective of nationalist and developmentalist politics, these overseas students were the means through which Nigeria could build a strong, skilled, internationally competitive workforce. Although exact numbers are hard to come by, various estimates can illustrate the extent to which the population of black Africans in Britain grew in the 1950s, and particularly the number of black African students. Hakim Adi estimated that in 1940 there were only about seventy West African students in Britain, but by the early 1950s that number had risen to more than two thousand.[51] A report by the Political and Economic Planning group of Great Britain enumerated 3,969 West African students in Britain in 1954,[52] the majority of whom were probably Nigerian given the population differentials of British West African colonies. Lambo estimated that as of 1957 more than five thousand Nigerians were residing in the UK for the primary purpose of seeking a degree.[53] The emphasis on the subgroup of Nigerian students within the larger group of Nigerian migrants can in some ways be explained in terms of the need to prevent attrition in the ranks of Nigeria's vanguard modernizers. Lambo was himself a beneficiary of overseas experience, having studied and worked extensively in the UK before returning to Nigeria to work for the improvement of understanding and treatment of mental illness in Nigeria. He certainly saw the value inherent in facilitating overseas education for young Nigerians.

Lambo's study was therefore meant to offer recommendations for the amelioration of the problem so that students would not be forced to abandon their studies over what might be preventable mental breakdowns. However, beyond this it was an opportunity for Lambo to engage with methods and concepts of transcultural psychiatry to argue for the deracialization of psychological and psychiatric theory. As discussed in chapter 2, the development of transcultural psychiatry in the years after World War II coincided with the decolonization of European overseas empires. In Nigeria, the development of psychiatric infrastructure by T. Adeoye Lambo in the 1950s was therefore bound up with practical and ideological processes of the times: promotion of national sovereignty and development; negotiating the preservation of tradition while simultaneously ushering in modernization schemes; and fighting against the vestiges of colonialism and racism. Such influences led Lambo to embrace a research and clinical practice agenda that focused on breaking down the racial barriers that ethnopsychiatry had constructed and to emphasize instead basic psychological similarities that human beings shared regardless of racial and cultural background. He believed that discovering ways to incorporate cultural particularities into a universalizing structure had the capacity to contribute to the development and modernization of Nigeria and to improve the scientific objectivity of psychiatry as a medical discipline. Examining the psychological problems of Nigerian immigrants in the United Kingdom served as an ideal way to synthesize all these goals in a single project.

Lambo argued that the key factors impinging upon the mental health of Nigerian students in the United Kingdom were the universal stressors associated with being both an immigrant and a student, regardless of racial or cultural background, coupled with the particular stressors of combating race prejudice. Like ethnopsychiatrists before him, Lambo believed that migration posed a serious psychological threat to Nigerians. Indeed, Lambo saw dislocation as a "threat to mental health so vast as to dwarf any other."[54] However, he believed that this threat was no greater for Nigerians than for other groups: it just so happened that Nigerians and other African groups were experiencing an ebb in migration patterns at the time. For Lambo, Nigerian overseas students, like all migrants, were "stripped of all the cultural and moral support to which [they were] accustomed"[55] at the same time that they were thrust into very stressful new life situations. Lambo emphasized this social dislocation, rather than the inability of Nigerians to cope with a "modern" environment, as a serious psychological stressor. In fact, Lambo noted in this report that "most of the African students in the United Kingdom came from urban environments and were completely 'detribalized'" (*SSH*, 14) before they even left home, a clear repudiation of any ethnopsychiatric claim about the inability of "primitive" Africans to adjust to "modern" European civilization. Furthermore, Lambo argued that the stresses of being a young person and a student were universal. By "taking the student world as a whole in various parts of the world," declared Lambo, "the problems of mental-ill health among students could easily be very loosely regarded as a vocational disease" (16). Adding to the stress of being a student came the normal stresses of young adulthood (e.g., individual responsibility, sexual exploration, and lifestyle and career choices), which many of the younger overseas students were also negotiating for the first time. The emphasis for Lambo was on the circumstantial peculiarities of being an overseas migrant and a student often at a particularly vulnerable point in life, not necessarily the psychological peculiarities of being from an African cultural background, as many of the repatriation files discussed above seemed to suggest.

Lambo did not wish to argue, however, that the international student experience was exactly the same for Nigerians as it was for immigrants from other areas. Certain social and financial stressors experienced by immigrants and students were definitely exacerbated for Nigerians. Financial strains and the insidious "colour bar" in the United Kingdom made it more difficult for Nigerian students to find reasonable and dignified accommodation than immigrant students from other European countries. Lambo noted that landladies often required black students to pay 40 to 45 percent higher rents for the same living spaces than whites, both as a discouragement to possible black tenants and as an insurance policy against the possibility that white students might "blacklist her house as 'blackdigs'" (*SSH*, 18). Under such conditions, the stresses on Nigerian and other black students could well be seen as in excess of those faced by native-born students or even nonnative white students. At the same time, it served as evidence of the extent to which Nigerian students might not feel welcome in their host country and, therefore, would make less of an effort to acculturate, increasing their sense of alienation and vulnerability to psychological distress relative to other migrant groups.

Financial strain was usually "the most significant and constant factor . . . in most cases of maladjustment," according to Lambo (*SSH*, 35). Some students traveling to the United Kingdom in the 1950s received government scholarships of one form or another. As of 1954, out of 3,101 students from the Western Region of Nigeria studying in the UK, only 400 were there on government scholarships. The remainder were "private" students who financed their educations on their own or, more likely, through significant assistance from family and friends. Lambo found that in 1952 more than 25 percent of the families of private students had borrowed money to help maintain their family members overseas (17). This posed many financial worries for the student because, as Lambo put it, "the financial transaction almost amounts to a 'contract' between the student and their parents and relatives. This 'contract' embodies the wishes of their (the students') parents, social prestige and future economic opportunities. Failure to accomplish their (the students') ambition implies that they could not very well go home. This way of thinking profoundly influences the students' attitudes to their courses overseas" (17). Even those students on government scholarships received too little to live comfortably in the UK, according to Lambo (17). He noted that more than 30 percent of Nigerian students also had the burden of providing some financial support to dependents back in Nigeria (18).

The result was that the majority of Nigerian students overseas had to be extraordinarily parsimonious simply to survive. This financial worry contributed to already high levels of academic stress and put students at greater risk of mental breakdown. The need to live economically also negatively affected Nigerian students' social lives while in the United Kingdom. They could not afford to engage in many recreational activities, thereby increasing the already pronounced sense of alienation felt by many. Some Nigerian students reported to Lambo that they nearly starved themselves out of the need to stretch funds, "forced to subsist for a whole day on a little gruel—and sometimes for weeks or months" (*SSH*, 19). Under such circumstances, students' physical health declined as well, contributing again to greater mental and emotional instability.

Given that the problems faced by Nigerian students were largely social in nature, Lambo considered them to be largely preventable as well. The study concluded that the solution to overseas migrants' psychological problems lay in *more* contact and interaction between British and Nigerian cultures, not *less*, as was stressed in so many of the repatriation files discussed above. While repatriation made sense as a short-term solution for severe individual cases, Lambo did not place any special emphasis on the desirability of returning mentally ill Nigerians to "familiar" surroundings, and certainly did not attribute the problems of mentally ill Nigerians in the United Kingdom to constitutional defects in Nigerian psyches. Instead, he argued that much of the problem stemmed from cultural ignorance of both Britons and Nigerians about one another. He noted that "problems of social integration" were sometimes exacerbated by "ignorance of the British public about life in Nigeria," which resulted in "unfortunate and hurtful comments" made to and about Nigerian students. Lambo excoriated the continued reliance on "old films and missionary propaganda" as the basis of information about Nigerians that "fostered misrepresentations and distortions of facts" (*SSH*, 33–34). Nigerians, for their part, knew too little about what to expect when they traveled to the UK. When reality did not meet expectations, Lambo argued, Nigerian students often became disillusioned, withdrawn, and despondent. Many Nigerian students were not prepared for the general aloofness they found among the British. This perceived indifference and unfriendliness often led Nigerians to assume race prejudice at play in cases where it probably did not exist. Lambo, for example, recounted the tale of a particular student in Aberdeen who "underwent some mental strain for the first two years of his career since he felt that the fact that he was not invited to eat with his landlady's family implied some kind of colour bar" (25). It was not until the student attended a symposium at the university that he learned this experience was common to "approximately 75–80%" of all students and simply an unexpected difference between Nigerian and British cultures (25).

Cross-cultural integration and understanding, rather than segregation, needed to be seen as the long-term solution to the problem of psychological maladjustment in Nigerian overseas students. In the short term, Lambo called for stronger support services for Nigerian students, including stronger efforts from the Ministries of Education and Health to develop both the professional and the interpersonal relationships with overseas students that would engender trust among students and, hopefully, result in more students' approaching relevant authorities when in distress. He also called for stronger financial support for Nigerian students on the part of the government and for a reassessment of screening practices for students that he believed should focus more on support for those with "stable personalities" than strictly those who demonstrated academic brilliance (*SSH*, 37).

Lambo also noted that psychological and psychiatric services for Nigerian students were not culturally calibrated and needed strengthening to address Nigerian students' concerns in culturally sensitive ways. He noted that many psychiatric experts in the United Kingdom themselves recognized that they did not have the cultural understanding necessary to engage Nigerian patients or to treat them effectively, particularly in cases where patients believed there was some kind of supernatural basis to their sufferings. This problem was not insignificant, as Lambo had previously found that an average of 90 percent of Nigerian students suffering mental instability in Britain believed their problems to have traditional, indigenous causes such as bewitchment.[56] Lambo's interviews with students revealed that 60 percent of Nigerian students claimed they would "much prefer to consult African doctors in respect of psychological and emotional disturbances," while 70 percent of those who had consulted British psychiatrists had done so "with great reluctance and at the stage when it was obvious they could not carry on with their normal social and academic activities" (*SSH*, 39–40). In light of such data, Lambo concluded that there was a strong need for the Nigerian government to post a Nigerian doctor to the Student Health Service so as to create a situation where students would be more likely to seek help earlier and in which the help provided might be much more effective.

Lambo also argued for long-term preventive strategies centered on better cross-cultural understanding between Britons and Nigerians. He urged the Nigerian government to engage in "propaganda work in Nigeria about life in Britain and the re-education and reorientation of the parents in Nigeria towards the appreciation of their children's social and academic difficulties" (*SSH*, 53). At the same time, Lambo tried to persuade the Nigerian government to undertake a propaganda campaign in the United Kingdom to "intensify the spread of information about Nigeria by the distribution of literature, films, etc. to portray Nigeria in its true perspective as a means of combating the prejudices prevalent among the British people" (53). He suggested that this might be accomplished in part by transmitting productions of the Nigerian Broadcasting Corporation in the UK to "help enliven Nigerian students here and enlighten the natives of Britain" (53). Cross-cultural understanding and tolerance were, after all, the bedrock principle upon which transcultural psychiatry itself relied.

There is an apparent irony between Lambo's approach toward treating psychological disorder in overseas students and his approach toward community therapy in the Aro Village Scheme discussed in chapter 2. While on the one hand Lambo argued that the benefits of Aro Village lay in immersing patients in familiar cultural surroundings, on the other he argued that this type of treatment would not be in the best interests of Nigerians residing overseas. At first blush, this may seem like a contradiction of sorts. However, from Lambo's perspective, different Nigerians might require different forms of treatment. In fact, Lambo designed Aro Village to treat patients primarily from rural, agrarian backgrounds; it was not culturally calibrated to meet the needs of urbanites or the significantly "detribalized." Since, as we have seen, Lambo considered Nigerians in the United Kingdom to be significantly detribalized, treating them in a rural, agrarian setting would not be conducive to their recovery. This in itself is an indication of the ways that Lambo saw a need to reconstruct the ways psychiatrists thought about the relationship between race, culture, and mental illness. All Nigerians did not have the same culture: they had different belief systems, different lifestyles, different goals and ambitions, and their psychological disturbances needed to be recognized as reflective of more idiosyncratic elements of their personalities and backgrounds.

Nevertheless, Lambo's study does not appear to have had a great immediate impact; it does not seem to have been widely distributed at the time of its production. Partly as a result, in 1970, the Nigerian psychiatrist Amechi Anumonye conducted an exhaustive investigation into the psychological problems of Nigerian students at Edinburgh University and found circumstances relatively unchanged. Immigration restrictions targeting Commonwealth immigrants came into effect in 1962 and were tightened in 1964, meaning that the general social atmosphere for Nigerian students in the United Kingdom was not particularly more accommodating in the postindependence era than in the 1950s. As a result, Anumonye's conclusions were very similar to those that Lambo had reached more than a decade earlier. For Anumonye, financial strain and unmet expectations were by far the most important factors contributing to psychological distress in Nigerian students. Anumonye found that 86 percent of the students he surveyed declared that their presence in the UK had placed significant financial strain on their families back home (*SSH*, 64). Like Lambo, Anumonye pointed out that racism could be in the eye of the beholder, noting "pecularities associated with insularity like shyness and self-consciousness sometimes make the British appear to be less hospitable than they actually are."[57] However, he also found the same accommodation problems that Lambo had identified as well. As of 1965 only 37 percent of landladies in Edinburgh were willing to rent to "coloured male students," and "some white students refused to share rooms with coloured ones."[58]

The extent to which Nigerian students saw their overseas education primarily as the means through which to facilitate good careers back in Nigeria also helped to explain some of the perceived social maladjustment of Nigerian students in Anumonye's view. However, whereas Lambo had found levels of social alienation to be high and distressing to Nigerian students, Anumonye found that most students in Edinburgh did not feel that a lack of extracurricular socialization affected their mental states. Many had no difficulty in establishing friendly relationships; many came with spouses, and, perhaps most importantly, most saw themselves as temporary migrants and, as such, had very little need to socialize since the goal was to work hard and return home.[59] Limited socialization could therefore be a choice, according to Anumonye.

One of the biggest problems that Anumonye identified was disillusionment with the British education system on the part of Nigerian students. Anumonye found that some Nigerian students were upset by the fact that the educations they received in the United Kingdom had very little practical application for the careers they would have when they returned to Nigeria. For example, Anumonye lambasted situations where "promising African young men and women are encouraged to spend three or four years specializing on such ridiculous subjects like the heat emission of glow-worms under simulated Arctic conditions or the digestive enzymes of the common parasites of the American potato beetle while tropical issues relating to the students' national needs are left unexplored."[60] Under such circumstances, the psychological impact of the privations that overseas students endured was exacerbated by concerns that the education they were receiving was not as valuable as they had hoped, in terms of either their personal professional development or their abilities to contribute to the development of their communities and country.

Like Lambo, Anumonye also found the greatest opportunity for reducing mental distress among Nigerian overseas students to be in preventive psychiatry. Anumonye focused most heavily on the need for "anticipatory guidance" of students heading to the United Kingdom. Anumonye believed that research conducted by Nigerian psychiatrists by this time had made the kinds of crises that Nigerian students would face in the UK quite predictable. If they were predictable, then students could be guided to anticipate them. If the crises were anticipated, then they would not be as difficult to combat. Anumonye borrowed this concept of "anticipatory guidance" from the United States Peace Corps, which used it to train its cadets to anticipate the culture shock they would feel at their posts abroad.[61]

The emphasis that Lambo and Anumonye put on preventive psychiatry based on intensification of cross-cultural interaction clearly conflicted with the psychological justification for repatriating Nigerian mental patients as a long-term strategy for dealing with the problem. However, repatriations of individual Nigerian migrants continued to occur in the 1960s, with more than eighty occurring between 1961 and 1964.[62] Over the long term, the perspective that providing culturally sensitive and easily accessible mental health services to immigrant populations was an approach far superior to repatriation became the mainstream perspective of transcultural psychiatry, and one that Nigerian psychiatrists championed as well. Repatriation could have psychological consequences itself, after all. As Lambo had noted, returning to Nigeria was often an undesirable outcome, particularly for students who would have to face their families as "failures." Anumonye seconded the undesirability of repatriation in a 1967 study of repatriated Nigerian students. While Anumonye argued that "where the patient does not respond" to treatment in the United Kingdom, "it may be necessary finally to repatriate him to his homeland,"[63] he emphasized this only as a last resort, noting, as had others before him, that returning a "failure" could, in fact, be detrimental to recovery.

To a certain extent, the development of psychopharmaceutical treatments that could help people to cope with stressful environmental circumstances and counteract the most severe symptoms of major psychotic disorders regardless of geographical or cultural surroundings aided the argument against repatriation. However, by the 1970s, studies were also beginning to suggest that repatriation did not provide positive therapeutic benefits as a general rule. Tolani Asuni conducted a study of eighty-two students repatriated to

Nigeria between 1961 and 1964 and found that, in general, "they do respond better to treatment at home than abroad, but the rate of relapse is high."[64] Of the eighty-two patients examined, twenty had to be readmitted to Aro Hospital after an initial discharge, five were known to have had relapses but not returned to Aro for treatment, four had returned to the United Kingdom and suffered relapses, and one had committed suicide.[65] Studies from the Caribbean in the early 1970s indicated that West Indians did not respond particularly well to repatriation either.[66] Even for those who might see great short-term benefits from repatriation, there was recognition that this needed to be balanced against the long-term consequences. As Philip H. Rack put it: "A difficult dilemma is provided by the overseas student who suffers an acute stress-related breakdown. Repatriation may relieve his symptoms instantly—indeed, in some cases he is quite well by the time he steps off the plane at the other end—but if this is achieved at the cost of his whole future career, it is a heavy price to pay."[67] Repatriation of Nigerians from the UK slowly declined over the course of the 1960s. Over the period from 1952 to 1959, an average of roughly seven repatriations occurred per year.[68] By 1970–76, the average had dropped to less than one.[69]

CONCLUSION

During the 1950s and 1960s, the problem of what to do with mentally ill black immigrants had medical as well as political implications, as the relationship between the United Kingdom and Nigeria changed from one of colonial master and colonial possession to one of independent and presumably equal sovereign entities. Evidence from the repatriation files of mentally ill Nigerians illustrates the extent to which the colonial psychiatric theories of the inferior "African mind" incapable of adaptation from "primitive" to "modern" cultural norms partially shaped perspectives taken by psychiatric authorities in the UK of their Nigerian patients in the 1950s. Psychiatric authorities in the UK regularly proposed repatriation from stressful "modern" surroundings to a more familiar "primitive" locale as in patients' best interests for future recovery and functionality.

However, these racialized perspectives overlapped with arguments coming out of transcultural psychiatry that urged cross-cultural integration and universal human psychology. Nigerian psychiatrists who embraced transcultural psychiatry as a means of combating the racist interpretations of black psychology that had dominated psychiatric theory and practice prior to the 1950s were less inclined to see repatriation as an attractive option. Lambo and Anumonye believed that the mental distress found in Nigerian overseas students was multivalent, but ultimately preventable. The problem for students, in particular, was not so much that their "African minds" were incapable of adapting to European "modernity," but rather that for many of these students, European modernity turned out to be less impressive and less incorporative than they had been led to believe. By recognizing these as the chief problems contributing to student distress, Lambo and Anumonye believed that much could be done long-term to improve conditions for overseas students short of repatriating them. The process of fostering cross-cultural interaction and understanding as a means of promoting mental health made sense both in the medical context of transcultural psychiatry and in the political context of decolonization, independence, and anticolonial nationalism that emphasized Nigeria's need to develop, modernize, and, in so doing, become an equal actor in the international community. The next chapter examines how this desire to de-link the psychological problems of Nigerians and other Africans from racial and cultural characteristics and to reformulate them in terms of universal biological, social, and psychological processes also characterized Nigerian psychiatrists' attitudes toward the diagnosis of psychiatric disorders.

4 Schizophrenia, Depression, and "Brain-Fag Syndrome"

Diagnosis and the Boundaries of Culture

THE DECOLONIZATION OF PSYCHIATRIC INSTITUTIONS in Nigeria during the 1950s and 1960s, as well as the subsequent incorporation of Nigerian psychiatrists like T. Adeoye Lambo into international networks of psychiatric research, created a new environment within which to examine the psychology of Africans, who, as the previous chapter showed, were increasingly recognized to be living beyond the ethnic, racial, and geographical boundaries that ethnopsychiatry had constructed to define them. This chapter uses three particular psychiatric disease entities—schizophrenia, depression, and "brain-fag syndrome"—to examine ways that Nigerian psychiatrists used their time and resources to engage in research that argued for the innate equality of "African minds" with all other racial and cultural groups in the world, thereby breaking down preconceived racial-cum-cultural boundaries. They did so by arguing that mental illnesses like schizophrenia and depression were universally present in all cultures, but that cultural factors influenced the way these universal mental illnesses presented in different cultures and, consequently, what the diagnostic criteria for identifying these disorders in African cultures should be. Simultaneously, they mostly rejected the notion that distinct cultural units had the capacity to create culturally specific mental illnesses that could not be classified within a universal construct. Hence "brain-fag syndrome," which is listed in the *DSM-IV* as a "culture-bound disorder," has been a diagnostic entity that many Nigerian researchers have rejected either completely or in part on the grounds that it is not, in fact, bound to any specific culture.

A note is needed about the usage of the term "culture" in this chapter. For the most part, the psychiatrists discussed in this chapter saw culture as a set of beliefs and values that informed how their patients experienced the world around them and, ultimately, how they expressed their illnesses. Nigerian psychiatrists made very little effort to delineate specific cultural boundaries, partly because they were not anthropologists and partly because, at the most basic level, they were interested much more in what they considered to be the underlying *similarities* present beneath the veneer of cultural difference. Nigerian psychiatrists like T. Adeoye Lambo believed it was important for psychiatrists to be sensitive to the cultures they worked in not because it would allow them to diagnose psychiatric illnesses distinct to these cultures (as many medical anthropologists would now hold), but because it would allow them to peel away the layers of cultural influence that masked universal psychiatric disorders. The overwhelming emphasis of Nigerian psychiatrists, therefore, was not on difference but on similarity. As a result, they tended to compare African groups to one another in ways that allowed them to continue to use the conglomeration "African" as a descriptive term, and they tended to compare "Africans" similarly to equally generic cultural units such as "Europeans," "British," "Judeo-Christian," and so on. They did this partly because they were engaged in a counterdiscourse to a colonial psychiatry that had constructed Africans as psychologically inferior, and Nigerian psychiatrists chose to focus their attention on the inferior part of the equation rather than the African. But they also did this partly because, at the end of the day, cultural differences between people were less meaningful to Nigerian psychiatrists—indeed, to transcultural psychiatry generally at this time—than the underlying psychological similarities that they believed characterized all humans regardless of culture.

The point of this chapter, then, is not to argue that in the absence of colonial racism the science of transcultural psychiatry was able to "get it right." In fact, debates raged about the scientific accuracy and clinical practicality of looking past cultural uniqueness to construct schizophrenia and depression as cross-culturally universal entities. Recognizing that these problems continue to plague diagnosticians, this chapter uses the changes in diagnostic practices since the 1950s to make three key points. First, for Nigerian psychiatrists, research into the nature of depression, schizophrenia, and brain-fag syndrome was inherently linked to anticolonial cultural politics emanating from the legacy of colonial-era ethnopsychiatry. Second, the research that Nigerian psychiatrists conducted locally fit naturally within international networks of transcultural psychiatry that were interested in asking the same types of questions about the relative universality of these illnesses. Third, Nigerian psychiatrists became influential participants in the transformation of psychiatric theory regarding the diagnostic criteria of schizophrenia and depression not only in their local environment, but also at a global level. This decolonization was grounded in Western psychiatric concepts, but in a way that incorporated formerly colonized peoples as cultural and psychological equals rather than as inferiors, irrespective of the scientific merits or demerits of doing so. This examination of the role of Nigerian psychiatrists in cross-cultural research on diagnostic processes therefore illustrates the extent to which it is impossible to de-link the global transformation in psychiatric theory and practice at this time from the local political conditions that were influencing psychiatric thinking in decolonizing environments.

SCHIZOPHRENIA

The Western psychiatric tradition has long recognized schizophrenia as one of the most universal psychiatric disorders. "Dementia praecox," as schizophrenia was originally called, became a preoccupying diagnostic entity for European psychiatrists from the early nineteenth century. Emil Kraepelin codified much of the accepted symptomatology of the disease in the 1890s, but it was given the name schizophrenia by Eugen Bleuler in 1908. "Schizophrenia" is actually a blanket term for a variety of psychotic disorders that can have very different symptom complexes and prognoses for recovery. Although these disorders may manifest differently, there are broad shared characteristics that have allowed psychiatrists to group them together, namely what Bleuler termed "primary" symptoms, most important of which is the deterioration of a patient's logical capacity, often resulting in a psychotic break from "reality." A variety of "secondary" symptoms are also common, including hallucinations, delusions, and emotional withdrawal. Schizophrenia has been broken down into several subtypes based on the symptom profile, including paranoid, catatonic, and disorganized, but all have in common a dissociation of the individual from the "real" world in terms of perception and social relations.[1]

Although most Western-trained psychiatrists have historically believed that social, cultural, and environmental factors all play a role in the manifestation, progression, and prognosis of schizophrenia, there has been widespread agreement since the 1940s that biological factors play a significant role in the development of schizophrenia. This has been proved scientifically through "twin studies" conducted since the 1940s that have consistently found that if one identical twin develops a form of schizophrenia, then the likelihood is statistically high that the other will develop a schizophrenic or schizophreniform disorder at some point as well.[2] Although many of the earliest twin studies evidenced a variety of methodological deficiencies, more recent studies have confirmed the general concept of a biological element in schizophrenia genesis, although with an increasingly strong recognition of the importance of environmental cofactors.[3] Environmental triggers have long been considered to impinge upon the development and presentation of the disease, and cultural norms influence the expression of symptoms and the boundaries of the diagnostic criteria, both of which have shown significant diversity over time and from place to place, as this chapter will show. While Kraepelin and Bleuler saw schizophrenia as primarily an endogenous disorder, Sigmund Freud and other psychoanalysts saw schizophrenia as rooted in psychological complexes related to early child development and psychosexual factors. Carl Jung incorporated schizophrenic symptomatology into his theory of the collective unconscious, arguing that, in essence, schizophrenics represented a primal human psychology, closer to nature and shorn of social filters.[4]

Such psychoanalytic concepts contributed to ethnopsychiatric notions that Africans, as innately more "primitive" people than Europeans, lived their everyday existences closer to the borderline between sanity and schizophrenia. It is not surprising, then, that schizophrenia became by far the most commonly diagnosed mental illness in Africans during the colonial era. In 1936, Horace Shelley and W. H. Watson found that 35 percent of all cases at Zomba Lunatic Asylum in Nyasaland had been diagnosed with schizophrenia, with the next most common diagnosis, "epileptic psychosis," diagnosed in 13 percent of patients.[5] In Kenya, J. C. Carothers identified more than 28 percent of all patients as schizophrenic,[6] and famously referred to schizophrenia as "par excellence the chronic form of insanity in Africans as in Europeans."[7] In Nigeria, R. Cunyngham Brown's 1938 survey of mental institutions revealed that roughly 20 percent of both asylum and home-care patients were classified as suffering from "dementia praecox."[8]

Many factors contributed to the high rate of schizophrenia diagnoses vis-à-vis other recognized mental illnesses in colonial Africa. As seen in chapter 1, colonial asylums were essentially prisons where little treatment took place. As a result, those who ended up on the asylum statistics sheet tended to be those whose behavior was so violent, uncontrollable, or unmanageable that they needed to be shut away from the rest of society, and a large number of these would have been easily classified as schizophrenics based on these behavior patterns. Furthermore, since the diagnosis of schizophrenia requires an inability on the part of the patient to express an appropriate engagement with "reality," it becomes extremely important that both the medical authority and the patient share a similar understanding of what "reality" is. This becomes much more complicated in cross-cultural dialogues, whereby values, beliefs, and even language can color the diagnoser's interpretation of the diagnosee's condition. In colonial African settings, it is very possible that many patients were diagnosed with schizophrenia on the basis that the things they said did not make any sense to the European making the diagnosis. Whether this was because the patient was schizophrenic or just expressing cultural idiosyncrasies in inarticulate ways may never be known.[9]

Colonial psychiatrists across Africa recognized that the prevalence of schizophrenia among indigenous populations could be explained in these very practical terms, but this did not prevent them from speculating that more insidious factors were also at play. It has been well established that ethnopsychiatric theory defined the "normal" African as much closer to psychotic than the average European.[10] From the perspective of ethnopsychiatric experts, "normal" Africans did not base their worldviews on "reality" to begin with. Colonial psychiatrists regularly defined "African culture" as placing a dangerous overemphasis on supernatural phenomena to explain the natural world. African cultures also privileged emotional rather than logical responses to stimuli and tended to deny individual responsibility for the circumstances of one's life, all elements that were also identified with the schizophrenic inability to logically delineate "real" cause and effect.[11] Such a situation caused Carothers to surmise in 1940 that "the normal African is not schizophrenic, but the step from the primitive attitude to schizophrenia is but a short and easy one."[12]

As with other forms of mental illness, colonial psychiatrists became obsessed with the possibility that detribalization was somehow causing an increase in the prevalence of schizophrenia cases in African populations. The unproven theory suggested that the intrapersonal disruption brought about by the clash of primitive and modern worldviews created irreconcilable conflict within the African psyche, resulting in many cases in a psychotic break. As evidence, some colonial psychiatrists noted that the typical symptom complex associated with schizophrenia, particularly paranoia and delusions of grandeur, tended to occur in patients that had attained a significant degree of "Westernization" (i.e., urbanization, European education, etc.).[13] Even Bleuler, the man who had named schizophrenia and considered it to be primarily biological in origin, believed that "Negroes . . . become insane in greater numbers the more they approach the manner of living of the whites."[14] Such a position was very open to debate, however. For example,

B. J. F. Laubscher, writing about South Africa, declared that such findings were an indication that cultural factors affected only the content, not the form, of schizophrenia.[15] Many colonial psychiatrists recognized that schizophrenia did, in fact, exist in rural communities relatively uncontaminated by European "civilization," thereby indicating that detribalization could not be the only cause of schizophrenia in Africans, if it was a cause at all. Carothers noted that in rural Kenyans, for example, schizophrenia was "common" and tended to manifest in delusions of persecution rather than the delusions of grandeur associated with classical schizophrenia in European cultures.[16]

Two questions, then, vexed ethnopsychiatrists in regard to schizophrenia. First, if schizophrenia was universal and existed in all societies, did it necessarily exist in similar ratios in all societies? While recognizing broad patterns that could be classified as schizophrenia in rural African societies, lack of resources prevented adequate collection of data to indicate whether so-called "primitive" Africans experienced schizophrenia at similar rates to "detribalized" Africans or to Europeans. Second, even if it was clear that cultural factors affected the symptom content of schizophrenics, it remained completely unclear whether this mattered in any way beyond the diagnostic process. Did the content of schizophrenic symptoms say anything about the cause or prognosis of the patient's psychosis or in any way affect how the patient should be treated?

When T. Adeoye Lambo took the helm of Aro Mental Hospital in 1954, he began almost immediately to engage what he saw as the deficiencies of ethnopsychiatric research on schizophrenia in Africans and to insert Nigeria into the increasingly cross-cultural dialogue on the nature of schizophrenia. Lambo's earliest scientific publications were concerned primarily with the problem of diagnosing schizophrenia in Africans, and particularly with the role that culture played in shaping the form and content of schizophrenia.[17] In these writings, one from 1954 and one from 1957, Lambo addressed many of the assumptions of ethnopsychiatry and found them wanting. While he agreed with Western psychiatric models that posited schizophrenia as a cross-culturally universal phenomenon linked to brain biology, he vehemently objected to the idea that the culture of the "normal" African exhibited psychotic tendencies that paved a short, easy path to a schizophrenic break. Reacting to the body of literature claiming that African beliefs in the mystical properties of things and of the omnipresence of supernatural forces represented the kind of "logical" break characteristic of European schizophrenics, Lambo noted that "primitive man's magic is no sign of a 'pre-logical' mentality . . . but of a 'pre-causal' (that is, pre-scientific) thinking."[18] He noted that the ritual activities of African healers relied to a great extent on a consistent logic; it just happened not to conform to the scientific logic that European scientists trumpeted as the only objective form of "reality" by which to judge sane behavior. "It would be a dangerous suggestion for scientific orientation to think that being different is being pathological," he concluded.[19]

Lambo also disagreed with the colonial psychiatric notion that rates of full-blown schizophrenia were probably lower among Africans in their indigenous cultures than among those detribalized Africans struggling to modernize. Whereas Carothers and others had argued traditional, rural African cultures were relatively undemanding of individuals, allowing borderline and mild psychotic cases to pass undetected and even function more or less "normally,"[20] Lambo believed that schizophrenic reactions were common in rural communities and that they reflected the "psychic stresses which are inherent in the tribal culture."[21] He argued that one of the main reasons colonial psychiatrists had assumed otherwise was because of their inability to identify schizophrenic symptoms when their cultural content differed from that found in Europeans.

In his own studies among his native Yoruba people, Lambo found that when significantly detribalized Nigerians developed schizophrenia, the form and content of their symptoms tended to conform to those seen in people from a European cultural background. However, the symptoms of rural schizophrenics tended to differ from the classical European model. Lambo identified an "atypical" set of symptoms more common in rural patients that included "anxiety state, neurotic depression, vague hypochondriacal symptoms, magico-mystical projection symptoms, episodic twilight or confusional states, atypical depersonalization phenomenon, emotional liability and retrospective falsification of hallucinatory experiences,"[22] representing a much broader symptom complex than that of the average European schizophrenic. A multiplicity of the atypical symptoms might be present in the rural nonliterate patient at any given time, and they had a tendency to be transitory, according to Lambo. When delusions occurred, those of rural nonliterate patients tended to exhibit content related to supernaturalism and ancestral cults, while literate, Westernized patients tended to express their delusions in the form of hypochondria more typical of Europeans.

However, despite the significant differences between the symptom complexes of the rural, the nonliterate, and the classical form of the disease, Lambo argued that this should not be seen as evidence of a "peculiar native psychosis," since all the symptoms could be explained within existing psychodynamic formulations. He noted that "aggressive excitement, restlessness and bizarre psychoneurotic features are not an uncommon accompaniment of all the principal forms of schizophrenia in any race or cultural group," and that "precipitating factors can be found if one looks for them in any environment," indicating similarities where others might focus on difference.[23] Indeed, the culturally specific features that Lambo emphasized existed "only in addition to thought disorder, passivity feelings, affective disturbances, disturbed association of ideas and other symptoms," which Lambo found to be "varying aspects of the fundamental schizophrenic order common to both [literate, urban; and nonliterate, rural] groups."[24]

The overall picture for Lambo was one in which schizophrenia was a universal disorder, the form and content of which was determined by cultural markers. In this way, the African psyche, regardless of its cultural background, functioned no differently than the psyche of any other human being whose reactions to stimuli were also culturally determined but not necessarily culturally caused. For Lambo, the fact that the manifestation of schizophrenia looked different in urban, literate and rural, nonliterate Nigerians was proof of the fact that the "innate psychological qualities" of Europeans and Africans did not actually differ substantially. If they did, it should be expected that Westernized Yoruba men would react differently to the stresses of modern civilization than Europeans because of differences in constitutional factors. That those Nigerians most acculturated to European ways exhibited similar form and content of schizophrenia to Europeans indicated that they assimilated cultural cues in much the same way that Europeans did and were therefore psychologically similar to Europeans despite their racial difference. Lambo believed that his findings went a long way toward disproving some of the more outrageously racist claims of colonial psychiatrists and declared that "on the basis of deeper psychological determinants, this investigation has shown that the aphorism 'the nature of men is identical; what divides them is their custom,' is a valid statement even at the level of psychotic regression."[25]

After a few years of using his new diagnostic criteria for schizophrenia in clinical practice, Lambo provided data from Aro Hospital indicating the significant levels of rural schizophrenia that had been uncovered through greater engagement with rural communities. By 1960, of 960 schizophrenic patients treated at Aro Hospital, only 370 were urban and literate, while 270 were rural, the remaining quotient being urban and illiterate. These numbers masked the reality that large numbers of rural schizophrenics were still not seeking treatment at psychiatric hospitals.[26]

While Lambo was adamant that the cultural impact on the form and content of schizophrenia in Africans was not an indication of differences in causality, he became increasingly interested in the possibility that cultural factors might have a significant effect on the prognosis of individual schizophrenic patients. By the early 1960s, Lambo had become aware that a "lack of complete regression and of severe chronicity" was "remarkably noticeable in African schizophrenics" compared to European patients. Of the 960 schizophrenic patients treated at Aro Hospital between 1954 and 1959, Lambo noted that 486 of them had improved to the point that they could go home and resume some, possibly all, of their normal responsibilities in their communities.[27] This was a remission rate of over 50 percent for Nigerian patients at a time when most Euro-American studies showed improvement rates between 20 and 40 percent.[28] He further noted that "permanent recovery . . . seems to occur much more readily in African patients, probably more often than has been generally supposed by experienced workers in Western culture."[29] Lambo attributed the lack of chronicity in African patients partly to "genetic and constitutional factors," but believed that environmental and cultural factors played a key role in this outcome. "Assuming that genetic endowment, especially in respect of predisposition to schizophrenia, is similar in all ethnic groups," he hypothesized that "the difference in the course and outcome of the disorders can only be found in the differential cultural conditioning to which these people have been subjected."[30] Lambo credited the cultural emphasis on community care in African healing systems, and his own reformulation of it at Aro Village, as the most apparent contributor to the recovery and reintegration of African schizophrenics into their societies and suggested that prolonged institutionalization in Western-style hospital settings might actually exacerbate chronicity in European and American patients.

Lambo was not the first or the only Western-trained psychiatrist to suggest that schizophrenia looked different in different cultures. Indeed, the type of work that Lambo was doing fit naturally into a growing network of cross-cultural psychiatry that was beginning to compile and share data on schizophrenia from across the world. In the 1950s and 1960s, a number of studies of schizophrenia from a variety of different cultural settings illustrated that although Western-trained psychiatrists were diagnosing schizophrenia in all racial, cultural, and social groups, the typical form and content of schizophrenia looked different in different places. For example, beginning in the late 1950s, the group of transcultural psychiatrists at McGill University in Montreal began trying to compile and synthesize data on the form and content of schizophrenia in various parts of the world. Using the network developed through the distribution of the *Transcultural Psychiatric Review and Newsletter*, Erik D. Wittkower, H. B. M. Murphy, J. Fried, and H. Ellenberger sent out questionnaires to psychiatrists working in different cultural environments to learn what their field experience taught them about schizophrenia in their respective territories. Respondents returned thirty-seven questionnaires from twenty-five different countries encompassing the six inhabited continents, including data from Nigeria.

By the early 1960s, the World Health Organization (WHO) had also begun the process of systematizing the compilation of epidemiological data on schizophrenia around the world. In 1959, WHO declared an interest in promoting cross-cultural psychiatric epidemiology and spent the next several years developing an effective methodology for a broad-based study. The result was the International Pilot Study of Schizophrenia (IPSS), launched in 1966 to test whether effective criteria for diagnosing schizophrenia cross-culturally could be determined. Nine centers across the globe were designated as catchment areas for the accumulation of data. Ibadan, Nigeria, was one of them.[31] From 1966 to 1971, T. Adeoye Lambo served as the chief collaborating investigator of the Ibadan group. Tolani Asuni also served as a collaborating investigator during this period before taking over as chief collaborating investigator for the period of 1971–76. The Nigerian catchment area accounted for a plurality of all the patients included in the data analysis, providing 145 of the 1,202 cases analyzed, slightly more than one-ninth of the study group.[32]

The findings of cross-cultural research into schizophrenia around the world tended to confirm the conclusions that Lambo had reached based on Nigerian circumstances. Studies conducted in Europe and Asia in the 1950s supported Lambo's contention that rural schizophrenia was not uncommon. Asian studies also found, similarly to Lambo, that the form of schizophrenia among non-Westernized individuals tended to follow the pattern of aggression, excitement, and confusional state following a course of acute onset but with a relatively benign long-term prognosis.[33] Cross-cultural studies also found, in concordance with Lambo, that symptom content varied culturally. The results of the McGill study in 1960 indicated that, at a broad level, psychiatrists the world over did agree on what the typical characteristics of schizophrenia were: namely, "social and emotional withdrawal, hallucinations and delusions, and flatness of affect."[34] However, beyond this basic agreement, results diverged significantly on the frequency of subtypes and symptom content. According to the responses, paranoid schizophrenia was common everywhere, but other subtypes of schizophrenia varied significantly across space. For example, catatonic schizophrenia was much more common among Japanese and Indian patients than among Euro-American ones. Furthermore, the content of specific symptoms varied greatly as well. While auditory hallucinations were generally common, visual hallucinations were much more common in African and Middle Eastern patients than other groups. Where delusions were common, their content was much more likely to be religious in nature in Christian and Muslim groups than in others. Japanese and Indian patients were characterized as experiencing flatness of affect more frequently than other groups.[35] In fact, in fifteen cultures, flatness of affect was categorized as an infrequent symptom despite being universally recognized as a basic characteristic of the disease.

Similarly, the IPSS noted in the publication of its first volume of results in 1973 that all nine catchment areas were able to consistently differentiate schizophrenia from major affective disorders, although there were some anomalies. For example, it was found, famously, that the American and Soviet definitions of what qualified as schizophrenia were significantly broader than those adhered to by the other seven research centers.[36] However, perhaps the most important finding of the WHO project came from a follow-up study conducted two years later. In the follow-up study, investigators tracked down patients from the original study to see how they were managing their illness. The results indicated that patients from non-Western backgrounds had a much more favorable long-term prognosis than those from Europe and the United States.[37] Of all the groups, the Ibadan patients had the best course and outcome, with 46 percent reporting full remission. Ninety-seven percent had stayed out of the hospital for at least three-quarters of the time since the initial study.[38] The findings of the follow-up study therefore confirmed the impressions that Lambo had noted twenty years earlier: that African schizophrenics were much less likely to develop chronic schizophrenia than Euro-Americans.

These cross-cultural studies ultimately raised more questions than they answered. Methodological complications and logistical issues allowed for significant criticism of the findings and little agreement on what the results meant. Clearly, psychiatrists the world over agreed that something called schizophrenia in the Western definitional sense *did* exist universally in human cultures, but there were clearly some significant differences in the ways that psychiatrists around the world were diagnosing it. However, what the cross-cultural syntheses of the 1960s and 1970s could not prove was whether these differences resulted from differences in the diagnostic judgments of individual psychiatrists or whether they actually arose from differences in the ways that cultural factors influenced the course of schizophrenia. It was not at all clear where the boundaries of any given culture should be set. Although responses came from twenty-five different countries in the McGill study, and nine different countries in the IPSS, the religious, ethnic, social, and cultural backgrounds were undoubtedly very diverse within and across these national boundaries. Psychiatrists themselves often did not share a cultural background with their patients, making issues of communication and bias more problematic in the diagnostic process. Ultimately, Wittkower, Murphy, and Ellenberger concluded that their 1960 findings indicated "a major barrier for transcultural comparison."[39] Cross-cultural psychiatrists also criticized the process of the IPSS, noting that it paid far more attention in its analysis to social indicators (e.g., marital status, education level, wealth, etc.) than to explicitly cultural factors. Others criticized the incomprehensiveness of the IPSS findings (it was, after all, only a pilot study) and its inability to provide a perfectly acceptable and encompassing definition of schizophrenia for universal application.[40]

Criticisms aside, transcultural psychiatric research on schizophrenia clearly provided an outlet and an opportunity for Lambo to achieve a broader agenda of reforming racialized conceptions of mental illness developed under colonial power structures. Presenting schizophrenia as a universal mental illness masked by pathoplastic cultural overlay promoted Lambo's cultural politics of equality. Cross-cultural evidence that cultural variation of schizophrenic form and content was universal promoted the concept of the innate equality of human psychological function. Data demonstrating that non-Westerners recovered more readily from schizophrenia suggested that Western psychotherapeutics had something to learn from non-Western cultures and healing regimens. Lambo's personal research suggested these conclusions at a local level in the 1950s; international networks of transcultural psychiatric research reinforced them at a global level in the 1960s and 1970s.

DEPRESSION

One of the oldest maladies in the Western medical tradition, the illness currently known as depression goes back at least as far as Hippocrates, who dubbed the term "melancholic" in the fifth century BCE to describe people who experienced prolonged despondency. Depressive illnesses have been known by a variety of different names in Western civilization over the last two millennia, but "depression" emerged in psychiatric discourse in the early twentieth century as the mainstream term for a variety of affective (mood) disorders characterized by sadness, loss of energy, and feelings of guilt and personal depreciation.[41]

Depression, like schizophrenia, has long been considered a condition that any person can conceivably develop. Indeed, it is a condition that virtually everyone will experience to a certain degree at various points in life.

Sadness, worry, and agitation are universal emotions that all cultures recognize as part of a "normal" individual's response to trying life circumstances. Unlike schizophrenia, which is primarily characterized by a recognizable distortion of *thought*, depression is historically characterized by *mood* responses that are disruptive to individuals' physical and social functionality. While a variety of different gradations and subtypes of depression have been recognized within psychiatry, the primary distinction for most of the twentieth century was between neurotic (reactive or exogenous) and psychotic (or endogenous) depression. Neurotic depression has been characterized as dejection precipitated primarily by external forces (loss of loved one, loss of career, general dissatisfaction with the path and outcome of one's life), while psychotic depression represents a dysphoria precipitated from within the individual and usually inexplicable in terms of one's environmental circumstances. Because of the extent to which neurotic depression can be considered a "normal" response to external stimuli, it has been abandoned as a psychiatric diagnosis since the publication of the *DSM-III* in 1980. However, it is recognized that bouts of "neurotic" depression can mask or precipitate the development of major affective disorders or a variety of other psychotic illnesses that are still recognized, including major depression, bipolar disorder, and schizoaffective disorder.[42]

Whereas colonial ethnopsychiatrists had believed schizophrenia to be by far the most common form of mental illness in Africans, depression was considered to be extremely rare among such "primitive" peoples.[43] Indeed, statistics from colonial mental asylums seemed to bear out the contention that depression was quite uncommon for Africans. As late as 1950, Geoffrey C. Tooth diagnosed only 6 out of 34 cases of affective psychosis as depressive in the Gold Coast. Carothers diagnosed only 24 out of more than 1,500 patients seen at Mathari Hospital in Kenya with depressive psychosis over a ten-year period from 1938 to 1949.[44] R. Cunyngham Brown reported only 0.3 percent of patients in Nigerian asylums suffering from "acute melancholia" in 1938, while an additional 7.3 percent had been diagnosed with manic depression.[45]

Several logistical reasons explained why colonial officials saw so little depression among Africans. First, most medical officials saw mentally ill Africans only in the context of their incarceration in an asylum. However, since asylums were reserved mostly for the maintenance of the dangerous and the violent, it was very unlikely that people with depressive illnesses would be found there, other than manic-depressives, whose manic episodes might necessitate custodial oversight. Furthermore, since little in the way of treatment was offered to African patients in colonial asylums, the overwhelming majority of people suffering depressionlike illnesses were undoubtedly treated by family, friends, and indigenous healers rather than at an asylum that offered them little hope for recovery. Colonial psychiatrists had no way of assessing what percentage of people underwent traditional therapies for symptoms enumerated in the European diagnostic entity of depression.

Colonial ethnopsychiatrists recognized these practical barriers to generalization about the rates of depression in African societies, but, as in other things, this did not prevent them from speculating that racial-cum-cultural characteristics of Africans probably prevented most Africans from developing depression at the rates that Europeans did. For Europeans in the first half of the twentieth century, the key symptoms necessary for a diagnosis of depression were despondent mood and an internalization of aggression in the form of feelings of guilt and personal depreciation.[46] General assumptions about the nature of African culture inclined ethnopsychiatrists to assume that it was impossible for Africans to feel endogenous sadness and guilt because they were incapable of taking personal responsibility for anything. Widespread beliefs in witchcraft and other supernatural causation for life's tragedies prevalent in African cultures led ethnopsychiatrists to the belief that Africans always sought out external blame for trauma, and were therefore able to exonerate themselves of guilt feelings by naming witches, gods, and fate as the culprits for life's misfortunes. Beliefs that Africans lived only in the present, without a care for the future, and that African communal culture made it impossible for Africans to think critically about the individual self were also seen by ethnopsychiatrists as reasons that Africans would be less likely to become depressed.[47] In European history since the Renaissance, melancholy had frequently been romanticized as a disease of genius, likely to afflict the most intelligent and creative members of society.[48] The preponderance of depression in Europeans became a marker of "civilization," a by-product of a culture that had inculcated values of personal responsibility, self-improvement, and progress-seeking ambition, and, therefore, a disease of prestige. The perceived lack of depression in Africans became one more piece of "evidence" indicating the relative inability of black cultures to produce highly insightful or intellectual individuals.[49]

The clinical picture of depression in Africa began to change as psychiatric facilities were decolonizing in Nigeria and other parts of Africa in the late 1950s and early 1960s. As in other areas of transcultural psychiatry, T. Adeoye Lambo was among the first to find that depression was much more common in Africans than had previously been believed. Early in his career, Lambo had very much accepted the notion that depression was rare in Africans, declaring in a 1956 article that "since beliefs and superstitions still pervade most of the aspects of African lives, even those of the westernized group to a certain extent, these factors must damp down depression."[50] Even at this point, however, Lambo was careful to note that this observation might be "more apparent than real," and that depression might exist at high rates in the general population but fall beneath the radar of both Western and indigenous health-care providers.

By 1960, however, Lambo had become certain that depression was far more common among Africans than had previously been suspected. Based on clinical findings from his work at Aro, Lambo concluded that many cases of neurotic depression had been misclassified as "neurasthenia" or a somatic complaint. Furthermore, many cases of psychotic depression had been classified simply as "intractable psychoneurotics." The reason for this clinical picture, according to Lambo, was a lack of understanding about the typical symptom complex that characterized depression in African patients. While depressed mood very often was a symptom, it rarely was the primary symptom, and was almost never the symptom of which the patient most complained. "The patient is invariably preoccupied with vague somatic complaints and looks more anxious and agitated than depressed," declared Lambo. Nevertheless, "insomnia of varying degrees is a most constant finding," and "a subjective feeling of difficulty in thinking may occasionally be complained of." The preoccupation with bodily complaints represented a "psychosomatic overlay" to the depression. Unlike classical European depression, Lambo found that "ideas of self-accusation or ruin, of fear for the future, of regret, and a profound sense of sorrow," were usually completely absent.[51] Lambo noted that colonial psychiatrists therefore frequently misdiagnosed depression in Africans because "in most instances the outward affective state by no means corresponds to the patient's real feelings."[52] With such diagnostic criteria to go from, Lambo enumerated 184 out of 3,975 patients treated at Aro for endogenous depression between 1954 and 1959. This accounted for 4.6 percent of all patients seen during this time period and, while still small proportionate to European rates, represented more than fifteen times what Brown had reported in Nigeria twenty years earlier.[53]

As was the case with schizophrenia, Lambo's findings became integrated into a growing body of cross-cultural studies on depression. By the early 1960s, psychiatrists working in a variety of different African environments had begun to question the rarity of depression in their populations, arguing that cultural ignorance had prevented earlier psychiatrists from recognizing depression in Africans. At the First Pan-African Psychiatric Conference organized by Lambo in 1961, several psychiatrists working in different African countries presented findings indicating that depression was far more common in Africans than previously believed. Most emphasized the extent to which somatic and hypochondriacal complaints dominated the symptom pool, while expressions of disturbed mood and guilt were uncommon.[54] The Cornell-Aro cross-cultural project that resulted in the report *Psychiatric Disorder among the Yoruba* found that in addition to the atypical symptom constellation, classical symptoms of depression were also common in Nigerians. The Cornell-Aro study found that, although patients did not volunteer that they experienced depressed mood, "many of the component symptoms of depression came up in one context or another: sapped vitality, a sense of 'dwindling,' crying continuously, extreme worry, loss of appetite, and lost [*sic*] of interest in life." The authors noted that "depression seems an unfamiliar concept, and there is linguistic difficulty in finding Yoruba words with which to describe the subjective feelings meant by the term."[55] When all the newly recognized means of understanding depressive symptomatology in Africans were considered, the Cornell-Aro project ultimately found that psychoneurotic symptoms of depression were actually somewhat more common among the Yoruba than among North Americans. Psychotic depression continued to present as somewhat more uncommon in the African population, and suicidal and guilt manifestations remained rare.[56]

Lambo's perspective on depressive symptomatology in Nigeria corresponded not only with findings emerging from other African environments, but also with studies appearing from across the world. Encouraged by the findings of their schizophrenia study, the McGill group conducted a cross-cultural study on depressive symptomatology in 1964.[57] Data came from questionnaires returned by sixty respondents in thirty different countries, including Nigeria, on six continents. Results indicated that "a mood of depression or dejection; diurnal mood change; insomnia with early morning wakening; diminution of interest in social environment," were "almost universally regarded as the core syndrome of depressive states."[58] However, strong variations in typical symptom presentation existed across a variety of cultural categories. The results indicated that Hindus rarely expressed diurnal mood change, Muslims were particularly unlikely to express feelings of guilt, and Japanese patients were less likely than other groups to experience loss of sexual interest or to express excitement and theatrical grief, while Africans frequently expressed excitement and "ideas of influence and of being possessed."[59] Overall, findings indicated to the group that cultural factors did not seem to affect the frequency of psychotic depression, which was universally present in all cultures, but clearly played a role in the symptomatology and, consequently, the diagnostic process.

Critiques of the extent to which depression in Africans could be found only by significantly altering the definition of the disease itself emerged by the late 1960s, but they did not come from Nigerian psychiatrists. Raymond H. Prince, for example, found it suspiciously coincidental that so much of the research indicating the commonality of African depression came in the context of decolonization and political independence of African countries. He called the theoretical turn in depressive symptomatology in Africa the "Independence Shift," raising the possibility that identifying somatic symptoms as the primary marker of depression in Africans was more politically than scientifically justifiable.[60] The second generation of Nigerian psychiatrists, however, overwhelmingly embraced the notion of depression as a universal disease entity that presented differently in different cultures. In 1973, Michael O. Olatawura declared that it "was no longer a debatable point" that "depression is not rare in Africans."[61] In 1981, G. G. C. Rwegellera indicated, "Though the form of depressive illness remains essentially the same from culture to culture, the content of these illnesses varies in certain respects in different cultures."[62] Similarly, A. Kalunta expressed the view that general agreement existed on the belief that "psychiatric syndromes or reactions, by and large, are similar in all races throughout the world. Environmental, constitutional and tribal cultural background merely modify the symptom constellation," including for depressive illnesses.[63] Nigerian studies in the 1970s had even begun to chip away at the notion that Africans expressed depression differently from Westerners. John C. Ebie found in a 1972 study that most Nigerian depressives would not volunteer mood symptoms. However, when questioned specifically about their mood, they would admit to sadness.[64] Rwegellera cited studies indicating that feelings of guilt were on the rise, and that suicide, while still uncommon in Nigeria, was being found to be much more common in other parts of Africa than had previously been indicated.[65]

In all these analyses, Nigerian psychiatrists were occupied with illustrating the extent to which cultural factors did not cause individuals to suffer different mental illnesses. People from all cultural backgrounds could develop the universal illness of depression; their cultures (African or other) simply had the capacity to affect how individuals would express their depression to others. Once again, Nigerian psychiatrists, invested in the cultural politics of antiracism and anticolonialism, had engaged with international networks of cross-cultural research in an effort to change mainstream psychiatric theory toward a more incorporative, egalitarian, and universalist model.

THE SO-CALLED "BRAIN-FAG SYNDROME"

While much of transcultural psychiatry was focused on universalizing Western diagnostic entities like schizophrenia and depression in the 1950s and

1960s, some psychiatric researchers were seeking to explain psychological disorders that seemed to be isolated to particular cultural communities and were not experienced universally across cultures. The presence of these "exotic" syndromes, particularly in non-Western societies, had long been noted,[66] but it was not until the 1960s that P. M. Yap coined the term "culture-bound syndromes" to imply that elements in the indigenous cultures were responsible in some way for the seemingly localized natures of these disorders.[67] One example of a presumably "culture-bound syndrome" is amok, a dissociative homicidal episode originally found in Malaysia that inspired the English idiom "running amok." Koro, found in a variety of cultures in south and east Asia, refers to an intense anxiety that the genitals (penis for men; vulva and sometimes nipples for women) are retracting into the body and that this will result in death; while ghost sickness has been described as a morbid preoccupation with death and the deceased among some Native American peoples.[68] Then there's brain-fag syndrome, defined in the appendix on culture-bound syndromes in the fourth edition of the *Diagnostic and Statistical Manual of Mental Disorders* (*DSM-IV*) as "a term initially used in West Africa to refer to a condition experienced by high school or university students in response to the challenges of schooling."[69] The place in West Africa where brain fag was first found happened to be southwestern Nigeria, its "discoverer" none other than Raymond H. Prince, the Canadian psychiatrist who had conducted more than a year of clinical work in Nigeria in the late 1950s and who served along with the Leightons, Savage, and Lambo as the psychiatric research team for the Cornell-Aro project discussed in chapter 2.

In 1957, Prince arrived at Aro Hospital in Abeokuta to begin work in the new outpatient clinics designed by T. Adeoye Lambo.[70] Within a few months, Prince became struck by what he perceived as a strong pattern in the demographic and symptomatological makeup of presenting patients in these clinics. Most were adolescent male students who complained of having lost the capacity to retain information that they read in books or heard in formal lectures. Furthermore, in a preponderance of these cases, the patients complained of physical ailments, most notably crawling or burning sensations in the head. Students described their symptoms as "brain fag," indicating their belief that their symptoms were caused by severe mental fatigue. Intrigued by these patients' consistency of symptoms, Prince conducted a series of interviews with presenting patients and a questionnaire of secondary school students in the Lagos area. In 1960 and 1962, Prince published two articles reporting his findings on the pattern, incidence, and possible causes of his newly discovered "brain-fag syndrome."[71]

Brain-fag syndrome (BFS), according to Prince, consisted of the following "distinctive cluster of symptoms" in Nigerian students and other "brain workers": "(1) unpleasant head sensations (burning, crawling feelings etc); (2) visual difficulties (blurring, eye pain, excessive tearing etc.); (3) inability to grasp the meaning of printed symbols; (4) poor retentivity; and (5) fatigue and sleepiness in spite of adequate rest."[72] The symptoms could be incapacitating. For example, Prince described the case of A.B., a twenty-eight-year-old unmarried male Yoruba teacher who was studying for an honors degree in classics by extension from the University of London. A.B. had begun to notice symptoms of BFS after writing a BA examination in 1953. At this point, he "felt weak and could not concentrate for about two weeks." Symptoms recurred three years later as he was studying for his classics exams, at which point "he began to have sharp pains in the head and could not grasp what he was reading. He slept more than usual, and had difficulty in forcing himself to go to school in the morning. When writing examinations, he felt that he knew the answers, but was unable to recall them; his mind was blank. His right hand was weak and shook so that he couldn't write."[73] A.B.'s difficulties prevented him from taking his classics examinations for two years.

Alarming about BFS was the supposed prevalence of the disorder. Prince suggested the extent to which brain fag had become something of a stereotype in late 1950s Nigeria, anecdotally noting that "one medical officer remarked to me, 'if a young man comes in with glasses and European dress, you may be sure that he will complain of burning in his head and inability to read.'"[74] Not to be convinced by such anecdotal evidence, Prince conducted a survey of six secondary schools in southern Nigeria to determine the relative incidence of BFS symptoms among Nigeria's Western-educated youth. Prince received 844 responses to his questionnaire and discovered that a shocking 54 percent of all respondents (458 students) complained of "symptoms associated with study."[75] Prince recognized that his survey did not indicate full-blown "cases" of BFS, but it did indicate to him a generally high risk for the possible development of brain fag in a significant proportion of the student population. BFS quickly became a common diagnosis for Nigerian psychiatric patients. Alexander Boroffka and A. A. Marinho reported that thirty-five of sixty-six total patients received at the psychiatric outpatient clinic attached to Yaba Mental Hospital outside Lagos had been diagnosed with BFS over the course of a year beginning in June 1961.[76]

Prince declared that the symptoms associated with BFS were quite uncommon in the West, where neurotics generally presented with "anxiety, depression, insomnia, palpitation, obsessive thinking, etc,"[77] and not with an inability to reason or think as seen in Nigerian cases. Although Prince provided no data to support this conclusion, the assumption based on it is clear: brain-fag syndrome was not a universal form of mental illness, but rather one that existed only in specific places. The question begged by this conclusion is, what caused brain fag to appear so much more often in Nigeria than in the West? Biological components seemed unlikely. There was no apparent correlation between age or perceived intelligence level and the onset or severity of brain-fag symptoms.[78] Prince found the disorder overwhelmingly in males, but this was chalked up mainly to the disproportionate male-female ratio in Western educational institutions at the time of the studies.[79]

The stress associated with earning a European education probably contributed to the development of BFS, according to Prince. As a European education became the avenue to wealth and prestige in Nigeria as a result of British colonial rule, it became increasingly important that young Nigerians, particularly males, earn a European degree. According to Prince, the education process often became a family affair, with many different family members contributing financially to the success of one bright pupil. This was done in the understanding that once the pupil earned his degree and began a well-paying career, he would distribute his largesse among his family, true to his communal roots. The importance of European education, according to Prince, was therefore much greater for the average Nigerian student, whose entire family depended upon his success, than for the average European student, whose education was more often an individual exercise. Prince indicated that the link between this cultural circumstance and BFS was "difficult to appraise," noting that patients "tended to minimize these factors." Nevertheless, Prince pointed out that two of his ten individual case studies declared that they would "rather die" than give up their studies.[80]

Adding to the stress felt by Nigerian students, according to Prince, was the fact that European educations were probably intrinsically more difficult for Nigerians to achieve because the individualized, book-centered curriculum of British schools clashed with the communal lifestyle into which Nigerians were inculcated. Indeed, although he could never find direct correlation, Prince was intrigued by the possibility that brain-fag sufferers were more likely to be the first generation of literates in their respective families. Although Prince's own data did not find a conclusive link with literacy patterns, he brushed this off by declaring that "parental literacy is of course accompanied in varying degrees by a whole cluster of Westernization effects," which "might have a considerably higher negative correlation with symptoms than literacy itself."[81] Such a speculative explanation could account for the preponderance of brain-fag cases in which parental literacy was high.

The stress put on Nigerian students was not strictly linked to learning a new medium of instruction, however. According to Prince, the long hours of isolated endeavor were anathema to the "Nigerian personality." The traditional Nigerian came from a "collectivistic society," which for Prince was characterized "by the extended family and shared family responsibilities . . . in this type of society there is a strong sense of identity with the group and a limited sense of individual identity . . . there is a remarked reluctance to assume individual responsibility in circumstances of choice and a distaste for isolated endeavor; there tends to be a blind acceptance of authority and established pattern but a 'paralysis' in the face of the new and a restriction of individual creativity." The collectivist Nigerian personality would find it difficult to adjust to an education system designed to suit the needs of an "individualistic society," such as had been established in Nigeria over generations of missionary influence and British colonial rule. As a result, Prince argued, "the circumstances of prolonged isolated book learning and the intense individual responsibility-in-isolation inherent in the western type of 'examination' system are of paramount importance in generating the painful feelings which result in this syndrome."[82]

Indeed, brain-fag syndrome, for Prince, was a subconscious rebellion of the Nigerian personality, which could not stand being put into a European box. "The student forces himself to sit before his book going through the motions of study but part of his mind will not assimilate, being in revolt against this fundamentally alien mode of isolated endeavour," declared Prince. "Some students may be seen sitting in the library before an open book, listlessly leafing the pages and 'cracking' their necks to release the tension generated by this conflict between conscious aim and more or less conscious revolt."[83] Brain-fag syndrome, as far as Prince defined it, was therefore a rejection of "modern" European education by the "traditional" African mind. His construction of the disorder was inextricably bound up with notions about the negative psychological consequences of "detribalization" that pervaded ethnopsychiatric thinking in the colonial period.

It would be unfair, however, to depict Prince as fully within the mold of colonialist ethnopsychiatry. Prince had come to Nigeria to work with T. Adeoye Lambo, one of the pioneering figures of transcultural psychiatry. Prince himself claimed his motivation for working in Nigeria was "specifically to study the effects of cultural factors on the forms of psychiatric disorder."[84] Prince was sincerely interested in researching the relationship between human psyches and specific cultural idioms in the Nigerian context. Working most extensively among the Yoruba of southwestern Nigeria, Prince produced numerous scholarly works on Yoruba perceptions of curse,[85] witchcraft,[86] and divination,[87] as well as on indigenous medical practices, both spiritual and pharmacological,[88] for diagnosing and treating mental disease. Furthermore, the idea that much of the psychiatric disorder appearing in Nigeria at this time was at least partly attributable to cultural dislocation was articulated on many instances by Nigerian psychiatrists like Lambo, as discussed in chapter 2. That said, the etiology of BFS, as defined by Prince, had direct links to the colonial ethnopsychiatry of the first half of the twentieth century insofar as it made claims about Nigerians' peculiar inability to internalize Western education and negotiate a perceived culture conflict in their own minds.

It should not be surprising, therefore, that many Nigerian psychiatrists were not impressed by the discovery of this supposedly culture-bound disorder. Debates have circled around the very notion of a "culture-bound syndrome." In order for a syndrome to be culture-bound, the symptom structure has to be unique to a particular cultural entity. This means that the symptoms must be dissimilar from symptoms of mental illnesses found in other cultures and that the cultural units to which these syndromes are bound can be identified by characteristics that make them distinct from all other cultural units. Neither of these criteria is easily met. The debate ultimately comes down to whether one wants to emphasize cross-cultural similarities or differences. With brain fag, the very definition of the disorder as in any way culture-bound had political implications linked to the histories of both Nigeria and psychiatry. However one wishes to view Prince's etiology of brain fag as essentially bound up in the "detribalization" problem, no psychiatrist in Nigeria has since denied the frequency with which patients present the symptoms associated with BFS. Indeed, neither Lambo nor Asuni, Nigeria's two most prominent psychiatrists of the 1960s, ever came out against BFS. However, since the 1970s Nigerian psychiatrists of the second and third generations have seriously questioned the extent to which the symptom cluster known as BFS represents a uniquely culture-bound entity. While Prince initially defined the disorder as precipitated by characteristics unique to the "Nigerian personality," the second and third generations of Nigerian psychiatrists did not find Prince's cultural boundaries or definitions compelling, and sought to recast brain fag as part of the universal spectrum of internationally recognized anxiety/depressive disorders, arguing that there was nothing particularly culturally determined about it.

Prince had called for studies to be done in other parts of the world to see if the symptom cluster he identified as BFS existed elsewhere. By the early 1970s, it was clear that BFS was by no means isolated to Nigeria. Studies in the late 1960s found cases of BFS in Uganda and Liberia,[89] and, more recently, in Tanzania,[90] Ivory Coast,[91] Swaziland,[92] South Africa,[93] and Ethiopian immigrants to Israel.[94] Such cross-cultural comparisons allowed Amechi Anumonye, a senior lecturer at Lagos University Teaching Hospital who would later write the only book on BFS, to declare that "similar somatisation reactions [to BFS] have been found in other less developed countries," leading to the conclusion that "the concept of the Nigerian personality is a myth."[95]

Further evidence of the flimsiness of the "Nigerian personality" hypothesis came from comparing Nigerian personality types to other cultures. In 1980, Olufemi Morakinyo of the Department of Medicine and Mental Health at the University of Ifé used two personality questionnaires commonly employed in Western psychological circles to examine thirty BFS patients in Nigeria. He compared the results with a control group of "healthy (normal)" Nigerians and with "known findings in British populations" to determine what, if any, personality characteristics were unique to Nigerian BFS sufferers.[96] If BFS was the result of something intrinsic to the "Nigerian personality," then presumably Morakinyo should have found significant differences in the personality types of Nigerians and Britons. He found exactly the opposite, however. The normal, healthy Nigerian population did not score significantly differently on the tests from British populations, and BFS patients scored higher than the healthy Nigerian and British populations only in neuroticism. Morakinyo therefore concluded that there were no inherent personality differences between Nigerians and the British and that the higher neuroticism score of BFS patients indicated a constitutional predisposition toward psychiatric illness, likely the result of being "highly strung and easily aroused" irrespective of their educational pursuits.[97]

The bulk of research on the subject by the 1980s tended toward an understanding that BFS, with its emphasis on specific somatic complaints, was really nothing more than masked anxiety and/or depression, universal conditions that had been increasingly associated with somatic symptoms in African patients since the 1950s. Although BFS did not fit perfectly within either nosology, mainstream psychiatry also recognized intrinsic links between anxiety and depressive states, so classifying BFS within the larger anxiety/depression matrix was perfectly feasible. In a 1973 article, Anumonye provided positive links between BFS and depression, arguing, "The similarity of the symptom-complex to depressive illness is remarkable. All the symptoms can in fact be explained on affective basis. In a culture where the word 'depression' does not occur and where somatization is common, this theory can be some part of the answer."[98] Anumonye soon came to recognize that anxiety and depression existed simultaneously in many BFS patients. Anumonye followed up on these claims with research into the treatment of BFS with antidepressive and antianxiety drugs. In 1975, he presented evidence that BFS could be treated effectively with the commonly prescribed antidepressants doxepin and diazepam (Valium).[99] Later studies by other psychiatrists seemed to confirm Anumonye's links between BFS and anxiety and depressive states.[100]

The intrinsic link Prince made between BFS and European-style education also came under scrutiny. In 1980, Morakinyo, for example, published an article declaring BFS to have a "multifactoral etiology" linked to the normal stresses that students experienced everywhere. Morakinyo concluded that BFS was, in fact, nothing more than "a stress reaction, in people with a nervous predisposition, induced principally by physical and psychological factors, *viz.*, sleep deprivation and drug abuse, which are self-imposed in order to ensure successful outcome of an enterprise,"[101] most notably European-type education. BFS was not an innate rejection of Western education, then, for Morakinyo; it was a normal stress reaction that had unfortunately been defined more by the context within which symptoms occurred than by the nature of those symptoms. Peter F. Omoluabi corroborated Morakinyo's findings in a 1986 study that linked BFS to test anxiety, a condition experienced frequently by students in the West.[102]

Of course, students were not the only Nigerians who experienced stress. Nigerian psychiatrists in the 1980s began to note similarities between BFS in "brain workers" and other forms of psychiatric disturbance in "non-brain workers." R. Olukayode Jegede of the Department of Psychiatry at the University of Ibadan provided case studies of non-brain workers with symptom patterns characteristic of BFS. One patient, a twenty-six-year-old woman dubbed Mrs. XY by Jegede, presented with "sleeplessness, heat in the head, crawling sensations all over the body especially the scalp, and vague aches and pains over the period of one year."[103] Although she was not a student, Mrs. XY's symptom pattern mirrored that of BFS patients. Her symptoms became so crippling that she had to be admitted to the Aro Village Community Mental Health Centre, where she was diagnosed not with BFS, as might be expected based on her symptom cluster, but with depressive neurosis, a much more appropriate diagnosis for "non-brain workers." Through psychotherapy it was determined that the likely cause of Mrs. XY's breakdown was an unhappy marriage. She responded positively to antidepressive medications and was discharged back to her family. The similarity between Mrs. XY's symptoms and BFS was not an anomaly, according to Jegede. He supplied data on the symptom patterns from twenty-five illiterate patients diagnosed with anxiety neurosis, noting that a significant number of them also complained of symptoms within the BFS cluster: five of the twenty-five experienced heat in the head, four had crawling feelings in the head, eight had heat in the body, seven had crawling sensations in the body, and ten complained of sleeplessness.[104] Clearly, according to Jegede, the symptoms that so distinguished BFS were not limited to students and other "brain workers" and therefore could not be explained in terms of a clash between Western education and the "Nigerian personality."

In 1985, Raymond H. Prince jumped back into the debate on BFS, arguing from a somewhat different perspective. Completely abandoning his earlier notion that BFS was a disease of "brain workers" caused by cultural particularities of the "Nigerian Personality," Prince was willing to recognize that "the majority of patients labelled brain-fag could be considered cases of anxiety-depression rather than any other Western psychiatric label,"[105] but he nevertheless concluded that BFS still merited the designation of a culture-bound syndrome because of what he considered its distinct symptom cluster and the presumed linkage between that symptom cluster and cultural circumstances unique to sub-Saharan African populations. The relevance of BFS as a culture-bound disorder depended on the perspective one took toward mental illness, according to Prince. From the standpoint of the psychopharmacologist whose job it is to treat mental illness, the cultural component of BFS was largely irrelevant, since the drugs used to treat it would be the same regardless. However, psychiatric epidemiologists might find the distinction useful because it would increase the accuracy of epidemiological reports if their compilers knew that they should include BFS cases with data on depression and anxiety cases. Finally, he argued that the fact that anxiety-depressive states manifest so differently across space would no doubt be of interest to psychological anthropologists researching the link between culture and psychology.

By this time, however, many Nigerian psychiatrists had declared the uselessness of BFS as a diagnostic label. Some argued that whether or not the diagnosis of BFS remained in place, it should be considered part of the constellation of anxiety and depressive states.[106] Others, however, argued for the entity to be stricken from the books. Jegede, for example, argued that psychiatrists continued to diagnose students with BFS "without any evidence that the constellation of symptoms do in fact constitute a different disease entity from those already known."[107] He concluded that "from the therapeutic point of view the B.F. syndrome is of little value,"[108] on the grounds that there was no real cultural basis for the diagnosis. Kalunta referred to BFS as "the so-called brain-fag syndrome" in 1981.[109]

Protestations from Nigerian psychiatrists did not prevent BFS from being included in the *DSM-IV*'s list of culture-bound syndromes in 1994. The

DSM-IV does, however, grant some credence to Nigerian concerns, suggesting that "'brain tiredness' or fatigue from 'too much thinking' is an idiom of distress in many cultures," not just Nigeria, and that at the very least it "resemble[s] certain Anxiety, Depressive, and Somatoform Disorders."[110] Debates have continued to rage about what, if anything, BFS actually means for psychiatrists.[111] However, the overlap between debates about BFS and those about schizophrenia and depression is evident. Colonial ethnopsychiatric theory inspired by racialist notions of the culture clash between "African minds" and "modern" European civilization was heavily critiqued by Nigerian psychiatrists who engaged in cross-cultural comparisons and research projects to illustrate the universality of this supposedly "culture-bound" disorder. The BFS case is also an illustration of the extent to which the universalist notions of transcultural psychiatrists like T. Adeoye Lambo and Tolani Asuni had, in fact, influenced the way that future generations of Nigerian psychiatrists conceived of the relationship between culture and psychiatric epidemiology. Where one sits on the issue of BFS is largely a matter of perspective: Those who want to emphasize cultural difference can find the evidence in BFS to make the argument. Those who want to emphasize cross-cultural psychological universality can argue to their point as well. The historical legacy of colonial psychiatry and the cultural politics of the postcolonial world, however, cannot be removed from the debate about brain-fag syndrome. Neither can the role that Nigerian psychiatrists have played in advancing this debate.

CONCLUSION

The research conducted by Nigerian psychiatrists after the 1950s helped to transform psychiatric theory about the nature of African minds in several specific ways. Schizophrenia, once seen by colonial psychiatrists as a universal disorder that Africans were particularly prone to developing, was recast as a universal disorder from which Africans were particularly good at recovering. Depression, once seen as particularly rare in black populations due to their cultural "primitiveness," was recast as a universal and relatively common disorder among Africans, although it tended to present with a different symptom structure among non-Westernized Africans. Brain-fag syndrome, originally considered to be a unique culture-bound disorder linked to the inability of Nigerian students to adapt to the rigors of the European education system, was dismantled and placed within the depression/anxiety family by Nigerian psychiatrists. All of these specific changes to diagnostic entities reflect one overarching belief on the part of the Nigerian psychiatrists engaged in diagnostic research: Africans experienced the same mental illnesses that other cultural groups in the world did. Secondarily, African cultures significantly influenced the presentation of mental illness in individuals, but this process was not unique to African cultures. Cross-cultural studies indicated that European cultures influenced the presentation of schizophrenia in Europeans, and Japanese culture affected the symptomatology of depression in Japan. Engagement with such cross-cultural research was instrumental in Nigerian psychiatrists' ability to influence psychiatric theory beyond a local level. It was also necessary for Nigerian psychiatrists to make a point that ethnopsychiatry had been unwilling to consider: namely, that Africans were not culturally or psychologically inferior to other people.

5 Gatekeepers of the Mind
Psychotherapy and "Traditional" Healers

With the advent of independence, Africans felt the need to rediscover their sociocultural identity; traditional medicine, an integral part of their heritage, benefited from this return to the fountain-head.

—Dr. C. Ramanohisoa, Regional Adviser,
WHO Regional Office for Africa, Brazzaville, Congo, 1983

Psychiatrists, after all, are just like chiefs, obeahmen, hunguns, voodoo healers, kali mai healers, and the whole variety of curanderos and other indigenous healers. That is to say, they themselves have a vested interest in the patients that come to them and they don't want to give up power, money, and responsibility.

—Phillip Singer, in an interview with T. Adeoye Lambo, 1977

ANTICOLONIAL NATIONALISM and transcultural psychiatric research dovetailed nicely in T. Adeoye Lambo's efforts to redefine mental illness in Africans in terms of a universalist construct that emphasized cross-cultural similarities in the forms of psychiatric disorder. However, diagnosis was largely a theoretical process. When transcultural psychiatrists turned their attention to the practicalities of treating patients, their efforts to define the healing process in universal terms turned out to be much more complicated. Although transcultural psychiatrists felt confident in their abilities to diagnose mental illnesses in non-Western cultures in terms of preexisting Western-derived categories, they were not nearly so confident about their ability to treat those diseases with preexisting Western-derived therapies. Just as transcultural psychiatrists felt the need to examine the culturally specific symptomatologies of mental illnesses around the world, so, too, did they become engaged in the ways that non-Western belief systems influenced how people in different cultures thought about treatments for mental illness.

This chapter examines how three transcultural psychiatrists thought about the relationship of "modern" psychiatry to "traditional" beliefs about mental health and illness in Nigeria. Over the course of the 1950s through the 1970s, Nigerian psychiatrists T. Adeoye Lambo and Tolani Asuni and

Canadian psychiatrist Raymond H. Prince produced an array of research and clinical experiments that sought to determine the similarities and differences between Western-derived psychotherapies and "traditional" healing systems in Nigeria. As they had done with diagnostic criteria, these transcultural psychiatrists tended to explain the "traditional" beliefs of Nigerian cultures and the activities of their healers in universal terms where possible, applying psychoanalytic and psychotherapeutic theories developed in the Euro-American context to practices in Nigerian, particularly Yoruba, cultures. This research built on the legacy of ethnopsychiatry, tending to define aspects of indigenous cultures as "primitive" in a culturally evolutionist sense, while simultaneously recognizing the important cultural advantage that traditional healers had over Western-trained psychiatrists in impressing upon their patients.

Referring to health systems as "traditional" is potentially fraught with interpretive problems,[1] but for our purposes, the adjective has value as an artifact of widely held colonial-era distinctions between European and African. While the traditional health systems in Nigeria were historically dynamic and often incorporative of nonindigenous ideas, they nevertheless had much deeper cultural roots in Nigerian societies in the mid-twentieth century than did the very recently imported psychiatric theories of Euro-American tradition. As a result, the beliefs and rituals associated with their healing processes were much more comprehensible and time-tested to Nigerians than were the psychotherapeutic beliefs and rituals of the West, and Western-trained psychiatrists knew this. Therefore, rather than "traditional" being defined as that which deviates from the "modern" Western norm, in this chapter "traditional" belief systems and the healers that practiced within them were for most Nigerians the "norm" with which Western-trained psychiatrists had to come to terms.

This basic truth meant that psychiatrists practicing in Nigeria in the late colonial and postindependence periods faced a crisis of legitimacy. Traditional healing systems often provided very different explanations than psychiatry for the cause of mental illnesses. Witchcraft, sorcery, spirit possession, supernatural affliction, and violation of taboo were frequently (although not always) invoked by different health-care providers in Nigeria as the underlying reason for mental distress. Traditional beliefs remained strong, and healers that treated mental illnesses within these etiological constructs have been and continue to be popular in Nigeria. Even Western-trained psychiatrists frequently noted that many traditional healing techniques achieved desirable results. Whereas Western biomedical interventions such as prophylactic and pharmaceutical treatment, inoculation, and even surgery correlated closely with long-established practices in many traditional health systems, the internalizing, individual-focused psychotherapies in which Western-trained psychiatrists were conversant had little similarity to prevailing cultural beliefs about the causes and treatments of mental illness in indigenous communities in Nigeria. Western-trained psychiatrists recognized that the cultural gap between themselves and their patients frequently affected their ability to communicate effectively and therefore impeded treatment. As a result, transcultural psychiatrists in the 1950s, 1960s, and 1970s were not able to invoke the inherent superiority of many of their psychotherapeutic methods.

The ways that Lambo, Asuni, and Prince addressed the relationship between their modern psychiatry and traditional healing techniques therefore had both political and professional implications. Lambo and Prince hoped to find psychotherapeutic allies in the traditional healers of Nigerian cultures and made strident efforts to redefine traditional healers within, rather than adjacent to, psychiatry. They hoped this process would allow traditional cultural beliefs to gain some dignity in a decolonizing and modernizing landscape by virtue of their association with scientific principles. The collaboration with traditional healers was also intended to legitimize psychiatric practice in Nigeria by bringing it into closer alignment with what most Nigerians considered to be "normal" therapeutic practice. Asuni, on the other hand, feared that incorporation might undermine traditional healers' power and contribute to a decline in the standards of clinical psychiatry.

In making distinctions about the relative therapeutic value of traditional beliefs and healing practices, Western-trained psychiatrists sought to establish themselves as gatekeepers, as the only people with the necessary skill sets to oversee cross-cultural interactions between the culturally relevant but scientifically imprecise practices of traditional healers and the supposedly medically superior but culturally alien techniques of Western psychotherapies. As they did with the symptomatology of psychological disorder discussed in chapter 4, transcultural psychiatrists sought to incorporate culturally specific healing systems into a universal structure based in the concepts and terminology of Western-derived theories of human psychology. They did so in ways that granted some dignity to African cultural practices previously seen as inherently pathological in colonial-era discourses. However, they also made it clear that their expertise as Western-trained psychiatrists with insight into Nigerian cultures put them in the best position to regulate and negotiate the relationship between Western medicine and traditional healing systems and in so doing contributed once again to the cultural politics of psychiatric modernization.

Since I am arguing that Western-trained psychiatrists' attitudes toward "traditional" healers were framed to a great extent in terms of legitimacy and competition, it makes sense at the outset to describe what these Western-trained psychiatrists considered traditional healing systems in Nigeria to be. For the most part, when psychiatrists referenced "traditional" healing systems, they meant any type of therapeutic practice that existed in Nigeria prior to the influx of the Euro-American psychiatric tradition. This included not only the healing processes of "indigenous" ethno-religious groups, but also Islamic medicine and charismatic Christian faith-healing practices. Of course, none of the traditional healing systems in Nigeria have been static or even particularly closed to external influence historically, and the dynamicity of traditional healing systems has been well documented in postcolonial critiques.[2] However, it is important to note that for our purposes, transcultural psychiatrists drew a rather sharp line between modern psychiatry and traditional healing, even if only for the ultimate purposes of blurring that line. This line was cultural in nature, dividing the healing traditions of Western psychiatric medicine from all other non-Western health systems.

I would like to outline the basic principles of one such traditional health system here, that of the Yoruba of southwestern Nigeria. Focusing on the Yoruba has some conceptual problems. In some ways it is too small of a group: it is unfair to extrapolate from Yoruba examples to generalize about the nature of all traditional healing systems in Nigeria. At the same time, it is in some ways too large of a group in that specific beliefs and practices, particularly about issues of health, disease, and medicine, differ somewhat from place to place and even healer to healer within Yorubaland.[3] As we have seen in previous chapters, defining the boundaries of a cultural unit is a matter of perspective. However, it makes sense to focus on something called the Yoruba traditional health system precisely because this is the scope from which psychiatrists like Lambo, Asuni, and Prince tended to see cultural difference. The Yoruba are one of the most ethnographically studied groups in sub-Saharan Africa, and this holds true within medical anthropological and psychiatric literature as well. Lambo and Asuni were both Yoruba, and all of Prince's ethnographic fieldwork took place among the Yoruba. Suffice it to say, when Western-trained psychiatrists talked about "traditional" health systems in Nigeria throughout the greater part of the period from the 1950s through the 1970s, they framed their discussion mostly around what they knew of Yoruba cultural beliefs and practices.

Health and healing within the Yoruba cultural tradition is intimately bound with Yoruba beliefs about the origin and nature of the cosmos. The supreme god of Yoruba belief, Olódùmarè, sent one of his fellow deities, Ọbàtálá, to create the world. While on the way to complete this task, Ọbàtálá became drunk from carousing with other gods, and Odùduwà, another agent of Olódùmarè, completed the job himself. Odùduwà descended from a chain into the universe and, using a shell full of soil and a five-toed cock, which spread the soil out on cosmic waters, created the world on the spot where the Yoruba sacred city of Ilé-Ifẹ̀ now stands. Odùduwà became the first god-king of Ilé-Ifè, and his descendants spread out to rule other parts of what is now called Yorubaland. Once the world was created, Olódùmarè sent somewhere between 201 and 401 gods known as *òrìṣàs* into the world along with sixteen spirit forces called *odù*, which contain all the sacred knowledge of the world. Individual òrìṣàs claim domain over specific attributes of the world: Ṣàngó is the god of thunder and lightning; Ògún of iron and war; Ọ̀ṣun of water; et cetera.[4] Although much of the literature on òrìṣàs written by Christian missionaries during the colonial era created a narrative in which some òrìṣàs are primarily good while others are evil, actually all òrìṣàs have the capacity to bring benefit or detriment to humans, depending on how humans interact with them.

Upon birth, humans are given an *orí*, or a destiny. *Orí* is also the Yoruba word for the body part known as the head, which the Yoruba see as the seat of one's destiny. The orí, which leads an individual through his or her life, can be revealed through divination. One of the primary òrìṣàs, named Ọrúnmìlà (or Ifá), is the god of divination, through whom humans can seek the cosmic wisdom of the odù at times of crisis and opportunity. Yoruba men and women consult Ifá at key points in life, for advice about marriage, travel, career, or anything about which they may have doubt. The wisdom of the odù will provide advice about the course an individual must take and, in particular, the sacrifices necessary to propitiate the gods to help one achieve one's orí. Naturally, those devout of the òrìṣàs also consult Ifá when their lives take an unexpected turn for the worse, such as a poor harvest, social dysfunction, or unexplained illness in the family. Many òrìṣàs also have cults into which individuals are initiated to serve specific gods and in turn be protected by that god, as we will see in the case of Sọ̀npọ̀nnọ́ below.

The healing system in Yoruba belief is conceptualized within this universe in which gods and other supernatural forces can directly and indirectly intervene in the affairs of man. Much of the Yoruba conceptualization of physical illness is naturalistic. Theories of hygiene, bodily imbalances, and heredity inform much of how the Yoruba think about many diseases and, consequently, their treatment. Herbalists (*oníṣègùn*), working within a complex indigenous pharmacopoeia, the knowledge of which is transmitted generationally through strenuous apprenticeships lasting years, can provide physical treatments to alleviate a wide variety of bodily misfortunes ranging from simple headaches to sexually transmitted diseases, malarial fever, and more culturally specific aliments such as *ẹ̀dà*, which is characterized by the vaginal canal of a woman being unable to hold in semen. Although the medicines of individual Yoruba herbalists might differ somewhat in terms of specific ingredients and their concentrations, Anthony D. Buckley has shown how herbalists' concoctions are grounded in conceptualizations of balance between colors, flavors, and temperatures designed to combat the physical imbalances perceived to be the root causes of the illness. Some herbal treatments require incantations to be activated, the power of which emanates from the odù.[5]

Not all illnesses have a physical cause treatable with material medicine, however. A wide variety of illnesses require spiritual intervention to heal. The Yoruba belief system holds that many illnesses, both physical and social in nature, can have supernatural roots. Belief that witchcraft and the machinations of enemies can cause misfortune is common. Sometimes humans might also offend gods or inadvertently cross paths with malevolent spirits, which could have negative consequences. Determining the root causes of many illnesses therefore requires the consultation of a diviner (*babaláwo*) who can seek cosmic wisdom and determine the required course of action to counteract the "bad medicine" or appease offended gods. Ifá divination is the most common form of divination in the Yoruba belief system, although a variety of oracles also exist. The Ifá diviner uses a set of instruments, including among other things a divining board, tapper, and sixteen palm nuts. The diviner casts the palm nuts between his hands multiple times, and, based on how they fall, the diviner is directed to a specific place in the *odù*, the 256-verse compilation of all Yoruba wisdom.[6] Learning the odù competently enough to divine effectively takes years in itself. But simply reaching the relevant odù is only part of the process. The diviner must have interpretive skills to determine how the odù is instructing the client on his or her specific problem. Once the odù has been effectively interpreted, the prescriptions for treatment are generated, and the client administers them as directed.

Mental illnesses are a well-established part of the traditional health belief system of the Yoruba. As with other types of illnesses, madness (*wèrè* in the Yoruba language) has a variety of forms and etiologies in Yoruba belief. The goal of the healer is to determine the cause of the madness and treat it. According to Roger O. A. Makanjuola, among others, etiology matters much more than symptomatology to traditional healers when determining the type of madness and its treatment. Causes of mental illness can vary significantly. Heredity is recognized as a major factor in the development of madness, contributing to widespread social stigmas associated with mental illness in the region. Some forms of headache, particularly the type known as *ọdẹ orí*, which is caused by an amorphous "worm" (*aràn*) that infests the head, can develop into madness (see conclusion). However, madness can also be the result of the malevolent actions of enemies as well as an affliction brought on by Sọ̀npọ̀nnọ́, the god of smallpox, or his spirit minions, discussed in more detail below.[7] As with other forms of illness, the treatment is closely related to the perceived cause of the illness, and may range from herbal treatments and the employment of antiwitchcraft protections, to propitiation of deities through sacrifices, or, in the case of Sọ̀npọ̀nnọ́, initiation into his cult of affliction.[8]

Efforts at cross-cultural translation of indigenous healing systems like that of the Yoruba have come in a variety of forms. Anthropologists of various stripes have shown that these systems are not "irrational" and unscientific, but work on an internal logic that must be understood in order to comprehend the nature of the healing strategy.[9] But whether there is an internal logic or not, the question remains of whether or how the more-or-less culturally specific healing system of the Yoruba relates to other healing systems. For the purposes of Western-trained psychiatrists, the primary comparison of interest was between indigenous Yoruba healing systems and that of Euro-American psychiatric medicine. Did the cultural specificity of the belief system mean that Yoruba healers who treated mental illness were actually using different knowledge than Western-trained psychiatrists, or, even more problematically, different *ways of knowing* than Western-trained psychiatrists could hope either to emulate or to displace? Or, were Yoruba healers using knowledge very similar to that of Western-trained psychiatrists, just articulating it differently?

Either of these questions could conceivably be answered in the affirmative, depending on the perspective one wants to take. Many medical anthropologists today would argue that attempting to medicalize the concepts and approaches of indigenous healing systems leads researchers to neglect the ways these systems may not be compatible.[10] But in the context of decolonization and the emergence of a transcultural psychiatry based on humanistic universalism, defining cultural approaches to psychological healing as intrinsically different was out of vogue. For Lambo, Asuni, and Prince to argue that Africans had psychologies similar to those of Europeans, indeed, similar to those of humans everywhere, they had to illustrate that African cultures shaped psyches in ways that could be explained in existing psychological terms. Furthermore, if they wanted to believe that their own brand of psychiatric training had any future in African settings, they needed to be able to articulate their own practices in terms compatible with local cultural beliefs, including beliefs in spiritual and supernatural processes. For Lambo and Prince, psychoanalytic theory offered a plausible structure within which to rationalize Yoruba cultural beliefs into a universal collective unconscious.[11] Psychoanalytic theory, however, had a cultural baggage of its own.

PSYCHOANALYZING "TRADITIONAL" BELIEFS

"Psychoanalysis" is the term coined by Sigmund Freud for both his theory of the nature of human psychological functioning and the therapeutic process through which psychic functions are revealed. At a basic level, Freud and his followers believed that irrational, unconscious processes mostly governed human beliefs and behaviors. Psychological disturbances, particularly neuroses, were the result of conflict between unconscious desires and resistances to them put up by the conscious, rational mind. For Freud, the unconscious was partly instinctual but also largely developed in early childhood. Psychological conflicts were mostly sexual in nature, and healing of psychological trauma occurred through the therapeutic relationship in which the analyst helped the patient to reveal unconscious desires and, in so doing, to resolve them.

Psychoanalysis has become a widely diverse and dynamic field of study in which different psychoanalytical theories about the nature of the relationship between the unconscious, the conscious, and society at large have competed for dominance. Adlerian psychoanalysis broke from Freudian analysis in its emphasis on the power of the ego to transform the self through conscious will. Carl Jung famously disavowed Freud's belief in religion as a delusionary coping mechanism and instead argued that the signs and symbols of religion reflected the processes of a collective unconscious of the human race much more essential and mystical than Freud acknowledged.[12] Kraepelinian psychiatrists, inclined to see psychological disorder in terms of physical processes, found psychoanalysis little more than a distraction. Racial, national, and class dynamics within Europe in the early twentieth century resulted in the extensive politicization of psychoanalysis even within Western psychiatric discourse. However, despite these and many other divisions, the basic principle that individual human behavior could be codified in terms of a psychoanalytic self, and that the domain of the unconscious was a central feature of human psychology, became highly influential in mainstream thought within Western civilization more generally during the twentieth century.

Questions about the universality of the unconscious and the effects of the spread of psychoanalytic theory globally have generated a great deal of debate. Psychoanalysis offered the possibility of a synthesis between non-Western and Western worldviews in a context of colonial denial and dissonance. For example, Girindrasekhar Bose's attempts to adapt Freud's theories and apply them to the psychic world and therapeutic needs of early twentieth-century middle-class Bengalis has been well documented.[13] Such engagement with psychoanalytic theory created a space in which the colonial subject could (re)present colonial elites as governing sovereign psychological selves, similar and related to the European bourgeois self, and therefore as legitimate candidates for citizenship and, potentially, political self-governance.[14] However, psychoanalysis has also been used to critique the colonial situation itself. Frantz Fanon and Octave Mannoni famously found the colonial state to be doing untold psychological damage to French colonial subjects in Algeria and Madagascar, respectively.[15] Ashis Nandy and Sudhir Kakar have used psychoanalytic concepts to describe the violent nature of colonial and postcolonial subjectivity.[16] The simultaneous development of psychoanalysis alongside European colonialism and its ideologies in Africa and Asia in the late nineteenth and twentieth centuries has led to an understanding that psychoanalysis has itself been in many ways complicit with the racial and gendered hierarchies of a late Victorian European mind-set. This has led to a postcolonial critique of psychoanalysis as a contributor to underlying ideologies of empire through its examinations of colonized peoples as exemplars of primitive psychology and its general co-optation of indigenous worldviews into a tautology that really reflects nothing more than a European bourgeois perspective.[17] Across the world, psychoanalytic theory has been a highly dynamic way of thinking about the relationship of self to other, functioning, as Warwick P. Anderson, Deborah Jenson, and Richard C. Keller have stated, in a "double act as colonial legacy and postcolonial critique."[18] This double edge of the psychoanalytic sword is evident in the ways Nigerian psychiatrists employed psychoanalytic concepts to explain the beliefs and behaviors of "traditional" African cultures.

Colonial-era ethnopsychiatry had drawn on the theoretical underpinnings of psychoanalysis to make comparisons about the "primitive" nature of African psychology. Freud's 1913 psychoanalytic treatise on supernatural belief systems, *Totem and Taboo*, in many ways framed the discourse on African health systems until well into the postcolonial era, arguing along cultural evolutionist lines that human belief systems had gone through three phases: the animistic, the religious, and the scientific. The animistic phase was characterized by the narcissistic belief of man that he could control the material world with his mental capacities. Belief in this "omnipotence of thought" negated the need for logical attribution of cause and effect. Beliefs in supernatural powers of a "demonic" nature that caused pain and misfortune held by animistic man were really an externalization of internal anxieties, an "objectification of fear," the true nature of which only psychoanalysis could reveal. Animistic man gave way to religious man, who, having come to terms with his inability to prevent death through sheer will, psychologically ceded some of his omnipotence to gods and spirits who could, nonetheless, be appeased and manipulated through the actions of man (through such practices as prayer, sorcery, etc.). Religious man developed into scientific man in the West, where humans had made amends with their weaknesses and resigned themselves "to death and the other necessities of nature."[19]

These three stages of belief were not mutually exclusive. Indeed, they blended into one another, and the vestiges of one remained present in its successors. However, overall, Freud held the view that the "savage tribes" of the "primitive" world continued to exhibit primarily the animistic and religious stages of development, while Western civilization had evolved into some semblance of the scientific. While Jung disagreed with Freud about the delusional qualities of religious thinking, he nevertheless also supported the notion that the psychoanalyst could see elements of more "primitive" ways of expressing the collective unconscious in non-Western cultures.[20] Both Freud and Jung recognized that elements of animistic thinking continued to pervade Western civilization. Freud, for example, compared "normal" adult "savages" with European children and obsessional neurotics. The idea that "savage" beliefs in the supernatural basis of illnesses and their treatments were irrational, pathological, and in need of the insight that psychoanalysis could provide is a trope that characterized much of ethnopsychiatric thought about African psychology.

A few ethnopsychiatrists attempted to apply psychoanalytic theory to their observations of the psychology of indigenous peoples in colonized African territories, although none did so in Nigeria prior to the 1950s.[21] Wulf Sachs's famous 1937 study *Black Hamlet* explained Africans' perceived inability to cope psychologically with the imposition of Western values in South Africa in terms of the Oedipal complex.[22] B. J. F. Laubscher's 1937 study of sexual mores among the Tembu in South Africa found schizophrenia in Africans to be organic in nature but also linked to libido regression. He noted that the permeation of the phallic cult among the Tembu was "almost an object lesson illustrating Professor Freud's theories," and declared that "the conceptions of psycho-analysis are not far-fetched" in application to Tembu belief systems. Laubscher also invoked Freud through constant comparisons of Tembu belief systems to what would be considered "infantile" and "neurotic" thinking among Europeans.[23] And in *Search for Security*, the anthropologist Margaret J. Field argued in 1960 that witchcraft beliefs among the Akan of the Gold Coast (Ghana) were often really externalizations of fear, anxiety, and depression, and that many of the people who visited shrines seeking aid from the machinations of witches were, in fact, mentally ill.[24]

The idea that African perspectives on mental illness based in ideas of supernatural causation were part of a universal human psychological pattern was quite attractive to transcultural psychiatrists, even if it contained some culturally evolutionist language. The first psychiatrist to take seriously the notion that ethnographic fieldwork into cultural explanations of mental illness in Nigeria would provide information important to the conduct of psychiatry was Raymond H. Prince, the "discoverer" of the brain-fag syndrome discussed in chapter 4. Drawing on ethnographic fieldwork conducted among the Yoruba of southwestern Nigeria over a seventeen-month period in the late 1950s, Prince produced many works over the course of the 1960s and 1970s analyzing what he saw as the fundamental beliefs about Yoruba conceptions of causation of mental illness. Although Prince's etiology of BFS had illustrated some of the tendencies of ethnopsychiatry to emphasize the stark differences between Nigerian and Western cultures, his research on Yoruba belief systems tended to focus on the psychiatric and psychoanalytic universals he thought they revealed.

Prince noted early in his work on the subject that Yoruba beliefs accounted for a variety of different causes of mental illness, both natural and supernatural. He found, for example, that heredity was seen as a major reason for the development of mental disorder, indicating an understanding of the role that biological processes could play. He noted that the Yoruba believed that types of mental illness could progress and change from one form to another, just as psychiatry suggested, and, in general, argued that Yoruba conceptions of mental illness fell fairly easily into the broad categories of "psychoses" and "neuroses," which formed the central diagnostic divide in psychiatric practice. For example, Prince claimed that the Yoruba disease entity *wèrè*, which was used to define chronic behaviors such as carelessness in dress, vagrancy, irrational speech, and experiences of auditory and visual hallucinations, was a disease that would easily be classified as a psychosis in psychiatric terms; while *àfọ́ta*, or hysterical blindness, was an example of a less severe or temporary condition that could be associated with the psychoneuroses. The comparisons were not exact, however, and Prince found that several diseases defined by Euro-American psychiatry as organic in nature, such as grand mal epilepsy and tetanus, were typically lumped into Yoruba definitions of mental illness.[25]

Prince was most interested, however, in uncovering the psychoanalytic basis of Yoruba beliefs in the supernatural causes of mental illness. Prince devoted an entire article to the prevalence of belief among the Yoruba in the power of curse and invocation to cause mental illness. Prince found such beliefs to be rooted in a Yoruba understanding of the "omnipotence of the word," very similar to Freud's enunciation of "omnipotence of thought." Prince linked the idea that spoken words could have tangible impact on the physical world to processes of childhood development. He argued that breast-feeding continued for the average Yoruba child "until at least the age of two years, often until three or four," so long that "many Yoruba can recall taking their mother's breast."[26] Such circumstances led Yoruba children to develop the idea that all they had to do was voice desires to have them come about: crying resulted in breast-feeding for so long that the power of vocalization of desires became an ingrained part of the adult Yoruba's worldview.

The ubiquity of belief in witchcraft as a major source of mental illness could also be linked to early childhood development. According to Prince, witchcraft in Yoruba culture was an inherently "feminine art" typically attributed to older women, although he noted that young women and girls could sometimes be implicated. Witches typically got their power through an "immaterial substance" that they either kept in a calabash in the roots of a tree or ingested and held in their abdomens. The power of witches was diffuse, including drinking blood; eating souls; interfering with reproduction, particularly by making men impotent; and causing a variety of illnesses including wasting diseases and psychiatric disturbances. Witches were notoriously fickle and might turn their malignant attention upon a man "for almost any reason—for some slight impoliteness, or because he accuses her of being a witch, or because he is getting too high in the world or even for no reason 'just because they are evil women.'"[27] Prince noted that many schizophrenic patients he saw attributed their illness to witchcraft, often accusing their own mothers or other close female relatives of bewitching them. While Prince saw such accusations as symptoms of the irrationality that characterized schizophrenia as a disease entity, the extent to which schizophrenics linked their problems to witchcraft created an important link between mental illness and witchcraft in the Yoruba cultural milieu.

Prince proposed a hypothesis that attempted to explain why witchcraft was such a prevalent idiom in Yoruba culture, and why women in particular were pathologized as witches. Explicitly citing the theories of Melanie Klein, the influential child psychoanalyst, Prince explained the persistence of witchcraft beliefs as a failure on the part of Yoruba culture to reach a key stage of early childhood development in which the child recognizes that the "good mother" who feeds and lavishes love and praise and the "bad mother" who disciplines and withholds are, in fact, the same person. "I do not think we would be distorting the Yoruba concept too much," he claimed, "to think of witchcraft as representing all the bad aspects of the mother or the female." Contributing to the paranoia surrounding witchcraft beliefs, Prince argued that in Yoruba culture the relationship between the mother and the child was extraordinarily intense, noting that "the Yoruba mother tends to be idealized and to a considerable extent the relationship between the mother and son is much more significant than between husband and wife." Because of this, "the mother tends to be on the one hand revered unrealistically and over-valued and on the other hand feared as a destructive entity in the background with all her witchly attributes."[28] This created a cultural environment in which not all women were considered to be witches, but because of their connections with motherhood, "all women are *potentially* witches,"[29] and therefore capable of causing mental illness in anyone who displeased them.

Like colonial-era psychoanalysts, Prince saw such beliefs as part of a basic human psychology held in all cultures, including Western European. However, he also tended to portray Yoruba beliefs as reminiscent of a distant past out of which the modern European had culturally evolved but in which the Yoruba remained trapped. Beliefs in curses and witchcraft could easily be found in "myths and fairy tales and from the Bible and Shakespeare in our own literature . . . in some of the thoughts and actions of our patients; not to mention in the more archaic areas of our own minds."[30] There was some pathologizing of Yoruba culture that went along with this analysis. Prince tended to produce case studies of psychiatric patients as proof of how "normal" Yoruba thought about things like witchcraft and curse. His Kleinian interpretation also equated normal psychological functions of adult Yoruba with those of European children.

Prince's ethnographic psychoanalysis of Yoruba cultural beliefs about health and illness, cause and consequence were part of the emphasis in transcultural psychiatry that focused on understanding the relationship between culture and mental illness. While he never claimed that any of the "traditional" cultural beliefs *caused* mental illness or predisposed the Yoruba toward certain types of mental illness, he certainly argued that cultural conceptions of mental illness affected the ways that individual Yoruba patients and Yoruba social groups understood psychological disorder and, by extension, how they expected to be treated for it. In this way, Prince was working within T. Adeoye Lambo's program to integrate psychiatry with indigenous cultures in ways that might prove effective both for the legitimization of psychiatry and for the mental health of the population at large.

Lambo himself had a love/hate relationship with psychoanalytic explanations of African "traditional" beliefs. He was certainly interested in any theory that sought to synthesize African with Western in a universal construct. In this sense, psychoanalytic theory provided a model that allowed for Africans to share innate psychological characteristics with Europeans. Early in his career, Lambo seemed willing to accept much of the psychoanalytic premise that African cultures represented a "primitive" state of human psychological functioning. "African culture, if one may be permitted to speak of an African culture," he declared in a 1962 lecture, "manifests in common with most nonliterate cultures, a sense of an intensely realized perception of supernatural presence but with a kind of adolescent impetuousness, and a fatuous, almost fanatical, faith in the magic of certain symbols to produce certain results."[31] This core belief in the magical and the supernatural "may be said to be a magical or mystical denial of the concept of causality and of the reality of their spatial and temporal relations."[32] He supported the notion that "traditional" rituals such as sacrifices were not a literal appeasement of the gods, but a means to relieve anxiety at either the individual or group level, thereby implicitly approving the psychoanalytical conception that ascription of supernatural agency was a human externalization of internal psychological tensions.

Although by the mid-1970s Lambo had come to the belief that psychoanalysis was a theoretical construct applicable to only Western cultural belief systems, in the 1950s and 1960s he believed that the application of psychoanalytic theory to African belief systems had the capacity to provide insights not only into the practice of psychiatry in Africa but into the understanding of human psychology in general. He argued that

> psychoanalytical treatments of many African mythological materials have helped us, with certain limits, to reconstruct the mode of thought which has produced superstitions that have long since vanished from among us. It has also enabled us to trace through the obscurity of the distant past those primordial forms of thought and feeling which determine the uniformity of the African

apprehensions of their world. There is no doubt that the Africans have held traditional beliefs similar to those which had occupied so noble a place among the speculations of antiquity.[33]

If psychoanalytic theory were used simply to incorporate African cultures into the global discussion about the nature of human psychology, Lambo had no problem with it. In fact, he believed that "of all human materials, there is perhaps none that presents to the historian of the human mind a deeper interest than African mythologies and there is certainly none that tells a better tale of the frustrations of human efforts and the futility of human hopes."[34] The problem with psychoanalytic theory came when psychoanalysts used the theory to suggest that Africans were very different from other human societies, inherently irrational or illogical, when, Lambo argued, psychoanalysis was itself intuitive and unscientific in nature.[35]

PSYCHOTHERAPY, PSYCHOPHARMACOLOGY, AND TRADITIONAL HEALERS

Transcultural psychiatrists quickly learned that the ability to explain traditional beliefs about the nature of mental illness in terms of psychoanalytic universals did not mean that treatment mechanisms could be so easily synthesized. The social psychiatry that transcultural psychiatrists like Lambo, Prince, and Asuni practiced promoted the concept of the "therapeutic community" and the idea that the patient must be an active participant in his or her healing process. In transcultural psychiatric terms, this meant that the treatment mechanism must to a certain extent conform to the patient's expectations of treatment. However, Western-trained psychiatrists and their Nigerian patients tended to have very different conceptions of the appropriate treatments for psychological disorder. For example, Lambo relayed in 1962 the story of an "English University–trained West African patient," who suffered an unspecified accident shortly after being promoted to a high-profile position in the Administrative Service. Afraid that his colleagues were trying to sabotage him "in a mysterious way," the man became "rather terrified," and sought treatment with Lambo for his anxiety. However, concurrent with his treatment, the patient had a dream in which his grandfather "assured him of long life expectancy, and also asked for a goat." The next day, the man bought a goat and sacrificed it, after which "he quickly recovered from his severe anxiety state." Although reticent to discuss the matter because of its embarrassing nature in reference to his very "modern" lifestyle and position, Lambo said the man "conceded the point that he believed there was something in this 'native thing.'"[36] The execution of a traditional ritual to treat an ailment brought on by what this man considered to be traditional means was apparently more effective than anything Lambo could provide.

This case was by no means isolated. Other psychiatrists frequently lamented the extent to which they found it difficult to reach patients who believed their ailments to be caused by magical and supernatural forces.[37] Lambo found early in his career that in addition to rural, "traditional" people, most highly Westernized Nigerian patients attributed their mental illnesses to supernatural causes like witchcraft or taboo. In a survey of Nigerian students who broke down while undergoing advanced education in the United Kingdom in 1957, Lambo found that more than 90 percent of them "offered clear-cut evidence of African traditional beliefs in bewitchment and machinations of the enemy" as the underlying cause of their problems.[38] This led Lambo to the conclusion that "under stress, emotional or otherwise, newly acquired and highly differentiated social attitudes and ideologies are more susceptible to 'damage' leaving the basic traditional beliefs and indigenous moral philosophy functionally overactive."[39] He found that in 1950 more than 60 percent of all patients admitted to a general hospital in Nigeria had consulted a traditional healer for their malady first,[40] and noted that for psychiatric conditions the percentage would undoubtedly be much higher.

Customarily, traditional healers had been responsible for the treatment of mental illnesses in Nigerian cultures. Good healers carried the cultural knowledge to determine the causes for mental disorders and the legitimacy to direct therapeutic regimens—be they physical, ritual, or otherwise—that were appropriate for the restoration of social balance between the suffering individual and his or her community. Even as of the 1960s, Lambo declared that most Nigerians considered psychological trauma to be "the exclusive responsibility of traditional medicine."[41] In order for Western-trained psychiatrists to provide effective therapeutic care for Nigerian patients, Lambo believed there was much they could learn from traditional healers. As part of this process, he brought twelve traditional healers into the operations of the Aro Village Scheme in the mid-1950s. These healers worked with the Western-trained psychiatric staff to help understand the maladies of the patients and provided direct treatments to desiring patients. Similarly, Raymond H. Prince examined the activities of many different traditional healers in Yorubaland and compared them to those of Western psychotherapists, finding many similarities in the underlying processes of each.

The belief that traditional healers might provide effective treatment for mental illnesses was not a new idea in the 1950s, but the willingness of

Western-trained doctors to believe they might learn something from traditional healers was a first for Nigeria. During the colonial era in Nigeria, the basic attitude of European officials and ethnopsychiatrists was that Western and traditional healing systems should remain separate and segregated. There is some evidence that traditional healers in Nigeria sought official interaction with the colonial psychiatric establishment but were largely rebuffed for their efforts. For example, in 1935 the Herbal Kingdom Society of Lagos wrote to the Lagos colonial government, requesting the government "to give us a trial treatment of the lunatic patients in the Yaba asylum."[42] Their request was denied without explanation.[43]

Ethnopsychiatrists who studied the Nigerian situation were more conciliatory to traditional healers, but still tended to see their practices as different from and inferior to those of Western medical science. R. Cunyngham Brown's 1938 report, discussed in greater detail in chapter 1, while remaining cautious about the efficacy of indigenous medical practitioners' methods, argued that "it is greatly to their credit that as a body they do their best for their patients according to their lights for small pecuniary reward, [and] meet with a certain measure of success notwithstanding the great defects of their practice and the employment of what, in other countries, would be deemed crude and even harsh methods."[44] Ultimately Brown argued that the colonial government should respect traditional medical practitioners "because of the public esteem in which they are held and because they at present and probably will for long fill with some success a great want,"[45] owing to the lack of Western-trained psychiatrists. J. C. Carothers went much further than Brown on this issue, arguing for the ultimate efficacy of traditional medical practitioners because of their local cultural understanding. Speaking of a particular practitioner who ran a private mental institution in a rural area, he concluded, "I am convinced that, within the framework of the rather highly developed indigenous culture of that area, this man is doing a necessary job of work as humanely and intelligently as possible, and it is even not improbable that some of the techniques that are practiced by him and others like him might be of general value."[46] In fact, Carothers argued, "mildly demented" and mentally defective conditions, whether due to "chronic and incurable organic illness, epilepsy or schizophrenia," as well as neurotic states "of recent onset and not of anti-social behaviour," were in his opinion best treated by traditional healers.[47]

Such declarations reveal a couple of strands of colonial-era thinking about the long-term relevance of traditional healers in Nigeria. On the one hand, Brown seems to have been taking an evolutionist stance, arguing that traditional healers were a necessary evil that might provide some valuable treatment but which ideally would be replaced in the long-term by proper European psychiatric experts. Carothers, on the other hand, seems to have been arguing much more strongly that indigenous medical practitioners were probably *more* qualified to treat most kinds of mental illness *because* of their cultural understanding of the forms and treatments of mental illness in their local communities. However, despite the superficial respect shown toward traditional healers, both Brown and Carothers were arguing at a basic level that indigenous approaches to treating mental illness were very different from, and ultimately incompatible with, European approaches. There is no discussion in their works of the possibility that traditional healers and Western-trained psychiatrists performed similar functions, that Western-trained psychiatrists might learn anything of value from traditional healers, or that traditional healers should be incorporated in any way into the official, Western-based medical system in colonial Nigeria despite the glaring inadequacies of the latter.

In the context of decolonization and the transition to transcultural psychiatry, however, the question of whether and how the activities of traditional healers related to the beliefs and practices of Western medicine became an area of increasing interest. With the emergence of transcultural psychiatry as a coherent field in the mid-1950s, psychiatrists began to show a concerted effort not only at diagnosing mental illnesses cross-culturally, but also of comparing treatment modalities. Studies done around the world began to find attributes of non-Western healing systems that could be explained in Western psychotherapeutic terms.[48]

Raymond H. Prince contributed most to the academic medicalization of traditional healers' approaches to mental illness in Nigeria. Based on observations made in the late 1950s of the activities of several Yoruba healers, Prince had no doubt that traditional healers did have the capacity to heal patients. He relayed the story of one patient he believed to have been aided by a skilled traditional healer. His illness had lasted for four years, and treatment by several practitioners, both "indigenous and Western," had been fruitless. However, after initiating treatment with someone Prince considered a "competent *babalawo*," who performed "several expensive sacrifices, a good deal of magical ritual, and initiation into the Ifa divination cult," the patient's symptoms cleared and he remained well for the duration of Prince's time in Nigeria, another thirteen months. Indeed, Prince was so impressed by traditional Yoruba healers that he concluded, "Western psychiatric techniques are not in my opinion demonstrably superior to many indigenous Yoruba practices."[49] The question was why Yoruba traditional healers were so successful.

The answer for Prince lay in the extent to which practices of traditional healers could be explained in terms of Western psychotherapeutic processes that he believed to be effective tools, namely those of psychoanalysis and social psychiatry. While Prince recognized that traditional healers used some psychopharmacological agents in their practices, he found their overall therapeutic value to be in the suggestive power of their activities and their revered position in Yoruba culture. The healer's ability to convince patients of the nature of the problem and then to convince them that he knew the proper treatment was itself instrumental in the patient's prognosis. Prince noted that this suggestive power was "the most important element in all primitive psychotherapies," and recognized that the power of suggestion was an element, even if undesired, of psychoanalytic therapy. He identified four factors in the healer-patient relationship in Yoruba culture that promoted efficacy of the treatment. They were:

1. The "omnipotence" of the healer through his dealings with the spirit world.
2. The healer's impressive performance. During divination the patient does not even tell the diviner what his problem is; the diviner learns it through his spirit contacts; the diviner is often a good intuitive psychologist and very much in tune with the peculiar stresses of his culture. He often makes impressive "blind" diagnoses.
3. His use of sacred and magical formulae, gestures, and paraphernalia.
4. The anxiety of the patient, which is often deliberately increased by the healer who may warn him of serious consequences should he fail to follow directions. The patient's anxiety is in marked contrast to the healer's confidence and optimism.[50]

Prince argued that diviners and other traditional medical men had the power to heal many cases of mental disorder by virtue of the fact that they were able to convince their patients that they had the power to heal mental disorder. Patients got better because they believed the healers were making them better, an idea that had explanatory power within prevailing psychotherapeutic models.

Prince also believed that traditional healing systems were able to positively influence the course of mental illnesses by strengthening relationships between patients and their social surroundings. Prince made this point most forcefully through examinations of the psychotherapeutic effects of possession cults in Yorubaland. Noting that anthropological literature had identified a variety of psychotherapeutic effects in possession cult activities cross-culturally, such as "attainment of high status through a cult role . . . acting out of aggressive and sexual behavior; reversal of sexual roles; and temporary freedom of responsibility for actions," Prince declared that these concepts applied to Yoruba possession rituals as well.[51] To prove this point, Prince produced multiple studies on the specific healing practices of the Sọ̀npọ̀nnọ́ cult. Sọ̀npọ̀nnọ́ was the name of an òrìṣà responsible for the spread of a variety of different illnesses, most catastrophically smallpox, but also some forms of mental illness.[52] Symptoms associated with these illnesses are explained in terms of the actions of the aggrieved spirit agents of Sọ̀npọ̀nnọ́ upon an individual. Physical weakness was the result of the blows of the spirits' clubs. Boils and carbuncles resulted from being struck by their spears, and rashes resulted from special arrows. Sọ̀npọ̀nnọ́ spirits could cause mental illness in several ways. Often spirits would blow a warm breeze on their victims that entered the blood and heated up the brain, resulting in madness. Prince also noted that mental illness could result from the fear of encountering Sọ̀npọ̀nnọ́ spirits in a vision. Mental illness could also be a symptom of being struck by Sọ̀npọ̀nnọ́ arrows.[53] Sọ̀npọ̀nnọ́ spirits typically attacked women, although men could also be victims. Typically, victims of Sọ̀npọ̀nnọ́ attacks were considered to be members of families that were historically linked to Sọ̀npọ̀nnọ́ worship. Regardless, if a diviner determined Sọ̀npọ̀nnọ́ to be the cause of an individual's mental illness, the most appropriate treatment was for that individual to appease the spirits by being initiated into the Sọ̀npọ̀nnọ́ cult, and in so doing to dedicate oneself to the worship of Sọ̀npọ̀nnọ́. Initiation into the Sọ̀npọ̀nnọ́ cult could take a variety of forms, but the main feature was the calling of the Sọ̀npọ̀nnọ́ spirits to possess the afflicted individual. The individual would then be possessed by the spirit that had "born" him or her, and through this process would both be healed of the affliction and become a devotee of Sọ̀npọ̀nnọ́, a member of the cult.

Prince found a variety of aspects of the spirit possession process potentially therapeutic. He identified several "abreactive" qualities in ceremonies performed not only by Sọ̀npọ̀nnọ́, but also by egúngún and Erinlẹ̀ cults, whereby the possessed was able to perform activities that would have been socially unacceptable under other circumstances. He relayed instances of "women acting in male roles as hunters or drummers and occasionally dressing in such male clothing as the uniform of a sanitary inspector; women who were normally polite and even obsequious to me becoming bold and defiant; women eating dirt, throwing themselves on the ground climbing trees, and so forth."[54] Such activities were conceivably cathartic in Western psychotherapeutic terms.

For Prince, possession cults were therapeutic not only for the afflicted individual who underwent possession. He claimed that possession cults provided "a tightening of the social structure" for the community at large. The basis for possession cult activities came from "an increase in social pathology [in the form of physical or mental illness], which leads the diviner to prescribe an increase in religious behavior, which in turn results in an increase in social contact, an increased strictness in abiding by taboos, a consolidation of lineage relationships, etc." Linking these activities to Western psychotherapeutic processes, Prince suggested that "if the theory linking social integration to mental health is correct, then this activity on the part of the diviner and the community should decrease the incidence of social pathology."[55] He also compared Christian faith-healing ceremonies involving spirit possession, in which "several women were possessed by the 'Holy Spirit' and very personal advice was dispensed to many of the members," to be "not unlike some kinds of Western group therapy."[56] For Prince, possession cults could be key providers of individual and community mental health services, and those services could be rationalized strictly within existing Western theories about how to provide effective psychotherapy.[57]

Although Lambo did not personally engage in the ethnographic examination of traditional Yoruba healers as Prince did, he tended to agree overall with sentiments about the psychotherapeutic efficacy of their treatments. While Lambo recognized that some traditional healers in Nigeria were "impostors or enthusiasts," many exhibited "extraordinary qualities of mind—common sense, great eloquence, great boldness, and their work displays great controversial dexterity."[58] Their powers of suggestion and their ability to manipulate local herbs for curative purposes illustrated a skill set "hardly equaled by the regular practitioners."[59] Lambo believed that traditional healers were particularly effective because they treated mental illness in terms that their patients understood. Deeply imbedded in the cultural atmosphere, traditional healers commanded a great deal of respect from their patients. He noted that "their methods embrace much that could be termed mystic doctrines, which exercise an extraordinary fascination over many minds. These methods seem to have comprised many traditions that have been long current among the tribes, mixed with much of the old doctrines of rituals, and with a large measure of pure naturalism," which Western psychiatry lacked.[60] He declared, "Institutionalized confessions, trances and primitive religious rites and ceremonies . . . are powerful psychotherapeutic measures."[61] He found Ifá divination rituals "integrating" for schizophrenics,[62] and believed that many native treatment centers could "claim greater success in the sphere of neuroses" than Western psychiatric institutions.[63]

For this reason, Lambo warned Western-trained psychiatrists that "primitive medicine, in spite of the associated religious tones and sentiments, 'is not a queer collection of errors and superstitions, but a number of living unities in living cultural patterns, quite able to function through the centuries.'"[64] Ultimately, Lambo was convinced from a very early point in his career that the activities of traditional healers were "as effective and scientifically sound as any I have seen practiced in Europe."[65] As we will see, Tolani Asuni disagreed.

GATEKEEPERS OF THE MIND

If many of the practices of traditional healers had real psychotherapeutic benefit, transcultural psychiatrists in Nigeria were faced with something of an existential quandary: What could they provide to their patients that traditional healers could not? As alien cultural imports, how could they provide an effective social psychiatry to populations that continued to have different beliefs about the cause, categories, and treatments of mental illnesses? The very legitimacy of psychiatry as medical practice hinged on how psychiatrists and their patients answered these questions. From the perspective of transcultural psychiatrists, there were two basic positions they could hold to attempt to enhance their legitimacy vis-à-vis traditional healers: incorporate or denigrate. In making decisions about whether and how traditional healers could or should be brought into the practice of social psychiatry in Nigeria, Lambo, Prince, and Asuni sought to establish themselves as gatekeepers, as the only ones with the appropriate balance of culturally specific knowledge and scientifically universal knowledge to determine what terms the relationship between the various healing systems should follow. Lambo and Prince firmly supported the position that the similarities between psychiatry and traditional healing systems were strong enough to merit an integration whereby the best qualities of both systems could be synthesized, while the worst elements could be discarded. In this way, both psychiatry and traditional healers could enhance their legitimacy through the greater success that would accrue from aggregating their knowledge. Asuni, on the other hand, took the position that the differences between psychiatry and traditional healers' methods were too pronounced to overcome through integration. In fact, he argued that both psychiatry and traditional healing systems would ultimately lose respectability by trying to bridge the cultural divide.

It was clear to Prince and Lambo that, although the basic healing processes were universal, specific treatments needed to be tailored to specific cultural circumstances. Prince believed that "psychotherapeutic techniques fit with the cultures in which they have developed and cannot cross cultural boundaries so successfully as can physical therapies."[66] For example, he found that even though psychoanalysis provided valuable explanations for traditional beliefs, it consistently failed as a therapeutic process for Nigerian patients because "this form of psychotherapy is not compatible with these cultures."[67] He argued that psychoanalysis, with its emphasis on deep personal insight and the taking of individual responsibility for behavior, was inappropriate for Nigerian patients because Nigerian cultures assigned very different values to independence and interdependence than Western cultures did. In order for psychoanalysis to work as a treatment mechanism, the individual undergoing it "must be capable of high mobility to be effective in his executive level occupation" and "capable of independent judgments and constant flexibility as well as a high level of competitiveness,"[68] since psychoanalysis was designed to strengthen the ego so that the individual could resume independent tasks and not be a burden on society. This was considered a necessary outcome in Western culture because, Prince claimed, "the extended family no longer functions, and the full burden of emotional support rests on the nuclear family; and economic support has been taken over by the state through tax and welfare systems."[69] Furthermore, in Western cultures, "the ideal man is self-determining and independent and capable of tolerating high levels of loneliness."[70] Prince declared that "psychoanalysis is part of this system and is geared to produce such personalities when families of origin fail to do so,"[71] unlike in Nigeria, where strong extended family ties and communal solidarity still held great value, even with highly Westernized individuals.

Western-trained psychiatrists were educated in environments that took these particular characteristics of Euro-American cultures for granted. To a great extent, according to Prince, they were not equipped, then, to provide psychotherapy to individuals coming from different cultural backgrounds with different value systems. By the 1970s, Prince was arguing that psychiatrists planning to practice in non-Western environments should not be trained in schools in the West. He believed that the training psychiatrists received was "so much bound up with the idiosyncratic world view of the West," that the non-Western psychiatrist "must jettison a good part of his training to successfully reintegrate into the world view of his homeland."[72] For this reason, from early in his career Prince had advocated the incorporation of traditional healers into psychiatric practice, the forging of "a liaison with official psychiatry"[73] that would better prepare psychiatrists for the kinds of therapy they would need to provide in order to treat Nigerian patients effectively.

Where Prince was arguing from a largely theoretical level, Lambo was actively involved in fostering direct collaboration between psychiatry and traditional healing systems through his incorporation of traditional healers into the Aro Village Scheme. Because traditional healers were so in tune with the cultural beliefs of their communities, beliefs that Nigerians were apparently maintaining in the face of widespread sociocultural change, Lambo believed that Western-trained psychiatrists could learn much from traditional healers. Since the rituals and practices of traditional healers were widely accepted as having therapeutic value, Lambo argued that "the modern psychoanalyst in particular, and the practitioner of modern medicine in general, may well find many points of congruence and may be tempted to take over some of the principles about causal relationships into his own body of beliefs," thereby expanding the knowledge base of psychotherapy. Even if this did not occur, Lambo argued, integration would ultimately be beneficial to Western medicine because it would make Western medicine more comprehensible and less alien to Nigerian patients. He argued that the arrogance of Western medicine in rejecting traditional healers "would seem to impede the total acceptance of western medicine by African societies as a meaningful substitute to beliefs and practices which have long satisfied certain basic human needs."[74] Along these lines, Lambo considered the participation of traditional healers at Aro Village to be an enormous success, claiming:

> Through their participation we have enriched our scientific knowledge of the psychopathology and psychodynamics of the major psychiatric disorders occurring in these exotic societies. We have also been able to accumulate a mass of data on the natural history and prevalence of many psychiatric disorders, in terms of cultural and social variables (variables that are ill defined and remain resistant to Western forms of categorization). Without the help of the "witch doctors" we would not have known how and where to look and what obstacles to skirt in searching for simple disorders like obsessional neurosis in the indigenous population of Africa.[75]

Beyond providing important data to Western-trained psychiatrists, traditional healers had a therapeutic impact as well, according to Lambo. Traditional healers were able to tap into "certain factors in the traditional environment and the village in particular [that] act as powerful buffers against social pressures and conflicts."[76]

The collaboration between traditional healers and Western-trained psychiatrists was not intended to benefit only the psychiatrists. Lambo and Prince also believed that traditional healers would benefit from access to knowledge emanating from the Western medical tradition. There were certain aspects of traditional healing systems that were unjustifiable in Western biomedical terms, particularly approaches to the physical treatment of patients. For example, Prince noted that some traditional healers practiced forms of physical abuse as part of their treatment regimens. He claimed to have seen scars on patients received in treatment centers, although he never personally witnessed physical abuse in any of the treatment centers he visited. Traditional healers often had to shackle their patients to control their movements, sedative drugs being largely unavailable to them. Prince noted that most traditional healers "take pride in the fact that their patients wear shackles for only a few days." However, he did point out that he had seen patients with "some severe 'bed sores' (or rather earth sores) as a result of prolonged shackling to a log." Such activities strengthened Prince's case for the need of collaboration so that psychiatrists, with their medical training, might bring about "as a secondary gain, some measure of salutary official control" over traditional health systems.[77]

Not all Western-trained psychiatrists in Nigeria agreed that the positives of working with traditional healers outweighed the negatives, however. The most vocal antagonist of the incorporation model in the 1960s and 1970s was Tolani Asuni, Lambo's second in command at Aro Mental Hospital and the man who took over operations there after Lambo left for the University of Ibadan in 1963. Asuni had firsthand experience with Lambo's incorporation of traditional healers into the Aro Village system. However, whereas Lambo was highly encouraged by the experiment, Asuni was less impressed. From the late 1960s, Asuni began to publish critiques of the incorporationist thesis. Not convinced by Prince's and Lambo's protestations of the psychotherapeutic value of traditional healing systems, Asuni asserted that claims about the efficacy of traditional healers in treating psychoneuroses "need to be verified" scientifically and not just anecdotally.[78] He noted that many patients at Aro Hospital had arrived only after multiple efforts by traditional healers to treat their ailments had failed. While he recognized that many patients also left Aro Hospital to seek alternative treatment with traditional healers, Asuni claimed this usually occurred "when the relatives were misdirected by other people, failed to carry out instructions, or held unduly high expectations,"[79] an indication that patients needed to learn more about psychiatric methods and not necessarily that psychiatrists needed to learn more about traditional beliefs.

Asuni clearly believed that the Western psychiatric tradition contained a far superior set of beliefs and practices to traditional healing systems in Nigeria, but, like Prince and Lambo, he recognized that Western-trained psychiatrists had a legitimacy problem. He argued that "since the traditional concept of psychiatric illness is that it is caused by curses, evil eye, violation of taboo, evil machination of malevolent agents, witchcraft, etc., most people in developing countries find it difficult to accept that modern psychiatry has much to offer . . . because it does not relate causation strongly and ostensibly enough to the traditional beliefs."[80] Using somewhat insensitive language, Asuni lamented how difficult it was for the Western-trained psychiatrist to "disabuse their [patients'] minds" of their erroneous explanations of their illnesses, "especially if it is shared by others in the same culture, and particularly the rest of the family."[81] For example, Asuni noted that it was "difficult to convince patients and relatives that reference to witchcraft is a symptom of depressive illness" in a culture where elderly women frequently accused themselves of the practice, thereby reinforcing the veracity of the notion.[82] For this reason, Asuni believed that traditional healers were likely to remain relevant in their communities for a long time. Indeed, Asuni made clear that this was not entirely a bad thing, noting that traditional healers should not "be condemned totally for they still fulfill a need in the face of the acute shortage of trained psychiatrists and doctors."[83]

As far as Asuni was concerned, Western-trained psychiatrists might be able to learn valuable information from traditional healers in the realm of local pharmacopoeia. Beyond that, he declared, "supplementing modern with traditional methods does not create much of a problem. It is integrating the two that is fraught with difficulties."[84] From Asuni's perspective, integration was impossible because the "philosophy, concept of aetiology and treatment" of traditional healers were all "at variance with those of modern medicine."[85] For example, Asuni pointed out fundamental differences in the treatments of delusions associated with depression between Western psychiatry and traditional healers:

> The traditional healers accept and confirm the false beliefs of the patient and sometimes elaborate on them. Quite often they even suggest to patients that their illness is caused by someone else, thus creating a delusion where it has not existed.
>
> Modern psychiatrists on the other hand accept the delusions only as a sign of illness and when the illness is abating, the patient is made to feel better and loose [*sic*] his delusions. It is considered necessary for the patient to realise that the delusions, even when

> they have subsided, are signs of illness. The establishment of this type of insight is necessary for secondary prevention. The patient having been made aware of the significance of his delusions, is asked to seek help as soon as he starts developing the delusions again, before they get established.[86]

He further argued that "the competent modern psychiatrist tries to make his anxious patient self-reliant, while the traditional healer tends to make the anxious patient forever dependent on him,"[87] by essentially exacerbating and possibly even creating psychiatric disturbance rather than healing it.

Asuni could not excuse the dangerous and counterproductive practices that he saw in traditional healers' methods as Prince had. He referenced the "inhuman practices" of some traditional healers who "flogged, purged and bled" their patients, and maligned the unscientific approach many traditional healers took toward herbal remedies, claiming that they made no effort to systematize the doses of highly potent psychoactive herbs, such as rauwolfia, that they gave to their patients. He relayed an anecdote about a visit he had made to a traditional healer's compound, where "a number of patients had been deeply sedated by a traditional healer and they were sound asleep on the floor. When I asked when they would wake up, the healer said perhaps tomorrow or the day after tomorrow. In the meantime, he could not do anything about clearing the air passage, catheterizing the urinary bladder, changing the position of the patients to avoid pressure ulcer, giving fluid by infusion, checking the electrolyte, etc.—the procedure which modern medicine would have followed."[88] Under such conditions, Asuni lamented, perhaps a bit hyperbolically, "we can never know how many of their patients sleep on to death."[89]

Because of these differences, Asuni believed that cooperation between psychiatrists and traditional healers was likely to be damaging to the integrity and respectability of both. He argued that allowing traditional healers to provide something called "psychiatric care" would "involve laying down a code of ethics different from modern medicine" in order to incorporate some of the nefarious practices of traditional healers. Simultaneously, the oversight of traditional healers that would have to occur within any official, legal psychiatric system would ultimately diminish suggestive powers by eroding their "image of omnipotence and consequently their psychotherapeutic effectiveness."[90] Asuni believed that even if integration were deemed desirable, it would be practically impossible to carry out because traditional healers did not have any particular code of conduct or professional organization to consult. Since Western-trained psychiatrists were not themselves experts in the practices of traditional healers, they would not be able to differentiate the legitimate traditional healers from charlatans.

Asuni's position was that as Western-derived psychiatric facilities and personnel expanded and Nigerians gained greater familiarity with their beneficial treatment options, "the traditional healers will be used less and less; just as with the increased provision of maternity centres less and less babies are being delivered by traditional methods,"[91] although he admitted that they would probably never disappear completely. Such an attitude mirrored that held by Brown and other psychiatrists of the colonial era who had suggested that as African cultures modernized, their traditional beliefs would lose their utility and slowly be discarded.

Even within the incorporationist model, however, it is important to note that Lambo and Prince ultimately believed that the categories and etiologies of the Western psychiatric tradition were superior and a closer approximation of the "truth" than those of traditional African belief systems and the healers who worked within them. Lambo and Prince did not believe that traditional healers were successful because their explanations of cause and treatment for mental illnesses were literally true. Indeed, Lambo frequently referenced the magical and mystical beliefs of traditional cultures as a denial of reality.[92] Traditional healers did not appease òrìṣàs or battle witches. Rather, the cultural idioms they employed represented underlying psychotherapeutic principles that could be explained in terms of Euro-American psychiatric theories. Traditional healers, despite their own belief systems, actually treated the disorders identified by Western-trained psychiatrists. There was dignity in Nigerian cultural beliefs about mental illness and in the practices that were employed to treat it, but that dignity could be articulated only in terms of how similarly those beliefs and practices could be compared to the more "scientific" norms of a universalizing psychotherapeutic tool bag emanating from a largely Western cultural tradition.

Illustrating this point, although Prince believed that psychoanalysis proved a poor therapeutic option for Nigerian patients, he ultimately believed that it provided a better means for effective recovery in Western patients than traditional healers' practices provided for African patients. Prince cited numerous occasions in which the therapeutic process functioned very differently for traditional healers than it would have for Western-trained psychotherapists. For example, although Prince saw spirit possession cults as psychotherapeutically valuable because of their social integration characteristics, he found them lacking in the insight and personal growth arenas, both of which were considered to be basic goals of psychotherapy in Western practice. He lamented that there was "very little evidence in Yoruba psychotherapy of any attempt to change the individual," noting that Sọnpọnnọ́ cults were explicit that the initiate never learn of their behaviors while under the influence of the spirit. To have such knowledge of unconscious desires and actions was seen to be dangerous among the Yoruba, where it was encouraged in Western psychoanalysis. While Western and traditional psychotherapies might both provide a net positive outcome, Prince argued that they might do so in very different ways. "Psychoanalysis and some other Western psychotherapies aim at insight (into psychodynamic factors) and independence," he claimed, whereas "religious psychotherapies" practiced by many faith healers, for example, "aim at belief and dependence. The religious convert gives up his freedom of behavior in exchange for divine favor and the social support of his fellow convert."[93] Prince made clear that the effectiveness of traditional healing methods among the Yoruba lay in making the individual dependent on others rather than functionally independent with a strong, stable ego. "The sense of protection and the sense of 'being watched over' by one's double, one's ancestors, and one's Orisha have, no doubt, profound ego-strengthening effects," argued Prince. However, he believed that "these factors do not increase the patient's inner strength in a mature way,"[94] as Western treatments supposedly did for Western patients.

While the beliefs and practices of traditional healers might be better for Nigerian patients than Western psychotherapeutic techniques, Lambo and Prince did not by any means see them as the equal of Western psychotherapeutic techniques in a general sense. Indeed, in terms of collaboration, it is clear that Lambo, Prince, and Asuni all saw the Western-trained psychiatrist as the primus inter pares. For example, Lambo made clear that in the Aro Village system, the Western-trained psychiatrist was in charge and traditional healers were there to serve the therapeutic needs of the psychiatric establishment. Lambo repeatedly emphasized that traditional healers at Aro always worked under "strict supervision"[95] and with the "guidance"[96] of the psychiatric staff. They were there primarily to enhance the ability of psychiatry to bypass the cultural illusions that traditional healers so successfully manipulated. In this way, even as Lambo and Prince argued for a space for traditional healing systems within the structures of "modern" psychiatry, they still sought to protect what they saw as the superior integrity of the Western medical knowledge production and implementation processes. In short, they still saw Western psychiatric explanations about the nature of mental illness as the baseline "truth" into which traditional health systems could be incorporated, and they saw themselves as the gatekeepers with the necessary qualifications to determine what knowledge to incorporate and on what terms.[97]

CONCLUSION

The amalgamation of "traditional" health systems with "modern" psychiatry has been messy and incomplete, with the result that universally diagnosed disorders like schizophrenia and depression could not be correlated with universally valid forms of psychotherapy across cultural boundaries. The problem of aligning universal diagnoses with culturally specific treatments remains a major concern of psychiatric practice in the twenty-first century in Nigeria as it does elsewhere. Interestingly enough, by the early 1980s it seemed that Asuni's position on the desired relationship between traditional healers and Western-trained psychiatrists was displacing the incorporative philosophy of Lambo and Prince. Asuni himself abandoned the practice of working with traditional healers in his community care system by the mid-1970s,[98] and by 1981, even the original Aro Village that Lambo had taken with him to the University of Ibadan had severed its ties with local traditional healers.[99] Although official efforts have continued to search for ways that traditional healing systems might cooperate with official psychiatric structures, the transcultural psychiatric literature on the subject in Nigeria has been overwhelmingly ambivalent: unsure about the efficacy of imported Western ideas, unsure about the value of retaining traditional treatments, and uncomfortable with the prospects for synthesis. This ambivalence reflects the ideological tensions of the transition from a world order based on the reality of European might and unassailability of Western scientific rationalism to one based on constant fluctuations in negotiations between anticolonial nationalism, modernization and development processes, and culturally relativistic identity politics. As we will see in the next chapter, a similar ambivalence pervaded Nigerian psychiatrists' attitudes toward drug therapy.

6 ⟿ The Paradoxes of Psychoactive Drugs

THE DECOLONIZATION OF NIGERIA and the emergence of indigenous psychiatric professionals in the 1950s coincided with what is often called the psychopharmaceutical revolution in psychiatry. Indeed, clinical trials for chlorpromazine, the first highly effective antipsychotic drug, were taking place in 1952–53, just a year before T. Adeoye Lambo took over the reins of Aro Mental Hospital. Historians of psychiatry have frequently depicted the development of chlorpromazine as the beginning of a drastic change in mainstream psychiatric thinking, away from the cultural and environmental explanations of mental illness promoted particularly by psychoanalysts and toward a new biological psychiatry that has focused on altering brain chemistry as the foundation of treating psychological disorder.[1] However, this turn toward the biological has had complications of its own, as the massive expansion of the psychopharmaceutical industry has found many detractors within the psychiatric profession and among layfolk, both in Western industrialized countries and in the developing world.[2] At the same time, Nigeria was also seeing increased importation of a variety of other psychoactive drugs, many of which were technically illegal but increasingly available for recreational or self-medicating use. This chapter examines the ways that Nigerian psychiatrists understood psychoactive drug use in Nigeria from the late 1950s to the early 1980s, paying particular attention to the ways that discourses about drug use were simultaneously illustrative of political and social concerns specific to the Nigerian context of decolonization, modernization, and independence on the one hand, and growing international concerns about the medical and sociological role of drugs in society on the other.

Drugs, a category of "substances taken into the human body for purposes other than nutrition,"[3] have served as mediators between human beings and their social and physical surroundings since the dawn of human existence. Psychoactive (or psychotropic) drugs, which affect consciousness, mood, or awareness, have historically served a broad range of ritual, social, and medical purposes.[4] Historically, societies have had to negotiate what drugs are permissible and impermissible, as well as what constitutes acceptable, healthy use of permissible drugs and what constitutes abuse of those drugs. As David Healy has put it, the primary question for psychiatrists since the onset of the psychopharmaceutical revolution has been one of "how to distinguish drugs that restored social order from drugs that subverted the social order."[5] However, in Nigeria in the 1950s, 1960s, and 1970s, psychiatrists were functioning on the recognition that the social order itself was in flux. As processes of urbanization and economic modernization in the postwar era were changing sociocultural relations for millions of Nigerians at a presumably rapid pace, so, too, were they making available to Nigerians a host of new psychoactive substances. Included in this list were not only the newly developed psychopharmaceuticals, whose importation and dispensation were heavily regulated, but also legal substances such as alcohol and illegal narcotics such as cannabis and cocaine, which while prohibited were increasingly ubiquitous, particularly in urban areas, from the 1950s.[6] All of these substances had the capacity to help Nigerians cope with the psychological tensions of the times, but in different ways and through different channels. In mid-twentieth-century Nigeria, psychiatrists had to determine the social and psychological implications of various types of drug use for the health not only of individual patients, but of Nigerian society in general.

Just as Nigerian psychiatrists were critical of the value of adopting Western methods of psychotherapy, so, too, did they show trepidation about the importation of psychotropic drugs—both illicit and medically regulated—into Nigeria; and to the development of "modern" drug cultures—both medical and nonmedical—that they portended. Balancing the perceived merits and demerits of psychoactive drug use meant addressing several paradoxes that these drugs posed to a society perceived to be in transition. Sociologically, Nigerian psychiatrists were faced with the question of whether and how the psychopharmaceuticals they prescribed were, in fact, different from any of the other illicit psychoactive substances that Nigerians used in nonmedical contexts. Were nonmedical drug users self-medicating or self-destructing?

Was habitual drug abuse a symptom of an abnormal inability to cope with social pressures or a normal response to social conditions that were themselves abnormal and possibly even pathological? Medically, Nigerian psychiatrists also had to question whether their own increasing reliance on psychopharmacotherapy was actually the best possible treatment for ailing patients or contrarily a professional panacea compensating for Nigerian psychiatrists' inability to provide other forms of psychotherapy. Nigerian psychiatrists recognized that the effects of psychoactive drugs on individual brain chemistry were largely similar across human populations regardless of race, religion, ethnicity, et cetera. In terms of cultural politics, the psychopharmaceutical revolution therefore served as an important piece of evidence for the basic similarity of human psychology that Nigerian psychiatrists embraced. However, most psychoactive drugs were recent imports into Nigeria, and had not historically been a significant part of the cultural fabric for managing psychological and social tensions. Nigerian psychiatrists were therefore suspicious about the long-term consequences of widespread use of psychotropic drugs, in either medical or nonmedical contexts, in much the same way that they were uneasy about the importation of other Western-originating therapeutic regimens.

The profundity of these paradoxes made it difficult for Nigerian psychiatrists to conclude that drugs, either collectively or in specificity, were generally good or bad. Indeed, Nigerian psychiatrists never had an overt debate on these subjects and never fully reconciled these paradoxes. Neither has the international psychiatric community more generally, however. For our purposes, this chapter uses the paradoxes of psychoactive drugs to reinforce three points about the transition from colonial to transcultural psychiatry in Nigeria and globally. First, the ways that Nigerian psychiatrists approached the paradoxes of drug use were inherently linked to Nigeria's colonial legacies. Concerns that Nigerian psychiatrists displayed about the role psychoactive drugs should play in Nigerian society, and their own role in regulating their use, were part of a political climate that sought, however imperfectly, to modernize but not to imitate, to integrate with international processes but not to rely on foreigners to solve Nigerian problems.

Second, as we saw in chapter 5, Nigerian psychiatrists posited themselves (in conjunction with Western-trained social scientists) as the most qualified professionals to conduct the cost-benefit analysis of the effects that psychoactive drugs were having on Nigerian society in general and psychiatric practice specifically. Just as they saw themselves as gatekeepers charged with negotiating the relationship between "Western" and "traditional" psychotherapies, they also saw themselves as gatekeepers who needed to stand between Nigerians and the foreign substances they put in their bodies. However, although Nigerian psychiatrists were by no means able to enforce their role as gatekeepers, their desire to do so illustrates a locally specific articulation of much more generalized international tensions attendant to the rise of a new biological psychiatry that thought about mental illness as primarily a physical problem that could conceivably be both exacerbated and mitigated through the implementation of psychoactive drugs.

Finally, Nigerian psychiatrists' general concerns about the increasing ubiquity of drugs in society and in psychiatric practice corresponded with dynamics taking place in international psychiatric circles, although specific articulation of those concerns was based on local observations. While previous chapters have argued that Nigerian psychiatrists were somewhat influential in helping to change research agendas and clinical processes in global psychiatry since the 1950s, this chapter argues that Nigerian psychiatrists tended to feel that they had very little control over the drug deluge that was coming to define their profession from the 1960s on. The reality that multinational corporations based in Western industrialized countries increasingly provided the research and development for virtually all psychopharmaceutical treatments sat poorly with Nigerian psychiatrists. Similar concerns came out of Western countries, where the antipsychiatry movement of the 1960s argued that antipsychotics were nothing more than a chemical straitjacket.[7] By the 1970s, many psychiatric researchers had started to recognize long-term negative consequences of prolonged psychotherapeutic care and increasingly criticized a psychopharmaceutical industry more concerned with the commercial viability of their products than with their capacity to heal.[8] Nigerian psychiatrists shared these concerns; however, they also saw increasing reliance on psychopharmaceuticals in clinical practice as a response to stagnating economies that did not allow for more time- and labor-intensive therapies. The influx of psychopharmaceuticals, as with illicit psychoactive drugs, was bound up with the failures of modernization to achieve the kind of robust psychiatric infrastructure that Lambo and others had envisioned in the 1950s. By the 1980s, the psychopharmaceutical revolution had come to represent for many Nigerian psychiatrists the entrenched geopolitical and economic dependencies that now characterize the age of globalization in so many critics' minds.

FOREIGN SUBSTANCES AND SELF-MEDICATION IN THE 1960S

In the early years of transcultural psychiatry in Nigeria, concerns about psychoactive drug use were overwhelmingly focused on the nonmedical use of illicit substances, which psychiatrists practicing in Nigeria saw as mostly recent imports with little to no traditional role in Nigerian cultures. As such, they came to be seen by psychiatrists as a product of Nigeria's modernization processes—as indicative of Nigeria's integration into the global economy and Nigeria's social and cultural transition to "modern" lifestyles. David T. Courtwright has identified five major objections that are typically raised about the effects of nonmedical drug use: (1) the harm drug users do to themselves and others in terms of both physical health and socially destructive behavior such as crime; (2) the social costs of drug abuse in terms of lost manpower and public expenditure to mitigate damage caused by drug users; (3) religious disapproval; (4) association of drugs with undesirable groups, often foreigners or racial and ethnic others; and (5) that use of drugs by members of the group weakens the overall group—be it an ethnic, national, or religious entity—making it vulnerable to internal decline and external infiltration (such as by the undesirable groups of #4).[9] Indeed, all but #3 apply to the perspective that psychiatrists practicing in Nigeria took to the perceived growth in availability of psychoactive substances in the context of decolonization, urbanization, and modernization of the Nigerian economy.

The earliest psychiatric studies of drug use in Nigeria concerned the psychological and social effects of cannabis. In the mid-1960s, Tolani Asuni, T. Adeoye Lambo, and Alexander Boroffka produced the earliest studies on the use of cannabis in Nigeria.[10] All three studies claimed that the appearance of cannabis in Nigeria dated to no earlier than the Second World War, but that its availability and consumption had been increasing dramatically since then. Lambo, for example, declared that "the problem of drug addiction in West Africa is a fairly recent phenomenon,"[11] and, although he could provide no data on the historical use of cannabis or other drugs in West Africa, he did provide some epidemiological data indicating that cannabis abuse was rampant at least in western Nigeria by 1960, noting that cannabis abuse accounted for 15 percent of all admissions to Aro Hospital in 1959–60 and 20 percent of admissions to the outpatient psychiatric clinic at the University College Hospital, Ibadan. Boroffka also noted dramatic increases in admissions at Yaba with a history of marijuana use, up from 8.1 percent of all admissions in 1961–62 to 21 percent of all admissions in 1964–65.[12]

Concerns about the psychoactive properties of cannabis had been an undercurrent of social and economic processes within the British Empire since at least the nineteenth century. Indigenous to the Indian subcontinent, cannabis had long been used for its psychoactive properties in medicines for a variety of illnesses and for inducing transcendental states for Buddhist mystics. British authorities, however, were most interested in the plant for its tough fibers, which they used to make rope for their powerful navy. For the British, the psychoactive elements of cannabis intoxication were always somewhat suspect. By the 1870s, studies of cannabis ingestion in India had linked the drug to increasing rates of insanity in Indian asylums. Although data linking cannabis to mental illness was later proved to be significantly flawed, the concept of its dangerous social and psychological effects became part of mainstream thinking both in Britain and internationally by the 1920s. In 1924 the Pharmaceutical Society of Great Britain added cannabis to its Poisons Schedule. In the same year, the Second Opium Conference, an international meeting of League of Nations member states, including Great Britain, passed restrictions on the trade in cannabis.[13] As a British colonial possession, legislation governing the importation and trafficking of such substances as opium, cocaine, and cannabis also applied to Nigeria.

These international attitudes toward cannabis were therefore clearly influential on Nigerian psychiatrists trained in contemporary Western medical conventions and familiar with British legal statutes. However, in the context of decolonization and Nigerian independence, Lambo and Asuni also saw the problem of cannabis availability in Nigeria as inextricably linked to Nigeria's colonial past and to its current entanglements in the global economy. Prior to the mid-twentieth century, the peoples of Nigeria had limited access to most psychoactive drugs, and, as a result, there was very little use of them in Nigerian societies. Notable exceptions were the kola nut, a mild stimulant used for social and ritual purposes in many parts of West Africa,[14] and alcohol in the form of indigenously produced palm wine and its distillate. From the sixteenth century, a limited supply of imported European liquors was also available to certain segments of many Nigerian societies.[15] This being the case, Asuni insisted that cannabis was not indigenous to Nigeria and had been introduced to the country only by Nigerian soldiers returning from deployments in the Middle East, Far East, and North Africa during the Second World War. Further supporting this theory, Asuni remarked that there was no traditional name for cannabis in indigenous Nigerian languages, and that compilations of indigenous plant life in Nigeria published prior to the war made no mention of it. Indeed, the most commonly used English name for cannabis in Nigeria at this time was "Indian hemp," indicating a belief in the foreign origin of the plant.[16]

Asuni and Lambo also linked the growing availability of cannabis in Nigeria to foreign demand and to Nigeria's export-oriented agricultural economy. Although not indigenous to Nigeria, once introduced the plant grew "profusely . . . with little or no care" in southern Nigeria's tropical climate, making it an attractive cash crop for local farmers, particularly once farmers learned of "the fantastic price paid abroad for a commodity which requires little effort to produce."[17] The move toward an economy centered in urban areas also brought about increased production of cannabis within Nigeria, according to Lambo. As young people migrated to the cities in search of gainful employment, the family members remaining in the rural areas were forced to find means of maintaining their agricultural revenues with less available labor. As a result, Lambo claimed, "while the young ones are on the move to sell their labour and become pedlars [*sic*], the older ones stay behind and explore other means of acquiring cash: many grow a cash crop, the cheapest with the greatest remuneration being cannabis."[18] Cash croppers had little difficulty finding foreign buyers since, as Asuni noted, "international trafficking of cannabis from Nigeria had also been facilitated in recent years by increased international communication and transport."[19] Lambo also connected the local cannabis economy to "tourists and seasonal workers," particularly in "urban areas, especially to new industrial centres with no infrastructure."[20]

Although the reasons for the increasing availability of cannabis could be directly related to foreign influences in Nigeria, they did not entirely explain why Nigerians themselves were ingesting a drug with which they had little to no prior experience. For Asuni, Lambo, and Boroffka, the answer to this question lay in the widespread social disruptions of the times, as Nigerian societies and individuals made the transition from rural, agrarian communities, with strong emphasis on extended family and kinship organization, to the increasingly urban environments characterized by large migrant populations dislocated from their families and communities of origin and striving to succeed in increasingly modern social, economic, and educational settings. All three studies found that cannabis smokers in Nigeria in the mid-1960s were overwhelmingly young, male, urban, and engaged in nontraditional sorts of work linked to Nigeria's modernizing economy. Asuni found that of twenty-six patients at Aro Hospital whose illness had been "definitely related to cannabis" over a period of eighteen months, all were male, and most (twenty-one) had lifestyles and occupations that Asuni considered to be representative of the "transitional" class of Nigerians—such as students, truck drivers, and clerks.[21] Boroffka reported similar data from Yaba Mental Hospital in Lagos, where students made up 10 percent of all admissions with a history of cannabis use, motor drivers and mechanics 21 percent, artisans and factory workers 20 percent, and clerical workers 13 percent. Only 7 percent of cases in Boroffka's assessment had occupations he considered "traditional."[22] Lambo found "young *migrant* workers," most of whom were male and urban, to be more prone to cannabis abuse than their "*non-migrant* elders."[23] Other demographic factors tended to be insignificant according to the studies. Women were less likely to abuse cannabis, according to Lambo and Asuni, because they were less likely to migrate and more likely than men to remain integrated into strong family units and kinship networks through marriage. All three studies found no correlation between ethnicity or religious background and cannabis use, indicating that the new processes of socioeconomic change tended to trump other factors of social organization. The same social transitions that caused cannabis to be increasingly available and marketable also made it increasingly consumable.

Explanations as to *why* the young, male, migrant, and urban demographic seemed to indulge in cannabis smoking more so than other groups were diverse and scientifically inconclusive, but did illustrate the preoccupations of the psychiatrists offering them. Asuni, Lambo, and Boroffka were willing to suggest that cannabis smoking was a means of redressing the social imbalance of such a stressful and alienating lifestyle. For those young, socially dislocated migrants, use of drugs was very much a process of self-medication. Lambo declared that "many young adolescent non-addict users of cannabis look upon the use of this drug as a means of . . . coping with their environment." Cannabis could be very effective for this purpose. Lambo himself conducted a study of seven patients who were prescribed twenty to twenty-five minutes a day of cannabis smoking over a nine- to sixteen-week period as a means to treat "severe non-rational anxiety." Lambo found that after six weeks of this therapy, "anxiety was markedly reduced with an appreciable relief of symptoms."[24] Similarly, Boroffka speculated that "Nigerians are traditionally closely knit into very intensive groups and communities and may suffer from loneliness after advancing into the western way of life and becoming urbanized and industrialized." He suggested that "one could theorize, they turn to Indian hemp in order to forget their homesickness and the good old times." As such, Boroffka concluded, "there is a strong suggestion that social factors play an important part" in individuals' decision to consume cannabis.[25]

Asuni also recognized that cannabis smoking was itself a social act, undertaken in some ways to provide a sense of inclusiveness that was often lacking for young people in urban settings. He provided the example of a young man's testimony of his first experience with cannabis at a nightclub:

> Eight of us occupied a table at one corner of the premises. There was a lady in our company.
>
> I hadn't met any of my table mates before, but we got along fine conversing on irrelevant subjects, commenting on the music and

the dresses worn by the beautiful women in attendance. . . . Suddenly one of them . . . got up, went to a nearby house and returned after a few minutes.

He handed a small envelope to the man sitting next to him. This man started wrapping something in the form of a cigarette. . . .

After wrapping the thing, he lit it, took a long draw, tightened his teeth, puffed his jaws, swallowed the smoke and passed the cigarette to the man next to him. He, too, did the same thing and passed it over to the girl, who took her turn. It dawned on me that they were not smoking the usual cigarette but Indian hemp. The odour was hideous, but I dared not show concern.

It next came to my turn and I politely refused since I had a cigarette in my mouth.

"Come on, have a go, boy!" one of the chaps loudly pressed me.

I always try novelties at least once, so I took a "pull" and handed it over to the next fellow. . . .

After five minutes of persistent coughing, I cooled down a little bit, opened my eyes and saw my newly-made friends laughing at me. . . .

I noticed thereafter that conversation at our table became more lively and my friends more jovial. The lady forgot convention and became more familiar with everyone, using obscene words.[26]

Here Asuni is clearly describing cannabis as an intensely social drug, one smoked for the purpose of facilitating sociability in a context where it would otherwise be lacking. The young acolyte, having no particular relationship with his tablemates at the beginning of the evening, considered them his "newly-made friends" as a result of the shared experience of smoking cannabis. In this sense, the people in question alleviated a symptom: social alienation, with a treatment: cannabis.

Despite the therapeutic value individuals might find in their indulgence, for Asuni, Lambo, and Boroffka, cannabis use portended a significant degree of social decay for Nigeria. Asuni believed that although the traffic in Indian hemp was a growing business, overall its use was insidiously destroying the Nigerian economy. He noted that cannabis smokers tended to be unemployed, or underemployed, and suggested that "even those who are employed tend to lose their efficiency, and tend to report late for work as their sense of time is often disturbed." He concluded that "the economic loss to the individual and to the nation is bound to be colossal" as cannabis intoxication undoubtedly wasted untold amounts of manpower. The studies found cannabis to have a similarly destructive effect on families. Asuni found that "those seriously involved in smoking cannabis are unable to fulfil their role as effective husbands and fathers" and often brought disgrace on their families through their "disruptive and irresponsible behaviour."[27] The use of cannabis among schoolchildren also threatened to destabilize family situations and to ruin a generation of productive workers. Asuni and Lambo linked cannabis use to all kinds of criminal behavior, from prostitution to political thuggery,[28] noting that cannabis afforded them "the assumed unconcern and disregard for society at large"[29] necessary to engage in such deviant behaviors. Asuni also linked cannabis use to traffic accidents, based on general knowledge that truck and taxi drivers often smoked cannabis because they thought it helped them to stay awake and alert for long hours on the road.[30]

It should be noted that the dire assessment of the sociological effects of cannabis smoking on Nigerian society provided by Asuni, Lambo, and Boroffka was almost entirely anecdotal, relying on local media reports and on vague references to "observation" lacking any scientific methodology. Interestingly, the arousal of social indifference presented as a negative result of cannabis consumption was also one of the major positive results of many antipsychotic agents like chlorpromazine. The ability to bring a state of calm indifference to excitable schizophrenics was primary evidence of the efficacy of psychopharmacotherapy at the same time that it was a sign of social decay when resulting from the nonmedical use of cannabis.

As psychiatrists, the most important question for Asuni, Lambo, and Boroffka was the relationship between cannabis and mental illness. Whereas the three scientists mostly agreed about the socioeconomic causes and effects of a growing cannabis culture, they were less conclusive about the psychological implications of cannabis abuse. The specific interactions that all three had experienced with cannabis smokers had come mainly in the context of official psychiatric treatment, meaning that their data on cannabis abuse came entirely from a subsection of the population that had experienced some form of psychological disorder. Was it just a coincidence that so many of those hospitalized for mental illness had a history of cannabis use, or were personalities that engaged in cannabis use predisposed in some way to psychological disorder? Was it possible that cannabis itself had caused their mental breakdowns, or did cannabis simply help to unmask preexisting psychiatric conditions? On these questions psychiatrists of Nigeria in the 1960s could reach no consensus.

Asuni tended to suspect that cannabis smokers were of a "personality type" predisposed to mental illness. For example, he pondered that transportation work, highly associated with cannabis abuse, by virtue of its "itenerant nature and the great opportunity it affords for emotional detachment," was attractive to "the particular type of personality prone to cannabis smoking."[31] He also suggested that many of the young men who migrated to the cities in search of employment and/or an escape from "the controlling influence of their small circumscribed communities" did so because of "their schizophrenic propensity," which made them more liable to a psychotic break in their new environments with our without the aid of cannabis.[32]

Lambo, on the other hand, tended to see cannabis use as not significantly related to mental illness at all. Lambo described the idea that drug addiction caused mental disorder as a "falsity" and declared that at best it could be seen as only one of many factors impinging upon individuals' psyches. Lambo preferred to view drug addiction "and many of its concomitant social manifestations, not as causes and effects, but rather as concomitant neurotic adjustment of individuals within changing or transitional social, cultural and economic systems."[33] In fact, Lambo lamented that one of the main challenges in attempting to treat or cure drug addiction in West Africa was that "the patient is usually a man in transition, and his problems—personal, economic, social or a combination of these—are invariably the same nature." Many West Africans simply had problems "with no clear guide as to how to solve them."[34] Under such circumstances, it was unclear to Lambo what the "normal" healthy response of these individuals to their life circumstances should be. Smoking marijuana was quite probably a perfectly reasonable, if potentially hazardous, coping strategy for otherwise psychologically healthy Nigerians, and there was very little that Lambo believed he could offer them in terms of better options other than to promote the long-term stabilization of Nigerian society and greater social support for people living on the margins.

Boroffka, on the other hand, tended toward the belief that cannabis could frequently be the primary cause behind the development of a mental illness. Like Asuni, he believed that people who used cannabis were, for the most part, "emotionally, mentally or socially unstable."[35] He claimed the idea that cannabis could directly cause mental illness to be "not well founded," although not conclusively impossible either. The idea that those with latent psychosis were more likely to be drawn to cannabis was equally difficult to prove in Boroffka's estimation because the symptoms associated with what he called "the hypothetical 'Indian Hemp Psychosis'" were indistinguishable from other types of psychoses, particularly types of schizophrenia. The result was that while cannabis was widely accepted to cause temporary psychosis in the "acute intoxicational state," there was no consensus on whether cannabis could cause or contribute to "protracted psychoses" like full-blown schizophrenia. Nevertheless, Boroffka indicated that at Yaba roughly half of the cases presenting with a history of cannabis use were diagnosed as "toxic psychosis," a tacit declaration of the belief that "the smoking of *Cannabis* can and does cause protracted psychoses which can be distinguished from other, especially schizophrenic psychoses."[36] Schizophrenic psychosis was the diagnosis for the other half of patients presenting with a history of cannabis usage. Boroffka provided no explanation for how either he or the other clinical staff at Yaba were able to make the distinction between such cases, however.

Assessing the direct psychological impact of cannabis abuse on individuals was a difficult proposition in circumstances where so many factors were operating. At the end of the day, Boroffka's conclusion that "Indian hemp constitutes a danger to the individual and consequently, if the habit spreads widely, to society as well,"[37] summed up the general attitude toward nonmedical or self-medicating drug use in Nigeria, although exactly how or in what way it was a cause of or contributor to individual psychopathology or social decay independently of other influences remained speculative. What is clear is that Asuni, Lambo, and Boroffka saw cannabis use as a recent, foreign, and decidedly negative phenomenon in Nigeria, and the bulk of their concern about drug abuse came from the fluctuating circumstances in which access to drugs was difficult to control and likely to spread, even with oversight from medical professionals like themselves.

ENTRENCHMENT OF THE DRUG CULTURE IN THE 1970S

From the 1970s, psychiatric studies of drug abuse began to diverge. Some Nigerian psychiatrists followed in Asuni's, Lambo's, and Boroffka's footsteps, emphasizing the links between rising levels of drug abuse and the rapid and recent increase in socioeconomic change taking place in Nigeria. For example, in 1976 Amechi Anumonye, then a physician specialist at Yaba, produced a synthesis study on alcohol and drug abuse in youth in Africa and Nigeria in which he, like those before him, blamed increasing drug abuse in Nigeria on foreign influence and socioeconomic change.[38] He declared that "for most workers in developing countries the association of drugs of abuse with industrialization, detribalization and urbanization is a reality."[39] He noted widespread abuse of a variety of drugs, including amphetamines, barbiturates, Mandrax (methaqualone), and cannabis, and lamented the massive increase in production of beer and liquor in 1970s Nigeria as governmental regulations on distillation loosened and state government breweries proliferated. Anumonye was also concerned, although for unclear reasons, that foreign whiskey and beer were displacing indigenous palm wine as the tipple of choice for many Nigerians, linking concerns with alcohol consumption to external socioeconomic influences.

Other studies followed up on Lambo's and Asuni's concerns that drug abuse had the capacity to severely undermine Nigeria's social stability and economic transformation. For example, Moses O. Akindele, of the Department of Psychiatry at the University of Ibadan, noted in a 1974 study on drug abuse among dropouts from Nigeria's universities between 1969 and 1972 that one of the primary consequences of drug abuse in Nigeria was "wastage of manpower,"[40] as it often forced students to abandon their university positions. This was particularly problematic for Akindele in "a developing country requiring highly skilled personnel" such as Nigeria because "dropouts cause wastage of University places and failure to utilize equipment and trained staff."[41] Akindele also noted that drug abuse tended to make people "irresponsible at work," which made it difficult for them to hold down jobs. When unemployed, drug users tended to devise means of obtaining money to purchase drugs by devious means. Members of Akindele's control group admitted that they "told lies, duped relatives, and . . . stole money or articles for sale from their parents or relations," all indicators of the social decay that the availability of psychoactive drugs caused.[42] Like Asuni, Lambo, and Boroffka, Akindele found that drug abuse, while initially undertaken by students as a coping mechanism, had decidedly negative long-term outcomes on the national economy and on family stability.

While such studies reinforced the concerns and findings of their predecessors by focusing primarily on young, urban populations undergoing the transition to "modernity" and having a significant degree of interaction with foreign products and ideas, other studies were beginning to complicate the epidemiological picture of drug use in Nigeria. For example, a 1976 study on cannabis abuse in Nigeria by V. Olufemi Oviasu, of the University of Benin Teaching Hospital in Benin City, corroborated many of the demographic characteristics emphasized by Asuni, Lambo, and Boroffka. Oviasu found most of his cannabis users to be young migrant males, mostly from urban areas and engaged in "transitional" occupations. He found that most were diagnosed with "toxic psychosis" upon admission to hospital, and that all had been released within six months after receiving a round of psychopharmacotherapy.[43] However, Oviasu also expanded on his predecessors' findings, adding a new occupation to the list of those particularly susceptible to cannabis abuse: soldiers. Oviasu recorded that 50 out of the 296 patients in his study were employed as soldiers, and many had served during Nigeria's bloody civil war of 1967–70. Many of the soldiers had joined the military, according to Oviasu "partly because of the prospects of excitement and partly because of the assured income,"[44] having previously had difficulty finding stable and remunerative work elsewhere. A connection to Asuni's idea that itinerant workers were predisposed by personality toward cannabis use could be made here; however, Oviasu was quick to point out that three-quarters of the soldiers in his study "were introduced to smoking Cannabis after joining the Army because under its influence fear and apprehension of unpleasant tasks were removed,"[45] suggesting more along the lines of Lambo that smoking cannabis was actually a coping mechanism for these soldiers as they sought to navigate extremely stressful circumstances. Significantly, here a Nigerian psychiatrist was eschewing a focus on the foreign nature of Nigeria's drug abuse picture and suggesting that the endogenous problems of postindependence Nigeria were themselves contributing to creating environments within which individuals felt the need to self-medicate with illicit psychoactive substances. Later, other studies would make tacit connections between the civil war and increasing levels of drug abuse as well.[46]

By the late 1970s studies were beginning to identify a significant amount of drug use in groups other than young, urban, migrant males. By examining levels of alcohol consumption, A. O. Odejide and Michael O. Olatawura of the Department of Psychiatry at University College Hospital, Ibadan, found that the use of psychoactive substances was fairly ubiquitous in Nigerian society regardless of geographical or sociocultural demographics.[47] Such findings had effectively complicated the drug-use picture in Nigeria by the 1980s. While it might be argued that urban, modernizing areas were more conducive to certain types of drug use and/or to certain types of unacceptable behavior attendant to drug abuse, it was no longer possible to suggest that urbanization, modernization, and migration should be seen as predominant *causes* of drug abuse. Such findings led John C. Ebie and Ona A. Pela, of the Department of Mental Health at the University of Benin, to declare in 1981 that the causative link between drug use and socioeconomic change was becoming increasingly tenuous as the epidemiological data deepened.[48] Ebie and Pela found relationships between socioeconomic status and drug abuse to be "contradictory," noting that "abuse of drugs has been reported in children of the rich and poor alike; in urban and in rural adolescents, and in highly literate and illiterate individuals." Reported factors impinging upon individuals' decisions to use drugs were equally diffuse, ranging from "curiosity, enjoyment, peer group pressure, conflict with parents, . . . academic pressure, loneliness and to a minor extent, as a means of fighting fatigue."[49] Ebie and Pela gave special attention to the vulnerabilities of adolescents struggling to integrate the "physiological self with the psychological self," and noted that this was conceivably more difficult in "modern society," where "stratification, individualism, intergroup tension, uncertainty and inhibitions predominate."[50] However, this perspective was presented as one of many factors and as more of a universal norm than a peculiarity of Nigerian circumstances.

Indeed, Nigerian psychiatrists were quick to point out the extent to which the drug abuse problem their country was experiencing was part of a global drug abuse problem that much of the world was experiencing. M. H. Ahmed and Moses O. Akindele, of the Psychiatric Unit at Ahmadu Bello University in Kaduna and the University College Hospital, Ibadan, respectively, chose to begin their 1974 study of drug abuse in Kaduna with the statement "The problem of Drug Abuse [*sic*] is worldwide. In Nigeria the problem exists like in other countries."[51] Odejide considered the existence of drug abuse in Nigeria to be evidence of "the universality of psychiatric disorders," noting that not only did drug abuse exist in both Western and non-Western cultures, but that "the etiological factors in the drug abuse subculture" were similar regardless of location or culture, centering mainly on "consequences of unhappy and poor background . . . , pressure to succeed in academic work . . . , influence of significant others (peer groups, parents, etc.) . . . , easy accessibility of drugs and . . . primary psychiatric illnesses."[52]

The scientific data on drug use patterns in Nigeria therefore unearthed no "truths" about the cause-and-effect relationship between drug abuse and psychological disorder in Nigeria. It did, however, reveal the preoccupations and anxieties of Nigerian psychologists and psychiatrists over the period from the 1960s to the 1980s. Original concerns about the recent explosion in abuse of foreign psychoactive substances linked to rapid socioeconomic change eventually gave way to concerns about the entrenchment of psychoactive drug use in the country and to the belief that in some ways Nigeria's drug problem was evidence of the extent to which it had entered the "modern" world. In the context of an entrenched drug culture, Nigerian psychiatrists were concerned about control and proper use of psychoactive substances that were clearly going to continue to be a part of the everyday reality of Nigerians for a long time. Nigerian psychiatrists saw themselves as the necessary mediator between the Nigerian public and the psychoactive substances that helped them cope with their environments. And while much of this concern centered on illicit drug use in nonmedical contexts, Nigerian psychiatrists also started to show concerns about the use of psychoactive drugs in psychiatric practice.

THE DOUBLE-EDGED PSYCHOPHARMACEUTICAL SWORD

The introduction of psychopharmaceuticals for specific treatment of mentally ill patients in Nigeria occurred more or less simultaneously with the growth in availability of illicit substances like cannabis. The psychopharmaceutical revolution of the postwar era was not the first time that psychiatrists had found drugs useful for the management of mental illness. Sedatives had long been used in Western psychiatric practice to make disruptive psychotic patients more passive, but these drugs had serious side effects that greatly affected normal psychomotor activities and levels of consciousness. The development of effective antipsychotics with less severe side effects came out of studies done on antihistamines in France in the late 1940s in the case of chlorpromazine, and in the isolation of active ingredients in the Indian plant *Rauwolfia serpentina* in India in the case of reserpine. Whereas Lambo and Asuni had considered the foreign origin of cannabis to be part of the danger associated with the plant, they found the integration of foreign antipsychotic psychopharmaceuticals into clinical practice at Aro Hospital in the mid-1950s to be a major boon to the psychiatric profession in Nigeria. "The cautious and judicious use of these drugs," declared Lambo in 1960, "has revolutionized the management of psychiatric disorders." In fact, Lambo gave psychopharmacotherapy a great deal of credit for the effectiveness of the Aro Village Scheme, noting that "without these drugs, which reduced tension, excitement, and aggression in many of our patients, this scheme could not have been successful."[53] This illustrated a common approach to the advent of psychopharmaceuticals in the 1950s and 1960s: the idea that these new drugs were not meant to be therapy in and of themselves but that they stabilized patients' moods and behaviors enough that psychotherapies like psychoanalysis, community therapy, or other forms of social psychiatry could have a better effect.[54]

The availability of "modern" pharmacotherapy was also evidence of the major strides that psychiatric practice was making over what had obtained under the colonial asylum system. Drug use for psychiatric care had been minimal and heavily controlled in colonial Nigeria, partly because of a lack of emphasis on mental health treatment in the colonial context and partly because of the general lack of effective psychopharmaceuticals until the 1950s. While traditional healers in southern Nigeria were known to use certain herbs containing psychoactive substances in their treatments for mental illness, particularly *Rauwolfia vomitoria,* an emetic used largely for its soporific effects (and a close relative of the Indian plant instrumental in the development of reserpine), it was also recognized that sometimes these drugs caused a variety of extrapyramidal side effects including twitching of the neck and other limbs and protrusion of the tongue (known as tardive dyskinesia in medical lingo), which made the drug unattractive for any kind of recreational purpose in the general population.[55] However, in the 1950s and 1960s, the ability to provide symptom relief with manageable side effects was therefore considered to be an unqualified improvement over prevailing options.

By the 1970s, however, many Nigerian psychiatrists were beginning to question their reliance on these drugs for use in Nigerian patients. Nigerian psychiatrists were wary of the extent to which medical professionals could misuse psychopharmaceuticals in their day-to-day operations. There was a growing concern in the Nigerian psychiatric community that drug therapy was being used excessively. Nigerian psychiatrists began to suggest that psychopharmaceuticals were serving as a stopgap measure to overcome staff shortages in Nigerian hospitals, which had not developed enough to meet the psychiatric needs of the population. Although Lambo had noted that psychotropic drugs had been instrumental in facilitating the community therapy program at Aro Village, Nigerian psychiatrists became increasingly frustrated with their inability to devote much effort to psychotherapeutic endeavors. Odejide declared, "The clinicians' workload gives minimal room for any other form of treatment than psychopharmacotherapy."[56] In 1979, Odejide noted that Nigerian psychiatrists were using a wide array of psychopharmaceuticals, including "chlorpromazine, thioridazine, triflouperazine, fluphenazine decanoate, and haloperidol," to treat schizophrenia; "imipramine, amitriptyline, trimipramine, chlorimipramine, and nortriptyline" for depression; "chlordiazapoxide, and diazepam" for neurosis; and "nitrazepam, butobarbitone, and secobarbital" for insomnia.[57] By the early 1980s, Nigerian psychiatric wards showed that most types of drugs on-site were used by less than 50 percent of the psychiatrists in attendance,[58] indicating a proliferation of available products tending toward overreliance. Those that were being used were prescribed in increasing quantities. O. O. Famuyiwa, of the Department of Psychiatry at the University of Lagos, found a "high frequency" of polypharmacy being practiced in Nigerian psychiatric institutions in the early 1980s, whereby patients received multiple daily doses of two or more psychotropic drugs. While this was increasingly common medical practice throughout the world by this time, Famuyiwa stressed the attendant dangers of such practice in a developing country such as Nigeria, "where there is a deplorably low nurse-patient ratio." Polypharmacy, Famuyiwa noted, "imposes an extra burden on the nurses," and in situations where nurses were already overburdened, "the risk of error increases as the need to complete tasks within a limited time increases."[59] Famuyiwa proposed replacing polypharmacy with single doses whenever possible as a means of mitigating this problem.[60]

Supporting Famuyiwa's contention that Nigerian patients were being overdosed with psychopharmaceuticals, Odejide and Ayinde found that reducing the dosage of neuroleptics from thrice daily to a single nightly dose after tissue saturation had been achieved resulted in effective symptom relief and a reduction of side effects.[61] Reducing the amount of psychotropic medication was deemed beneficial to the patient because "there is less bother in terms of time, there are fewer tablets to take, fewer and [more] mild side effects."[62] From the perspective of the psychiatrist, reducing dosages meant reduction of costs, as fewer drugs were needed, less manpower was necessary to administer treatment, and there was less need for prescriptions designed specifically to counter the side effects of certain psychotropic drugs.[63]

Overburdening caseloads, minimal staff, and a preponderance of available pharmaceutical substances created a perfect-storm situation in which psychiatrists could appear to be improving the condition of patients without making precise diagnoses or providing optimal care. At Aro Hospital in 1980, Odejide found that the vast majority of patients were on multiple-drug therapy. Furthermore, nearly 35 percent of patients were taking both antipsychotic and antidepressant drugs of various combinations, indicating, in Odejide's opinion, that "these diagnoses were not made in confidence."[64] Psychiatrists were apparently throwing drugs at problems and hoping they would go away. The findings of Odejide, Ayinde, and Famuyiwa are indicative of the pervasive feeling that psychotropic drugs were being poorly used in Nigeria by the 1980s.

In many ways, the concerns that Nigerian psychiatrists showed were consistent with the worries about the increasing reliance on psychopharmacotherapy that was taking place in the West as of the late 1960s as well.[65] The first generation of psychopharmaceuticals had been seen as a breakthrough in the ability to treat severe mental illnesses in Western countries, allowing psychiatrists to treat patients without confining them to the asylum space. However, by the 1960s, serious backlash to the psychopharmaceutical revolution was taking place within both psychiatric circles and the public at large. The antipsychiatry movement of the 1960s and 1970s argued that psychopharmaceuticals simply replaced the physical prison of the asylum with a chemical one. And over time, the long-term effects of some pharmaceutical treatments became clearer. Tardive dyskinesia proved to be a common side effect of many neuroleptic drugs and ultimately became a major public relations liability for psychiatric practice in Western countries in the 1970s, as many patients on long-term neuroleptic treatment developed these symptoms irreversibly.[66] By the late 1970s, it had become increasingly clear to many psychiatrists practicing around the world that a large number of the physical and behavioral problems of their patients were likely to be the result of overmedication rather than undermedication. Delineating symptoms caused by illness from symptoms caused by treatment became more difficult as patients were on more and more drugs for longer and longer periods.[67] As minor tranquilizers like Valium became the most prescribed drugs in the world by the early 1970s, many psychiatrists and laypersons began to fear that the commercialization of psychopharmaceuticals had the capacity to pathologize human experiences and behaviors once considered more or less normal.[68]

The "magic bullet" theory of psychopathology was proving to be a mirage, but critical psychiatrists and antipsychiatrists found themselves marginalized in a medical industrial complex that increasingly relied on the research and marketing of multinational pharmaceutical corporations to determine the most viable courses of treatment. Yet, even as such concerns were increasingly voiced, biomedical psychiatry doubled down. As many critics have noted, the 1980 publication of the *DSM-III* marked the triumph of the biomedical approach to psychiatry, establishing a broad-based classification system focused on diagnostic criteria for specific disorders for the first time. The *DSM-III* undermined the blurred spectra between normal and abnormal behavior, endogenous and exogenous forces, and constitutional and environmental causes that had historically characterized psychiatry, while allowing pharmaceutical companies to proclaim that their products treated specific disorders. As Rick Mayes and Allan V. Horowitz noted, "The DSM-III unintentionally positioned psychopharmacology on a growth trajectory that various institutions—insurance companies, managed care organizations, pharmaceutical companies, and the government—propelled significantly in subsequent years as they responded to the DSM-III's new diagnostic guidelines and the research incentives that it fostered."[69] The high reliance on psychopharmacotherapy was becoming a matter of global significance, and was in many ways a direct outgrowth of the emphasis on the universality of psychopathology that Nigerian psychiatrists of the 1950s and 1960s had so championed.

Nigerian psychiatrists were aware of these turns in broader psychiatric thinking about the drugs used in clinical practice. However, Nigerian psychiatrists' concerns about psychopharmacotherapy in the 1970s and early 1980s were also clearly linked to circumstances specific to the Nigerian geopolitical and socioeconomic contexts. The original embrasure of synthetic psychopharmaceuticals that Lambo expressed in the late 1950s gave way somewhat to concerns about the inappropriateness of Western-derived drugs for treatment in Nigerian patients. For example, Michael O. Olatawura seriously questioned whether psychiatric professionals in developing countries like Nigeria should be relying on psychopharmaceutical dosage recommendations based on Western clinical studies, which, of course, were the only clinical studies. Olatawura showed concern in two studies that individual responses to psychotropic drugs could be related to dietary habits and climate, both of which were very different for most Africans from those of most Westerners.[70] "Just as it is true that the effectiveness of psychoactive agents in general has been demonstrated in all populations," he argued, "so it is true that the effectiveness and adverse effects of the medicaments may not have received adequate attention in all parts of the world."[71] Olatawura argued that malnutrition, which was more prevalent in developing countries than in the industrialized West, had been shown in many studies to effect physiological attributes such as the pH of urine, vitamin deficiency, and serum ion levels, all of which could affect the way psychotropic drugs were metabolized in the body. Although Olatawura could not provide specific evidence that Nigerian patients had experienced anxiolytic and antidepressant drugs any differently than other groups, he suggested that this was primarily because of a lack of clinical trials of psychotropic drugs on African and Nigerian populations. He did note two studies indicating "excessive drowsiness and weakness" as side effects of chlorimipramine in Nigerians, and suggested that this might be an indication that "African populations might be better off on lower doses than recommended by manufacturers."[72] He also suggested that the better response of a group of Nigerian patients to injections of the drug than to pills might have been the result of a placebo effect brought about by cultural beliefs in the greater efficacy of injections.

The idea that Western drugs and theories about how to regulate their use were not as universally applicable as originally conceived in some ways mirrors Nigerian psychiatrists' concerns about the cultural inappropriateness of psychoanalytic psychotherapy discussed in previous chapters. Nigerian psychiatrists increasingly showed fears that the supposedly universal psychopharmacotherapies heralded not just a form of medical drug dependence for patients but a socioeconomic dependence of psychiatrists in developing countries on the products and theories coming out of wealthy and influential corporations in the West. For example, Lambo explained that when examining the effects of drugs on patients, African psychiatrists sometimes had to consult Western psychiatric literature filled with "psychological data based upon individuals in an entirely different society." In order to use the theories and practices of the Western psychiatric tradition, Lambo claimed they had to be manipulated to apply to African settings. The result was that "the application of these theories and concepts . . . to the African society by *ad hoc* investigators has sometimes been without the support of critical appraisal of the original research, and often by inference from an investigation designed for an entirely different purpose."[73] Lambo rejected the attitude that "the transfer, pure and simple, of methods employed in highly developed countries"[74] could effectively address the problems of drug use and abuse in African settings.

Amechi Anumonye also argued that the existing information available to less developed countries on drug dependence was "not always accurate," and lamented that "what is often handed down as authoritative information has in fact emanated from foreign countries"[75] without effort to ensure that the conclusions also applied to local circumstances. Even if the findings were accurate and transferrable, it did not necessarily mean that they represented the best possible approach to handling drug-related issues. "Must we follow the developed nations?" he queried. Anumonye made frequent reference to the ways things were done in the "over-developed" West, indicating a belief that Western development patterns were not necessarily the norm that Nigerians should be striving to achieve. Nigerian psychiatrists' perspective on their ability to control the use of psychopharmaceuticals was therefore linked in some ways to broader geopolitics and global economies, in which the promises of modernization of the 1950s and 1960s were giving way to patterns of underdevelopment, dependency, and neocolonialism by the 1970s.

By the early 1980s, Nigerians psychiatrists were also linking the crisis of psychopharmaceutical ubiquity to the failures of effective modernization in Nigeria. After years of political instability and mismanaged economies, Nigerian psychiatrists were perhaps more concerned about the effects of social decay on the general population in the 1980s than they had been in the 1960s. It was clear by this time that synthetic psychotropic drugs were no longer the highly regulated medical tools they were intended to be. Just as Nigerians had obtained greater access to a broad array of illicit drugs in the 1950s and 1960s, so, too, were they increasingly able to self-medicate using potent psychopharmaceuticals without the oversight of qualified medical practitioners. Nigerian psychiatrists showed a serious and repeated concern over the extent to which psychotropic drugs were being smuggled out of hospitals and used in nonmedical contexts. A study by Odejide of 691 civil service workers in Ibadan in 1982 showed that more than 95.5 percent of them had used a drug of one form or another without a prescription from a medical doctor. The most commonly used drugs were mild painkillers like paracetamol and aspirin, but much more potent analgesics were also well represented, such as codeine, which 32.5 percent of the study group claimed to have used. Psychotropic drugs were also well represented on the list, particularly tranquillo-sedatives. More than 40 percent of the civil servants questioned had used Valium without a prescription, 21.8 percent Phenergan, 14.4 percent Librium, and 3.6 percent Largactil (chlorpromazine).[76]

Nigerian psychiatrists blamed the use of psychotropic drugs without prescriptions on many different factors. Like other psychoactive drugs such as cannabis and alcohol, Nigerian psychiatrists saw popular abuse of prescription drugs as part of a broader sociocultural context of self-medication. Odejide noted that the vast majority of his subject group (94.6 percent) claimed to use these drugs only irregularly, "when they feel ill or tired." Only small minorities claimed to use the drugs for social purposes, a significant difference from cannabis or alcohol, but still supporting the notion that "self-medication is almost the norm in Nigerian society."[77] Olayiwola Erinosho, a sociologist from the University of Ibadan, linked desire for self-medication to mass-media advertisements of various drugs, "which are more or less given misleading captions" and directed toward an "illiterate population,"[78] thereby creating inappropriate desire for these drugs. However, the most despicable cause of all was the easy availability of these drugs without prescription. Nigerian psychiatrists lambasted the "indiscriminate sale of pharmaceuticals by pharmacists and medicine shop owners and vendors,"[79] lamenting that even though laws had existed since colonial times restricting the access and sale of medicines, "the society lacks the necessary machinery needed to enforce the rules and regulations which should govern access to these drugs."[80] As a result, "a Nigerian can literarily [*sic*] buy any kind of drug from any of the drug stores in the country."[81] Anumonye even implicated medical doctors, criticizing "the indiscriminate dispensing of medication by medically qualified doctors many of whom have private clinics and hospitals,"[82] and would presumably do anything to turn a profit. Erinosho proclaimed that the failure of the government to effectively control access to drugs was indicative of the lack of law and order in Nigerian society as a whole by the early 1980s.[83] This is another example of the extent to which by this time experts were beginning to suggest that foreign influence and rapid social change were no longer sufficient causative factors to explain drug abuse in Nigeria. Increasingly, experts were seeing the failures of the postindependence state as contributing to Nigerians' desire and ability to engage in illicit psychoactive drug use.

Psychiatric discourses about drug use in Nigeria changed from the 1950s to the 1980s, just as they changed in international spaces. An early hope that psychiatrists had found the "magic bullet" to treat psychological disorders gave way to concerns that too many people, many unqualified, were using those bullets to shoot too many people for the wrong reasons. Just as Nigerian psychiatrists saw themselves as the proper mediators to figure out how to develop "modern" psychotherapies for use on Nigerian patients in a time of transition, so, too, did they see themselves as suitable gatekeepers to stand between Nigerians and the psychoactive drugs that would help them cope with their surroundings. In establishing themselves as gatekeepers over mind-altering substances, it is important to note that their conceptions were idealistic: at no point did Nigerian psychiatrists ever control access to psychoactive drugs. Indeed, this was one of their chief complaints, particularly as the strong links between modernization, internationalization, and governmental development planning that had characterized the transition from colonial to transcultural psychiatry began to erode in the context of political instability and economic underdevelopment that occurred in Nigeria simultaneously with the rise of biomedical psychiatry and multinational pharmaceutical corporations.

However, examining the ways that Nigerian psychiatrists positioned themselves reveals patterns expressed throughout this book regarding the tenuous, negotiated space that they inhabited between indigenous and Western, between traditional and modern, and between arguing for the universal similarity of human psychology and understanding the particular social and cultural landscapes within which human psyches functioned. The paradoxes of psychoactive drug use were a ripe ground for such mediation, given the simultaneity of rapid political, social, and economic change in Nigeria with the psychopharmaceutical revolution within the psychiatric discipline. Nigerian psychiatrists recognized drug use, medical or otherwise, as a recent phenomenon in Nigeria inextricably linked to these changes but nevertheless increasingly entrenched in Nigerian medicine and society. And while Nigerian psychiatrists saw the influx of drugs as clear evidence of the ways the outside world was transforming Nigerian society, for better or worse, they also were aware of the extent to which Nigerians were themselves becoming a part of the outside world, with all the psychological consequences that entailed.

Conclusion

Nigerian Psychiatrists and the Globalization of Psychiatry

I WANT TO OFFER BY WAY OF CONCLUSION a brief explication of how sociopolitical factors came to shape the way that some psychiatrists around the world thought about the basic nature of mental illness from the mid- to late 1970s. At this time, the tenets of modernization and its universalizing tendencies were unraveling in the context of political and economic instability throughout the developing world, of which Nigeria was a part. At the same time, postmodernism, and with it postcolonial critiques of Western medicine and psychiatry, was on the ascendant in social and cultural studies. Transcultural psychiatry itself underwent a schism, as a new generation of anthropologically minded scholars began to reveal the contradictions and marginalizations that took place when applying the Western psychiatric rubric to non-Western peoples. Such critiques had always existed in transcultural psychiatry, but they became increasingly mainstream in an intellectual setting that now preferred splitting to lumping. The shift was not complete: it did not eradicate the universalizing tendencies of transcultural psychiatry, but it provided a new set of options for thinking about comparative psychiatry. The implications of this postmodern, postcolonial emphasis on contingency and cultural particularity have affected not just transcultural psychiatry, but also the way that scholars have thought about the history of psychiatry in non-Western places since the 1980s, with narratives of colonial power and indigenous resistance transforming into analyses of the complex negotiations of scientific knowledge, cultural categories, and individual subjectivities in the 2000s. I conclude by suggesting that an appreciation for connectivity and interrelatedness, rather than artificial categories like Western and non-Western, traditional and modern, opens new arenas of understanding the complexity of the globalization of psychiatry, by which our Nigerian psychiatrists were shaped and to which they most certainly contributed.

ỌDẸ ORÍ, OGBANJE, AND THE LIMITS OF UNIVERSALISM

As the previous chapters have indicated, the development of transcultural psychiatry both in Nigeria and internationally was linked to political and social commentaries about the relationship between race, culture, and human egalitarianism in the context of global movements for decolonization and civil rights. The incorporation of Africans into professional psychiatric theory and practice—both as practitioners and as patients—on equal terms was part of a broader struggle to bestow political rights and social dignity on all people universally, regardless of racial or cultural background. In this context, the differences that had been so accentuated in a geopolitical system based on racism and social evolutionism were repudiated and replaced by a newfound emphasis on the basic psychological similarities of all peoples. It did not work perfectly: the first generation of transcultural psychiatrists recognized the frayed edges and incongruities in the universalist model. For example, transcultural psychiatrists of the 1950s–1970s had been highly critical of the value of employing Western psychoanalytic techniques on non-Western patients who had different personal beliefs about the nature of their illnesses. And by the late 1960s, Raymond H. Prince was already questioning the extent to which cultural politics might be influencing new findings that depression was much more common in Africans than had previously been assumed.[1] Nevertheless, Nigerian transcultural psychiatrists like T. Adeoye Lambo, Tolani Asuni, and others believed that the Western-derived diagnostic categories of psychiatry were basic and "real," and that non-Westerners absolutely did experience schizophrenia, depression, anxiety, senility, et cetera, if in somewhat diverse ways that needed to be accounted for in the official criteria.

By the 1980s, however, some Nigerian psychiatrists were starting to question seriously the universality of those diagnostic categories. For example, in a 1982 article, Peter O. Ebigbo and U. H. Ihezue, of the Department of Psychological Medicine at the University of Nigeria, Enugu, conducted a study of the use of Western-derived psychiatric labels on patients with identical symptom classifications at the local hospital over the period from 1970 to 1979. They found that overall, "similar symptom clusters attract widely different diagnostic labels even in a single institution."[2] They were unable to determine if this diversity in diagnosis reflected "uncertainty on the part of the users of the labels" or "the inadequacy of these labels."[3] Either way, it suggested that psychiatric diagnostics were not being conducted in a universally similar way. These findings were confirmed by later studies that reinvigorated the debate about culture-bound syndromes in Nigerian populations. Although many Nigerian psychiatrists continued to argue against the culture-boundedness of brain-fag syndrome because of its etiological construct associated with detribalization and culture clash, some began to point out the explanatory power of some indigenous illness categories that predated the influx of European modernity and the extent to which they did not effectively fit the diagnostic categories upon which transcultural psychiatrists relied.

Two examples of Nigerian psychiatrists' renewed interest in culture-bound syndromes will suffice to illustrate this point. In 1987, Roger O. A. Makanjuola, of the Department of Mental Health at the University of Ifè, brought attention to the apparent incompatibility of ọdẹ orí with the categories and treatments of transcultural psychiatry. *Ọdẹ orí* is a widely recognized disease entity in Yoruba culture. Translated as "hunter of the head," it is characterized by a set of core symptoms, notably "a sensation of an organism crawling through the head and sometimes also other parts of the body, noises in the ears and palpitations," often accompanied by a variety of other somatic complaints. Traditional Yoruba healers claimed the cause of ọdẹ orí to be an *aràn*, a "worm, bug or relatively unformed organism" that entered the head of the victim and, from there, could migrate to other parts of the body. General consensus was that the worm was usually, but not always, put in the victim's head through the employment of supernatural powers.

For his comparison, Makanjuola identified thirty patients who had been admitted to the local hospital between 1982 and 1985, all of whom had been previously diagnosed with ọdẹ orí by a traditional healer. Of the thirty, five were male and twenty-five were female. Their mean age was thirty-six years within a range from sixteen to eighty. They were from a variety of different professional and educational backgrounds, from agricultural workers lacking formal education to professional and skilled workers with high European-education levels. All, however, were ethnically Yoruba.[4] Makanjuola found that the thirty patients complained to Western-trained psychiatrists of a great variety of symptoms. The following somatic symptoms were recorded in the test group: crawling sensations (25); noises in ears (22); palpitations (19);

peppery sensations (10); darkened vision (10); dizziness (9); and headaches (7). Accompanying somatic symptoms were a variety of psychological symptoms that the diagnosing psychiatrist was able to identify: depressed mood (25); tension pains (21); adverse evaluation of one's own physical health (20); insomnia (20); anxiety (18); fatigue (16); and worrying (12).[5]

The result of thirty years' worth of transcultural psychiatric research indicating that somatic symptoms in Africans were merely a masking effect for deeper psychological turmoil resulted in Western-trained psychiatrists' focusing much more heavily on the psychological symptoms to diagnose these patients. However, when it came to diagnosing these thirty patients, it became clear to Makanjuola that the supposedly universal categories in the psychiatrist's tool bag did not account very well for sufferers of ọdẹ orí. Although Raymond H. Prince had found it reasonable to classify ọdẹ orí as an example of a Yoruba "psychoneurosis,"[6] Makanjuola found that individuals in his test group received widely divergent diagnoses, both within and across the psychotic-neurotic divide. Overall, the thirty patients racked up ten different diagnoses among them: major depressive episode (10); schizophrenia (4); generalized anxiety disorder (4); atypical anxiety (3); atypical psychosis (2); dysthymic disorder (2); atypical depression (2); schizophreniform disorder (1); manic episode (1); and agoraphobia (1). The astounding lack of consensus about these patients, Makanjuola argued, came from an overvaluing of the psychological above the somatic symptoms in the diagnostic process, and, as a result, Makanjuola was forced to conclude that "the condition termed 'Ode Ori' by Yoruba traditional healers does not fit into any particular Western diagnostic category but rather consists of a syndrome of somatic, auditory and visually related symptoms which may occur in the context of a variety of Western clinical entities."[7]

The imprecise nature of the diagnoses resulted in fairly poor response to Western-derived psychotherapies as well. Makanjuola declared that some patients who were treated for mood disorders such as anxiety or depression with psychopharmacological agents saw their mood symptoms dissipate over time, but most patients, regardless of their diagnoses, continued to experience their somatic symptoms long after obtaining psychiatric care. Of the thirty patients, only nine saw a "complete disappearance of symptoms" after initial treatment, with at least seventeen of the remaining twenty-one continuing to complain of the primary somatic symptoms that defined ọdẹ orí. A one-year follow-up showed that only five out of the seventeen patients consulted no longer experienced symptoms of ọdẹ orí.

Makanjuola was well aware of the universalizing trend in transcultural psychiatry that had dominated diagnostic procedures, noting that since psychiatry in the Euro-American tradition had been practiced in West Africa in earnest after the Second World War, "the clinician's approach has been largely that of applying Western concepts of mental disorder to his clinical practice." He noted that with "few exceptions," indigenous symptom patterns had been "neatly fitted into Western-style diagnostic categories, any differences in symptomatology being explained away as culture-influenced modifications." He even noted the extent to which the supposedly culture-bound brain-fag syndrome had been reconceived as a variant within the more universal anxiety-depression spectrum. However, the failure of Western-derived psychotherapies to alleviate the somatic symptoms of ọdẹ orí led Makanjuola to make a startling suggestion. While he recognized that "it could be argued that the persistence of 'Ode Ori' symptoms represented merely persistence of residual depressive/anxiety symptoms," he found it "difficult to see why only the somatic symptoms would persist in those circumstances." Taking a bold leap, Makanjuola suggested that "it is just as feasible, though perhaps less acceptable to the Western trained psychiatrist that the depressive and anxiety symptoms found in these patients are secondary to an underlying disorder—'Ode Ori'!"[8] Makanjuola was clearly suggesting that there was no particular reason to believe that the categories used by transcultural psychiatrists represented basic, universal, cross-cultural "truth."

Another example that Nigerian psychiatrists employed to illustrate the important ways that cultural peculiarities were not accounted for in the universalizing discourse of transcultural psychiatry was the ogbanje/àbíkú concept held by many different groups in southern Nigeria. In essence, an *ogbanje* is a spirit that enters a woman's womb and is born as a human infant. The infant then dies and the spirit once more reincarnates in the woman's womb, repeating the process again and again. The constant loss of children causes serious psychological turmoil for the afflicted family, and some have argued that it has psychological implications for the surviving children in the family. In a 1990 article, Sunny T. C. Ilechukwu, of the Department of Psychiatry at the University of Lagos, came to the conclusion that those who believed themselves afflicted by ogbanje/àbíkú should be considered to be suffering from a culture-bound syndrome characterized by a variety of physical, psychological, and social symptoms, including "rapidity of progression of a physical condition or unexpected slowness of recovery from a minor ailment . . . unusual physical symptoms such as paralysis, blindness and non emotive weepiness said to be resistant to orthodox medical treatment; conduct disorder in children or adolescents; and rapidly changing social or economic circumstance,"[9] as well as visual hallucinations and dreams involving spiritual entities or physical objects associated with them. Ilechukwu noted that patients who reported to hospital wi[th a] history of ogbanje could often be effectively treated, although they elicited widely divergent diagnoses. At the same time, however, Ilechukwu recognized that "most of those who have easy access to the traditional remedies and faith healing services did not show up in hospital," indicating that these sources were probably quite effective at treating the illness in culturally appropriate ways. Overall, Ilechukwu concluded that ogbanje/àbíkú should be considered a culture-bound syndrome because "more sense seems to be conveyed by considerations of local beliefs about causation" than the etiological constructs of transcultural psychiatry.[10]

As these studies indicated, by the 1980s some Nigerian psychiatrists lacked confidence that their discipline had the capacity to treat certain culturally specific manifestations of mental illness. They simply could not be integrated seamlessly into transcultural psychiatry. This led to something of a reassessment of the relationship between psychiatrists and traditional healers. Makanjuola had noted that ọdẹ orí did not respond very well to psychopharmaceutical treatment. While Ilechukwu noted that ogbanje could be addressed in Western medical terms somewhat successfully, he argued that as a discreet entity it was probably better treated by traditional healers. Ebigbo and Ihezue believed that a significant part of the reason behind diagnostic confusion was that patients themselves internalized different concepts of mental illness, having been exposed to multiple cultural belief systems in their lives. In these cases, understanding of the cultural background of the patient mattered not just in providing a reasonable diagnosis, but also in the treatment plan. Unlike Lambo, Prince, and other transcultural psychiatrists of the previous generation who struggled to integrate traditional health systems with modern psychiatry, Ebigbo and Ihezue seemed to treat the two as separate but equal. They argued that the Western-trained psychiatrist "should not hesitate to send a patient to a traditional healer if he becomes too unsure of the symptom presentation."[11] Makanjuola criticized the efforts of transcultural psychiatrists like Prince, who had tried to explain the practices of "traditional healers" as essentially psychotherapy without insight, arguing that "while it is likely that psychological (or 'psychotherapeutic') factors do play a role in traditional healing, it would appear presumptuous to explain away the traditional healer's practice in this manner."[12] The idea that traditional healers might deserve more respect because of their differences from rather than similarities to Western-trained psychiatrists was part of a new turn in transcultural psychiatry that was much less idealistic about the notions of modernization that had dominated the period from the 1950s to the 1970s.

POSTMODERNISM, POSTCOLONIALISM, AND "THE NEW CROSS-CULTURAL PSYCHIATRY"

The reemphasizing of cultural particularities and probing of the limits of universal constructs that developed from the 1970s should be seen as embedded in two interrelated contexts. First, while the universalizing tendencies of transcultural psychiatry in the 1950s–1970s had been imbued with an optimism and idealism that non-Western societies were destined for "modernization" once freed from the shackles of racism and colonial oppression, the 1970s saw a slow but steady erosion in the belief that modernization based on the adoption of universal principles in their Western-derived forms was feasible. In Nigeria, the obvious failures of modernization had consequences in terms of the state's capacity to safeguard mental health—both through widespread political and economic instability and through the continued underdevelopment of the country's psychiatric service sector. Internationally, the recognition of the plights of countries like Nigeria and so many others in the Third World led to a serious intellectual critiquing of modernization and universalism in general. The emergence of postmodernism and postcolonialism eschewed the notion of a universal, objective reality through a focus on the interpretively compromised nature of knowledge production. Second, the rise of the postmodern and postcolonial critiques coincided with an increased emphasis on cultural differences within transcultural psychiatry known as "the new cross-cultural psychiatry." I do not mean to suggest here that any of these factors caused another, but that all were developing simultaneously, influencing and influenced by one another both in Nigeria and elsewhere.

To say that Nigeria has experienced serious political and economic instability in the postindependence era is an understatement. The efforts to forge a pluralistic, multicultural federation have proved extremely difficult. Rather than developing a strong Nigerian national identity, ethnic and religious identities have hardened, resulting in political strife and violence that have characterized much of the period since 1960 in many parts of the country.[13] Most disastrously, the civil war of 1967–70 revealed the fundamental differences that a great many Nigerians felt separated them from one another.[14] Divisions within the country have fueled political instability at the national level. As a result, Nigeria has been governed by military dictatorships for twenty-nine of its first fifty-two years since independence. Corruption, inefficiency, and unaccountability have been defining characteristics of most regimes, civilian and military, since 1960.[15] Mismanagement of resources and an increasing reliance on petroleum revenues resulted in a political economy that was significantly indebted to foreign interests and dependent on international markets by the late 1970s.[16] Debt crises and structural adjustment processes in the 1980s resulted in increasing rates of poverty throughout the country as social services declined.[17] Urbanization continued unabated, and, without a social service sector that could effectively coordinate and provide education, employment opportunities, health care, and other valuable resources, the social problems that Nigerian psychiatrists associated with the transition to "modernity" in the 1950s and 1960s had been exacerbated rather than alleviated by the 1980s.

The economic problems of Nigeria certainly caused a great deal of strain on the mental health of Nigerians, but beyond this, from the perspective of Nigerian psychiatrists, the poor economy hampered their own ability to provide mental health services to large numbers of people. High inflation and increasing unemployment rates meant that the majority of Nigerians did not have the expendable income necessary to acquire orthodox biomedical services of any kind, let alone psychiatric services. At the same time, the health service sector remained chronically underresourced throughout the postindependence period.[18] As time went on, availability of psychiatric services did not keep pace with the growing population of Nigeria. Nowhere is this more evident than in the fate of the Aro Village Scheme that had brought so much acclaim to Nigeria. By 1981, only the main Abule Aro village was still in operation out of the original four villages organized by Lambo in the 1950s.[19] By 2000, Boroffka noted that even this village had "disappeared."[20] Efforts have continued to expand services into state and local areas,[21] but it is clear that the modernization of psychiatric services in Nigeria has not come to pass in the way Lambo, Asuni, and others had envisioned.

Nigerian psychiatrists made frequent references to the effects that the resource crunch had on their ability to provide optimal psychiatric care by Western standards. They also made oblique references to the political and social problems of Nigeria. They occasionally referenced Nigeria as a country in "turmoil," and made clear that urbanization, poverty, and poor governance contributed to the psychological burdens that Nigerians carried.[22] Surprisingly little has been said about the effects of the two-and-a-half-year civil war that ravaged the country between 1967 and 1970, in which the Eastern Region of Nigeria attempted to secede from the federation and become the independent Republic of Biafra. However, when psychiatrists have mentioned the civil war, it has indubitably been to note its negative psychological impact. Ebie and Pela argued that the war led to increased drug abuse among soldiers as a means of coping with the conflict.[23] Benjamin O. Osuntokun and Alexander Boroffka identified what they considered to be a peculiar form of deaf-mutism that often developed in soldiers after the war. They compared it with the post-traumatic disorder that came to be known as "shell shock" in the post-WWI context in Europe and the United States.[24] Interestingly, I have found only one study that examined the psychological effects of the war on the civilian population. In 1971, S. Ejiofo Mbanefo conducted an epidemiological survey of refugees in Onitsha and found that roughly two-thirds of his test group qualified as "cases," the overwhelming majority of whom he diagnosed as experiencing depression of one sort or another. He further found that "the war did significantly upset the functional efficiency of approximately 48 percent of the respondents,"[25] a claim that had clear implications not only for the mental health of individuals but also for the development prospects of the country as a whole. A. Kalunta, of the Psychiatric and Nervous Diseases Hospital in Aba, reported anecdotally in 1981 that suicide rates had increased significantly during and after the war.[26]

The problems that Nigeria experienced in its first two decades of independence were systemic throughout much of Africa. By the late 1970s, modernization was falling out of vogue. Political economists and historians, including Andre Gunder Frank, Walter Rodney, and Samir Amin, produced influential scholarly works arguing that the package linking economic development to specific social, cultural, and political institutions based on Western models was a farce. The universalist discourse of modernization, they argued, had proved itself to be nothing but a neocolonialist agenda to keep the Third World dependent upon the West through the rigging of a perpetually uneven playing field.[27] Simultaneously, postmodernist critiques in the humanities began to focus on undermining notions of universal truths. They argued for all knowledge to be seen as contingent and constructed. Postcolonialist critiques from the late 1970s on equally sought to decouple ideas about the nature of knowledge production and consumption from their Western universalist underpinnings.[28] Solutions-oriented scholars argued that struggling countries needed to stop looking to apply Western models as cure-alls and instead focus on finding local solutions for complex local problems. At this time, histories of colonial psychiatry began to illustrate the nefarious relationship between knowledge about the human mind and the power of predominating, particularly Western, political and social structures.

Using similar theoretical reasoning, medical anthropology, which had previously claimed much of its relevance in terms of helping the implementation of public health interventions by bridging "modern" science with "traditional" cultures, took a relativist turn, with researchers increasingly interested in understanding discreet health systems on their own terms.[29] Although the notion of cultural relativity in anthropological interpretation dates back to Ruth Benedict's work in the 1930s, its impact on notions of psychiatric epidemiology was not strongly felt until the 1970s with the "birth" of the "new cross-cultural psychiatry," in which medical anthropologists began to emphasize the cultural rather than the biological basis for understanding the nature of health and illness. As Byron J. Good has stated, the work of Arthur M. Kleinman, a clinical instructor in the Department of Psychiatry and a lecturer in the Department of Anthropology at Harvard, both "sparked—and paralleled" developments in what Good calls the "meaning centered" approach to medical anthropology, in which "disease is not an entity but an explanatory model."[30] Anthropological works attempting to understand health systems, including Western biomedical ones, in terms of culturally constructed representations and interpretations began to fill the pages of the journal *Culture, Medicine, and Psychiatry* from 1977.

These shifting tides in intellectual inquiry had directly influenced developments in transcultural psychiatry by the late 1970s.[31] In "Depression, Somatization and the 'New Cross-Cultural Psychiatry,'" Kleinman articulated the concerns of cross-cultural psychiatrists at the time of the postmodern and postcolonial turn. He argued that unlike the "old transcultural psychiatry," which had focused on "a breathless search through large amounts of data from different societies looking for 'universals,'" the "new cross-cultural psychiatry" centered on "an interdisciplinary framework drawing off both anthropological and more recent psychiatric investigations of culture and illness."[32] Whereas the old transcultural psychiatry minimized cultural differences, the new cross-cultural psychiatry embraced in-depth analysis of "the ways culture influences the perception, classification, process of labeling, explanation, experience of symptoms, course, decisions regarding, and treatment of sickness."[33] Kleinman's primary argument was that the old transcultural psychiatry had committed a "category fallacy" in adopting preexisting disease entities in the Euro-American psychiatric tradition as the "natural" norms into which all other cultural expressions of mental illness must be fitted. Kleinman argued that Western disease constructs were themselves culture-bound and therefore poor fits for explaining the diverse ways that people expressed and experienced psychological distress around the world. By defining the criteria for diagnosis in strict terms with specified symptom clusters, transcultural psychiatrists had predetermined that they would always "*find* what is 'universal' and systematically *miss* what does not fit its tight parameters."[34] In other words, the old transcultural psychiatrists could find universals by diagnosing based on only symptoms that they recognized and ignoring or dismissing anything that did not fit their models, as in the ọdẹ orí cases examined by Makanjuola above.

As an anthropologist, Kleinman found this approach self-defeating. Sickness, he argued, was a product of two interrelated phenomena: *disease*, "the malfunctioning or maladaptation of biological or psychological processes"; and *illness*, "the personal, interpersonal, and cultural reaction to the disease."[35] Even in places where a universal "disease" could be identified (and Kleinman was by no means convinced that most psychiatric disorders fit this criteria), patients would experience illness differently. Both disease and illness needed to be addressed in order for patients to be effectively reintegrated into society. However, Kleinman argued that to date transcultural psychiatrists had cared about culture only as a mirage that they needed to see beyond in order to identify and "cure" the underlying disease. As a result, psychiatry had a poor record of "healing" the illnesses that different cultures—Western and non-Western—manifested in relationship with the disease. This approach exacerbated misunderstanding about the relationship between disease, illness, and culture; and fostered distrust and resentment of psychiatrists on the part of ailing patients, their families, and therapeutic communities. The new cross-cultural psychiatry's renewed focus on cultural particularities was meant to counter the universalizing aspects of biomedical structures and open new doors in comparative research and clinical practice.

Research using the methods of the new cross-cultural psychiatry in cultural settings around the world began to seriously complicate previously held notions of the universality of a wide range of psychosocial phenomena. Cross-cultural psychiatrists of the new school argued that all cultures, and even therapeutic communities within cultures, categorized and interpreted sicknesses in unique ways. Sometimes these categories and interpretations overlapped with those of Western biomedicine, but often they did not. Differences in definitions of health and illness across cultures were often linked to differing conceptions of the nature of the self vis-à-vis the larger community. While Western biomedicine had tended to see sickness as residing within the individual, other cultures sometimes assumed a collective responsibility for sickness. Such a conception affected therapeutic regimens, as collective healing was often necessary for overcoming an illness. Different cultures had different conceptions of range of emotion, and translations from language to language were recognized as far from perfect. In these medically plural environments where communication between cultural health systems was so fraught, patients made decisions about which treatment modalities to accept based on a wide range of layered knowledges, not just a lack of access to Western medical facilities.[36] Such being the case, Roland Littlewood argued that the only universal in psychotherapeutic terms was that of "a universality located in context-dependent meaning rather than in universal process."[37] The new cross-cultural psychiatry was coming down on the position that while biological "diseases" might affect human bodies in relatively universal ways, the ways that people expressed illness—whether biological or social—could indeed be fundamentally different across cultures and, as a result, were not likely to be better understood by force-fitting them into universal constructs. Such perspectives reflect the attitudes taken by Makanjuola and Ilechukwu regarding ọdẹ orí and obganje/àbíkú, respectively, by the mid-1980s.

The complexities that the new cross-cultural psychiatry emphasized were not new knowledge per se. Followers of the old transcultural psychiatry had been well aware of the imperfections in its universalist model. However, whereas followers of the old transcultural psychiatry had faith that over time and through sound research techniques the anomalies and unknowns could be accounted for, proponents of the new cross-cultural psychiatry argued that it was time to move on. In a sociopolitical context that had seen difference as inherently unequal, an emphasis on universal similarities made sense. Because of the success of the old transcultural psychiatry in eroding hierarchical notions of the psychology of human races and cultures, the new cross-cultural psychiatry was no longer as encumbered by the racist legacies of colonial ethnopsychiatry, and was in a position to argue that thirty years of research had not, in fact, tied up the loose ends that the old transcultural psychiatry had chosen to ignore in pursuance of a larger goal. For the new cross-cultural psychiatry, Western-derived psychiatric methods were not proving particularly more effective for classifying and treating mental illness in non-Westerners. Maybe cultural healing systems could not be fully integrated into one another, and maybe that was okay, even good. The new cross-cultural psychiatry certainly had its critics,[38] and most practicing psychiatrists continued to rely heavily on the universal categories laid out in the *Diagnostic and Statistical Manual of Mental Disorders* (*DSM*), the third edition of which was released in 1980, with a fourth edition following in 1994 and a fifth in 2013.[39] While the new cross-cultural psychiatry did not transform the practice of psychiatry in general, it did bring to the fore some of the concerns that had always lingered beneath the surface of the old transcultural psychiatry. It created a space within psychiatric discourse to talk about the ways that disease and illness categories were themselves socially and politically constructed and that, as a result, these categories were likely to be distinctly different as social and political circumstances changed across space and over time.

NIGERIAN PSYCHIATRISTS AND THE GLOBALIZATION OF PSYCHIATRY

The postmodern and postcolonial repudiation of the objective reality of Western-derived knowledge constructs has been reflected in more than just the development of the new cross-cultural psychiatry that Nigerian psychiatrists were engaging with by the 1980s: it is also the single most important theoretical influence on the history of psychiatry in non-Western parts of the world since this time. However, as important as the postcolonial critique has been to our recognition of the interrelatedness of psychiatric knowledge production and the political and social ideologies of European colonialism, it has tended to minimize the debates that emerged in transcultural psychiatry and, more important for our purposes, of non-Western contributors to them in the postcolonial context. The narrative emphasis on unidirectional power/knowledge flows emanating from the West and resisted or assimilated by the rest has resulted in something of a historical lacuna in which the characteristics and categories of colonial psychiatry have too often been used to describe the processes of the global networks of psychiatric knowledge production and dissemination that have developed since the 1950s.

In essence, critiques of these global networks of psychiatry are similar to critiques of economic and cultural globalization that emerged in the 1990s, which argued that the unipolar geopolitics of the post–Cold War era was producing a homogenized, Westernized world at the expense of any and all cultural uniqueness.[40] In the same way that critics of globalization argued that the emerging global consumer culture has provided a vapid, shallow set of values and symbols designed to appeal cross-culturally to a lowest common denominator, critics of psychiatry have argued that the spread of so-called "Western" psychiatric principles are redefining what were once culturally meaningful expressions of illness in terms appropriate to the values and symbols of a Western-dominated "globalization." One such example of this kind of analysis is Ethan Watters's journalistic treatment of the "globalization of the American psyche."[41] For the most part, Watters treats psychiatry in the contemporary context as a distinctly American thing: hence its globalization is considered to be an example of the Americanization of the world. Watters critiques the rising influence of multinational psychopharmaceutical companies and the intermittent cultural insensitivity of disaster relief agencies effectively, but to consider such entities as representatives of a solely American health system reinforces the notion that Westerners are the only ones who produce and disseminate psychiatric knowledge, and that non-Westerners, with their "traditional" cultures, are simply the recipients of that knowledge, and to their own detriment at that. Such contemporary critiques of the "globalization" of psychiatry thus elide over the transformations to knowledge, theory, and networks that occurred in the period of decolonization and political independence in order to construct an anachronistic Western psychiatric behemoth that is both culturally alien and mostly destructive.[42]

But this book has presented Nigerian psychiatrists as a thread in the tapestry of scholarship that seeks to decouple notions of psychiatric globalization and universalism from a geographically and ideologically constrained "Westernity." The discourse describing globalization as a binary conflict between the West and the rest has been seriously complicated in the first decade of the twenty-first century, in both historical and social-scientific terms. While the explicit study of "globalization" as a distinct phenomenon emerged among social scientists in the post–Cold War setting, historians have now shed light on the extent to which the processes used to describe the new "age of globalization"—rapid technological change, increased capital flows, international and transnational connectivity, and so on—were by no means new phenomena in the 1990s, although their scale may have been.[43] Debates about the appropriate definition, chronology, and central characteristics of globalization rage, but suffice to say, it is now recognized as a phenomenon that encompasses not only the spread of Western knowledge, values, and products around the world, but also the integration of non-Western tastes and perspectives into complex, multidirectional transnational flows.[44] Likewise, histories of psychiatry in non-Western parts of the world have begun to examine postcolonial contexts and to illuminate the highly complex relationships that characterize the construction of postmodern and postcolonial subjectivities in times of widespread transition, transformation, and disorder.[45] Along these lines, I hope to have shown here that while it is reasonable to consider psychiatry in the twentieth century to be "universalizing" or "globalizing," it was not "Western," "Euro-American," or "orthodox" in its totality; in fact, psychiatry was becoming less these things all the time through the incorporation of non-Western political, cultural, and professional realities into its knowledge production and dissemination processes.

Recognizing the ways Nigerian psychiatrists engaged with local, national, and international dynamics as well as universalist discourses is important not only for how we conceptualize the history of psychiatry in more global terms; it is important for how we conceptualize the histories of Nigerians, Africans, and all non-Westerners in relation to global processes more generally. The linking of psychiatric knowledge production and implementation to a strictly Western agency reinforces tautological notions in world history that Euro-American cultures have the capacity to impact the rest of the world but not the other way around. Perhaps more disturbing for historians, it implies that only Western cultures are capable of frequent and endogenous change, while non-Western cultures remain static until threatened by exogenous forces. In this context, non-Westerners can be posited in only one of two ways: either as passive accepters of an overwhelming force or as valiant resisters in the struggle against racism, oppression, and imperialism. Both options are interpretively fraught in terms of the global perspective. If non-Westerners engage with "Western" values, global processes, or universalizing discourses, then they contribute only to the "Westernization" of themselves and their cultures, not, for example, to the "Yorubazation," "Nigerianization," or "Africanization" of the West or the world. Conversely, if they are presented primarily as resisters then they can serve only a particular constituency: a cultural, racial, or national group depending on the narrative scope and not the interests of a global humanity or universal science. Non-Western impact beyond the local environment remains obscured if this narrative structure prevails.

This book has sought to complicate the dynamics of professional psychiatry in Nigeria and the rest of the world in the second half of the twentieth century, as global power structures shifted, as ideologies of Western imperialism were challenged and transformed, and as non-Western voices sought incorporation into universal narratives on equal rather than hierarchical terms. I do not want to suggest in any way that psychiatry as a medical discipline is not deserving of the postmodern and postcolonial criticisms that have been leveled at it; rather, I want to suggest that those criticisms reflect broader problems of representations of peoples and cultures that transcend psychiatric discourse. For more than twenty years, histories of medicine and psychiatry have sought to break down artificial dichotomies between colonizer/colonized, traditional/modern, and science/belief at local and national levels, and are now beginning to bring the fruits of those interpretive approaches to international and global subjects. The examination of Nigerian psychiatrists in the contexts of decolonization and postcolonial experience illustrates possible ways that a deprovincializing of non-Western histories of psychiatry and an engagement with the transnational, international, and global processes of psychiatric knowledge production can help to restructure the frameworks through which we write histories of postcolonial psychiatry.

Notes

INTRODUCTION: COLONIZING, DECOLONIZING, AND GLOBALIZING THE HISTORY OF PSYCHIATRY

Epigraph: Quoted in T. Adeoye Lambo, ed., *First Pan-African Psychiatric Conference, Abeokuta, Nigeria* (Ibadan: Government Printer, 1961), 11–12.

1. Ibid., v.

2. Ibid., 15–16.

3. Ibid., 20.

4. Ibid., v.

5. The terms "transcultural" and "cross-cultural" are often used interchangeably to describe this subfield of psychiatry. I have chosen to use the term "transcultural" in this book as a reference to the group of psychiatrists at McGill University in Montreal who in the 1950s founded the *Transcultural Psychiatric Research Newsletter,* which later became the *Transcultural Psychiatric Research Review,* the first academic journal dedicated specifically to comparative cross-cultural psychiatric research. "Cross-cultural" is used to reference a split that occurred within transcultural psychiatry in the 1970s between those who believed in the universalizing elements of the discipline and those who thought that universal application of Western psychiatric categories had actually resulted in the undermining of the important role that cultural factors played in the specific form and presentation of mental illnesses. See the conclusion in this book for more on the development of the new cross-cultural psychiatry.

6. Lambo, *First Pan-African Psychiatric Conference,* 1.

7. Frederick Cooper, "Conflict and Connection: Rethinking Colonial African History," *American Historical Review* 99, no. 5 (1994): 1517.

8. This literature focuses a lot on epidemic diseases and control measures instituted by colonial governments ostensibly to prevent their outbreak and spread, many of which had devastating social consequences. See, for example, Megan Vaughan, *Curing Their Ills: Colonial Power and African Illness* (Stanford, CA: Stanford University Press, 1991); Terence Ranger and Paul Slack, eds., *Epidemics and Ideas: Essays on the Historical Perception of Pestilence* (Cambridge: Cambridge University Press, 1992); David Arnold, ed., *Imperial Medicine and Indigenous Societies* (Manchester: Manchester University Press, 1992); and Myron J. Echenberg, *Black Death, White Medicine: Bubonic Plague and the Politics of Public Health in Colonial Senegal, 1914–1945* (Portsmouth, NH: Heinemann, 2002).

9. For example, Philip D. Curtin, "Medical Knowledge and Urban Planning in Tropical Africa," *American Historical Review* 90, no. 3 (1985): 594–613; see also Echenberg, *Black Death, White Medicine.*

10. As in, for example, Randall M. Packard, *White Plague, Black Labor: Tuberculosis and the Political Economy of Health and Disease in South Africa* (Berkeley: University of California Press, 1989); and Maryinez Lyons, *The Colonial Disease: A Social History of Sleeping Sickness in Northern Zaire, 1900–1940* (Cambridge: Cambridge University Press, 1992).

11. See, for example, Philippa Levine, *Prostitution, Race, and Politics: Policing Venereal Disease in the British Empire* (New York: Routledge, 2003).

12. Megan Vaughan, "Idioms of Madness: Zomba Lunatic Asylum, Nyasaland, in the Colonial Period," *Journal of Southern African Studies* 9, no. 2 (1983): 218–38.

13. Leland V. Bell, *Mental and Social Disorder in Sub-Saharan Africa: The Case of Sierra Leone, 1787–1990* (Westport, CT: Greenwood Press, 1991); Jock McCulloch, *Colonial Psychiatry and "The African Mind"* (Cambridge: Cambridge University Press, 1995); and Jonathan H. Sadowsky, *Imperial Bedlam: Institutions of Madness in Colonial Southwest Nigeria* (Berkeley: University of California Press, 1999). Also on Nigeria's asylums, see Alexander Boroffka, "A History of Psychiatry in Nigeria," *Psychiatry* 8 (1985): 709–14; and Boroffka, "The History of Mental Hospitals in Nigeria," *Psychiatry* 8 (1985): 37–43. On South African asylums, see Harriet J. Deacon, "Madness, Race and Moral Treatment: Robben Island Lunatic Asylum, Cape Colony, 1846–1890," *History of Psychiatry* 7 (1996): 287–97; Julie Parle, "The Fools on the Hill: The Natal Government Asylum and the Institutionalisation of Insanity in Colonial Natal," *Journal of Natal and Zulu History* 19 (2001): 1–40; and Sally Swartz, "Colonizing the Insane: Causes of Insanity in the Cape, 1891–1920," *History of the Human Sciences* 8, no. 4 (1995): 39–57. On Zimbabwe, see Lynette A. Jackson, *Surfacing Up: Psychiatry and Social Order in Colonial Zimbabwe, 1908–1968* (Ithaca, NY: Cornell University Press, 2005). For the Maghreb, see Richard C. Keller, *Colonial Madness: Psychiatry in French North Africa* (Chicago: University of Chicago Press, 2007). Other historical works on Algeria's asylums include Jean-Michel Bégué, "French Psychiatry in Algeria (1830–1962): From Colonial to Transcultural," *History of Psychiatry* 7 (1996): 533–48. For a compilation of a variety of different contexts both within and beyond Africa, see Sloan Mahone and Megan Vaughan, eds., *Psychiatry and Empire* (New York: Palgrave Macmillan, 2007).

14. Sadowsky, *Imperial Bedlam.*

15. Michel Foucault, *Madness and Civilization: A History of Insanity in the Age of Reason,* trans. Richard Howard (New York: Vintage, 1965); and Frantz Fanon, *The Wretched of the Earth*, trans. Constance Farrington (New York: Monthly Review Press, 1978), first published 1961. Fanon's ideas about the psychological impact of racist ideologies on colonial subjects are also central to his earlier work, Frantz Fanon, *Black Skin, White Masks,* trans. Charles Lam Markmann (New York: Grove Press, 1967), first published 1952. His argument that only through revolution could colonial subjects free themselves of the "primitive" label that they had been given and embrace an indigenous "modernity" is best elaborated in Frantz Fanon, *A Dying Colonialism,* trans. Haakon Chevalier (New York: Grove Press, 1965), first published 1959.

16. Keller, *Colonial Madness,* 83–120.

17. Jonathan H. Sadowsky, "The Confinements of Isaac O.: A Case of 'Acute Mania' in Colonial Nigeria," *History of Psychiatry* 7 (1996): 91–112.

18. See Jean Comaroff and John L. Comaroff, "The Madman and the Migrant: Work and Labor in the Historical Consciousness of a South African People," *American Ethnologist* 14, no. 2 (1987): 191–209.

19. Steven Feierman, "Struggles for Control: The Social Roots of Health and Healing in Modern Africa," *African Studies Review* 28, nos. 2–3 (1985): 73–147.

20. As any history of psychiatric institutions in European contexts can easily demonstrate. See, for example, Roy Porter, *Mind Forg'd Manacles: A History of Madness in England from the Restoration to the Regency* (Cambridge, MA: Harvard University Press, 1987); and Andrew Scull, *Social Order/Mental Disorder: Anglo-American Psychiatry in Historical Perspective* (London: Routledge, 1989).

21. For this interpretation, see, for example, Thomas S. Szasz, *The Manufacture of Madness: A Comparative Study of the Inquisition and the Mental Health Movement* (New York: Dell, 1970). Szasz's more famous work, *The Myth of Mental Illness: Foundations of a Theory of Personal Conduct* (New York: Hoeber-Harper, 1961), is also a useful example.

22. Shula Marks, "What Is Colonial about Colonial Medicine? And What has Happened to Imperialism and Health?," *Social History of Medicine* 10, no. 2 (1997): 205–19.

23. David Arnold, *Colonizing the Body: State Medicine and Epidemic Disease in Nineteenth-Century India* (Berkeley: University of California Press, 1993).

24. Daniel R. Headrick, *The Tools of Empire: Technology and European Imperialism in the Nineteenth Century* (Oxford: Oxford University Press, 1991).

25. Richard Grove, *Green Imperialism: Colonial Expansion, Tropical Island Edens and the Origins of Environmentalism, 1600–1860* (Cambridge: Cambridge University Press, 1995); Richard H. Drayton, *Nature's Government: Science, Imperial Britain, and the "Improvement" of the World* (New Haven, CT: Y ale University Press, 2000); and Michael Adas, *Machines as the Measure of Men: Science, Technology, and Ideologies of Western Dominance* (Ithaca, NY: Cornell University Press, 1989).

26. Discussed in more detail in chapter 5. See Warwick P. Anderson, Deborah Jenson, and Richard C. Keller, eds., *Unconscious Dominions: Psychoanalysis, Colonial Trauma, and Global Sovereignties* (Durham, NC: Duke University Press, 2011).

27. Keller, *Colonial Madness*, 121–60.

28. Ashis Nandy, "The Savage Freud: The First Non-Western Psychoanalyst and the Politics of Secret Selves in Colonial India," in *The Savage Freud and Other Essays on Possible and Retrievable Selves* (Princeton, NJ: Princeton University Press, 1995), 81–144; Sudhir Kakar, *Culture and Psyche: Psychoanalysis and India* (New York: Psyche Press, 1996).

29. Alice Bullard, "Imperial Networks and Postcolonial Independence: The Transition from Colonial to Transcultural Psychiatry," in Mahone and Vaughan, *Psychiatry and Empire*, 197–219.

30. Didier Fassin, "Ethnopsychiatry and the Postcolonial Encounter: A French Psychopolitics of Otherness," in Anderson, Jenson, and Keller, *Unconscious Dominions*, 223–46.

31. Sloan Mahone and Megan Vaughan, introduction to *Psychiatry and Empire*, 3.

32. Warwick P. Anderson, "Where Is the Postcolonial History of Medicine?," *Bulletin of the History of Medicine* 72 (1998): 522–30.

33. A point emphasized by Frederick Cooper in *Colonialism in Question: Theory, Knowledge, History* (Berkeley: University of California Press, 2005).

34. See, for example, Tracy J. Luedke and Harry G. West, eds., *Borders and Healers: Brokering Therapeutic Resources in Southeast Africa* (Bloomington: Indiana University Press, 2006).

35. As discussed throughout Anderson, Jenson, and Keller, *Unconscious Dominions*.

36. Byron J. Good, *Medicine, Rationality, and Experience: An Anthropological Perspective* (Cambridge: Cambridge University Press, 1994), 25–64.

37. John M. Janzen, *The Quest for Therapy: Medical Pluralism in Lower Zaire* (Berkeley: University of California Press, 1978); and Arthur M. Kleinman, *Patients and Healers in the Context of Culture: An Exploration of the Borderland between Anthropology, Medicine, and Psychiatry* (Berkeley: University of California Press, 1980).

38. As in João Biehl, Byron J. Good, and Arthur M. Kleinman, *Subjectivity: Ethnographic Investigations* (Berkeley: University of California Press, 2007); and Mary-Jo DelVecchio Good, Sandra T. Hyde, Sarah Pinto, and Byron J. Good, eds., *Postcolonial Disorders* (Berkeley: University of California Press, 2008).

39. Cooper, "Conflict and Connection," 1517.

40. For a background on the history of modernization theory and its critics, see Colin Leys, *The Rise and Fall of Development Theory* (Bloomington: Indiana University Press, 1996).

41. Dipesh Chakrabarty, *Provincializing Europe: Postcolonial Thought and Historical Difference* (Princeton, NJ: Princeton University Press, 2000).

42. Cooper, *Colonialism in Question*.

43. On Africanist historiography, with particular emphasis on developments in Nigeria, see "African Glories: Nationalist Historiography," in Toyin Falola, *Nationalism and African Intellectuals* (Rochester, NY: University of Rochester Press, 2001), 223–60.

44. Eric J. Hobsbawm and Terence Ranger, *The Invention of Tradition* (Cambridge: Cambridge University Press, 1983).

45. Foundational works in this field include Feierman, "Struggles for Control"; and Janzen, *Quest for Therapy*; as well as their coedited volume, Steven Feierman and John M. Janzen, eds., *The Social Basis of Health and Healing in Africa* (Berkeley: University of California Press, 1992). A more recent elucidation of the shifting sands of "traditional" health systems and "modern" medicine can be found in Karen E. Flint, *Healing Traditions: African Medicine, Cultural Exchange, and Competition in South Africa, 1820–1948* (Athens: Ohio University Press, 2008).

46. A primary point of Flint, *Healing Traditions*.

47. See H. B. M. Murphy, "The Historical Development of Transcultural Psychiatry," in *Transcultural Psychiatry*, ed. John L. Cox (London: Croom Helm, 1986); Jatinder Bains, "Race, Culture and Psychiatry: A History of Transcultural Psychiatry," *History of Psychiatry* 16, no. 2 (2005): 139–54.

48. Flint, *Healing Traditions*, 25.

49. See, for example, Adell Patton Jr., *Physicians, Colonial Racism, and Diaspora in West Africa* (Gainesville: University of Florida Press, 1996); and John Iliffe, *East African Doctors: A History of the Modern Profession* (Cambridge: Cambridge University Press, 1998).

50. Frederick Cooper has even argued that the nation-state as a construct is an extremely recent development in Western Europe, considering how long most of them were, in fact, imperial states whose identity politics were bound up with transnational phenomena for most of the "modern" history of Europe. See Cooper, *Colonialism in Question*, 22–24.

51. Murray Last, "Introduction: The Professionalisation of African Medicine: Ambiguities and Definitions," in *The Professionalisation of African Medicine*, ed. Murray Last and G. L. Chavunduka (Manchester: Manchester University Press, 1986), 10.

52. Leys, *Development Theory*.

53. George Basalla, "The Spread of Western Science," *Science* 156 (1967): 611–22.

54. David W. Chambers and Richard Gillespie, "Locality in the History of Science: Colonial Science, Technoscience, and Indigenous Knowledge," *Osiris* 15 (2000): 221–40.

55. Kapil Raj, *Relocating Modern Science: Circulation and the Construction of Knowledge in South Asia and Europe, 1650–1900* (New York: Palgrave Macmillan, 2007).

56. See Grove, *Green Imperialism*; Drayton, *Nature's Government*; and Headrick, *Tools of Empire*.

57. For more on this, see the historiographical discussion of networks in the British Empire in Alan Lester, "Imperial Circuits and Networks: Geographies of the British Empire," *History Compass* 4, no. 1 (2006): 124–41.

58. Joseph M. Hodge, *Triumph of the Expert: Agrarian Doctrines of Development and the Legacies of British Colonialism* (Athens: Ohio University Press, 2007).

59. Penny M. Von Eschen, *Race against Empire: Black Americans and Anticolonialism, 1937–1957* (Ithaca, NY: Cornell University Press, 1997); Thomas Borstelmann, *The Cold War and the Color Line: American Race Relations in the Global Arena* (Cambridge, MA: Harvard University Press, 2001); James H. Meriwether, *Proudly We Can Be Africans: Black Americans and Africa, 1935–1961* (Chapel Hill: University of North Carolina Press, 2002); and Kevin K. Gaines, *American Africans in Ghana: Black Expatriates and the Civil Rights Era* (Chapel Hill: University of North Carolina Press, 2006).

60. Dipesh Chakrabarty, "The Legacies of Bandung: Decolonization and the Politics of Culture," in *Making a World After Empire: The Bandung Moment and Its Political Afterlives*, ed. Christopher J. Lee (Athens: Ohio University Press, 2010), 47.

61. Kristen S. Tassin, "'Lift Up Your Head, My Brother': Nationalism and the Genesis of the Non-Aligned Movement," *Journal of Third World Studies* 23, no. 1 (2006): 147–68. See also the chapters in Lee, *Making a World After Empire*.

62. The importance of having a universal set of signs and symbols to the spread of "Western" science is one of the key arguments of David N. Livingstone, *Putting Science in Its Place: Geographies of Scientific Knowledge* (Chicago: University of Chicago Press, 2003), 135–78.

CHAPTER 1: COLONIAL INSTITUTIONS AND NETWORKS OF ETHNOPSYCHIATRY

Epigraphs: J. C. Carothers, *The African Mind in Health and Disease: A Study in Ethnopsychiatry* (Geneva: World Health Organization, 1953), 8; and C. E. Marlow, Acting Secretary (Health), File note, 26 March 1957, Nigerian National Archives, Ibadan (NNAI) MH 3313, 69.

1. Megan Vaughan, *Curing Their Ills: Colonial Power and African Illness* (Stanford, CA: Stanford University Press, 1991), 125.

2. Jonathan H. Sadowsky, *Imperial Bedlam: Institutions of Madness in Colonial Southwest Nigeria* (Berkeley: University of California Press, 1999), 30.

3. Ibid., 26–47.

4. On the systems of colonial administration set up in Nigeria, see I. F. Nicholson, *The Administration of Nigeria, 1900–1960: Men, Methods, and Myths* (Oxford: Clarendon Press, 1969).

5. See, for example, Margery Perham, *Native Administration in Nigeria* (London: Oxford University Press, 1937); and Robert Heussler, *The British in Northern Nigeria* (London: Oxford University Press, 1968).

6. Adiele E. Afigbo, *The Warrant Chiefs: Indirect Rule in Southeastern Nigeria, 1891–1929* (London: Longman, 1972); Harry A. Gailey, *The Road to Aba: A Study of British Administrative Policy in Eastern Nigeria* (New York: New York University Press, 1970); Elizabeth Isichei, *A History of the Igbo People* (London: Macmillan, 1976), 140–60; and Nicholson, *Administration of Nigeria*, 82–124.

7. Nicholson, *Administration of Nigeria*, 54–55. On colonial administration in Lagos, see, for example, Tekena N. Tamuno, *The Evolution of the Nigerian State: The Southern Phase, 1898–1914* (London: Longman, 1972); and Robert S. Smith, *The Lagos Consulate, 1851–1861* (London: Macmillan, 1978).

8. See, for example, Adiele E. Afigbo, "Sir Ralph Moor and the Economic Development of Southern Nigeria: 1896–1903," in *Nigerian History, Politics and Affairs: The Collected Essays of Adiele Afigbo*, ed. Toyin Falola (Trenton, NJ: Africa World Press, 2005), 185–212.

9. Frederick Lugard, *The Dual Mandate in British Tropical Africa*, 5th ed. (London: Archon, 1965); and Perham, *Native Administration*. For a more critical perspective, see Nicholson, *Administration of Nigeria*, 124–79.

10. Director of Medical and Sanitary Services, Lagos (DMSS) to Chief Secretary to the Government, Lagos, 18 September 1926, NNAI MH 59, vol. 1, 203A.

11. Director of Medical and Sanitary Services, Lagos, to Secretary, Southern Provinces, 25 January 1926, NNAI CSO 26/1 01507/S.2, 28.

12. DMSS to Chief Secretary, NNAI MH 59, vol. 1, 203A.

13. Secretary, Northern Provinces, Kaduna, to Chief Secretary, Lagos, 17 February 1925, NNAI MH 59, vol. 1, 137.

14. Secretariat, Northern Provinces, Kaduna, to Director of Medical and Sanitary Services, Lagos, 26 August 1926, NNAI MH 59, vol. 1, 202.

15. Sadowsky, *Imperial Bedlam*, 31–32, 99–100.

16. Secretary, Southern Provinces, Lagos, to Chief Secretary to the Government, Lagos, 23 August 1928, NNAI CSO 26/3 26973, vol. 1, 15.

17. H. L. Ward Price, Acting Resident, Abeokuta Province, Abeokuta, to Secretary, Southern Provinces, Lagos, 1 October 1928, NNAI CSO 26/3 26973, vol. 1, 36.

18. Acting Chief Secretary to the Government, Lagos, to Director of Medical and Sanitary Services, Lagos, 24 July 1928, NNAI CSO 26/3 26973, vol. 1, 7.

19. Secretary, Southern Provinces, Lagos, to Chief Secretary to the Government, Lagos, NNAI CSO 26/3 26973, vol. 1, 16.

20. Director of Medical and Sanitary Service, Lagos, to Chief Secretary to the Government, Lagos, 19 May 1930, NNAI CSO 26/3 26973, vol. 1, 78.

21. Ibid., 98.

22. Toyin Falola, *Development Planning and Decolonization in Nigeria* (Gainesville: University Press of Florida, 1996), 13.

23. Director of Medical and Sanitary Service, Lagos, to Chief Secretary to the Government, Lagos, 24 March 1931, NNAI CSO 26/3 26793, vol. 2, 127.

24. Director of Prisons, Southern Provinces, to Secretary, Southern Provinces, Enugu, 21 July 1934, NNAI CSO 26/1 01507, vol. 4, 526.

25. Sadowsky, *Imperial Bedlam*, 102.

26. R. Cunyngham Brown, *Report III on the Care and Treatment of Lunatics in the British West African Colonies: Nigeria* (Letchworth, UK: Garden City Press, 1938).

27. Ibid., 54–55.

28. Ibid., 59, 62.

29. Ibid., 63, 64.

30. Ibid., 64.

31. Director of Medical Service [DMS], Lagos, to Chief Secretary to the Government, Lagos, 2 February 1939, NNAI CSO 26/1 01507/S.1, 14.

32. Ibid.

33. J. C. Carothers, "A Report on the Psychiatric Services of Nigeria," (1955) NNAI MH 59/S.9, 18.

34. Ibid., 4.

35. Ibid., 31, underline in original.

36. Ibid., 23.

37. Carothers expands on what those requirements should be for each region in pages 44–51 of his report.

38. Acting Permanent Secretary to Southern Acting Secretary, 27 December 1957, NNAI MH 59/S.11, 113–14.

39. Ibid., 114.

40. Memo, C. E. Marlow to Permanent Secretary, 15 July 1957, NNAI MH 59/S.11, 83.

41. Joseph M. Hodge, *Triumph of the Expert: Agrarian Doctrines of Development and the Legacies of British Colonialism* (Athens: Ohio University Press, 2007), 126–43. In Nigeria, European education was seen as particularly disintegrating in that it created a class of colonial subjects who no longer saw the legitimacy of the "traditional" political institutions through which the British governed indirectly. See Perham, *Native Administration*, 357–60.

42. Brown, *Report III*, 9.

43. Ibid., 8.

44. Ibid.

45. Carothers, "Report," 27.

46. Ibid., 44.

47. Ibid., 45.

48. Ibid., 47.

49. Jock McCulloch, *Colonial Psychiatry and "The African Mind"* (Cambridge: Cambridge University Press, 1995). McCulloch makes clear that ethnopsychiatry occupied a "small and uncomfortable niche between the disciplines of psychiatry and anthropology" (1) and was made up of a variety of different types of specialists. "Some were qualified psychiatrists who worked directly with psychiatric patients, others physicians with an interest in psychological medicine but little clinical experience, others were psychologists, and still others gifted amateurs with a passion for a particular school of thought such as psychoanalysis of Adlerian psychology" (3).

50. Carothers, *African Mind in Health and Disease*, 87.

51. Ibid., 8.

52. Ibid.

53. Geoffrey C. Tooth, *Studies in Mental Illness in the Gold Coast* (London: His Majesty's Stationery Office, 1950), 40.

54. Although they were not completely abandoned. For example, Carothers went so far as to opine, without specific evidence one way or the other, "The African stock diverged from the European at least 30,000 years ago. Their common ancestors could be described as grandfathers at least a thousand times removed. It would be surprising if no divergent evolution had occurred in so many generations." Carothers, *African Mind in Health and Disease*, 72.

55. Ibid., 53.

56. S. Davidson, "Psychiatric Work among the Bemba," *Rhodes-Livingstone Journal* 7 (1949): 5, quoted in Carothers, *African Mind in Health and Disease*, 106.

57. Although at times some African societies were seen to be "more civilized" than others. Nevertheless, in such circumstances, the "more civilized" society was seen as deviating in a positive way from what were otherwise considered African norms. See, for example, Vaughan, *Curing Their Ills*, 129–54, in which Vaughan describes Baganda fear of syphilis as evidence of their superior civilization relative to what Europeans considered the "unnatural" social toleration of the disease typical of African societies in general.

58. J. C. Carothers, "A Study of Mental Derangement in Africans, and an Attempt to Explain Its Peculiarities, More Especially in Relation to the African Attitude of Life," *Journal of Mental Science* 93 (1947): 584.

59. Ibid.

60. Tooth, *Studies in Mental Illness*, 63.

61. Horace Shelley and W. H. Watson, "An Investigation Concerning Mental Disorder in the Nyasaland Natives," *Journal of Mental Science* 82 (1936): 704.

62. Carothers, *African Mind in Health and Disease*, 125.

63. Union of South Africa, *Annual Report of the Commissioner of Mental Hygiene* (Pretoria: Government Printer, 1950).

64. See McCulloch, *Colonial Psychiatry*, 9–46, for comparative perspectives on mental asylum facilities in different African colonies.

65. P. Gallais and L. Planques, "Etudes sur la deficiences mentale dans les terretoires d'outre mer: Perspectives ethnopsychiatriques dans l'Union francaise," *Medicine tropicale* 11 (1951): 5, translated and quoted in Carothers, *African Mind in Health and Disease*, 130.

66. Of course, detribalization was not necessarily the product of achieving a European education. Large numbers of African migrants moved to colonial urban centers in search of employment opportunities without the benefit of a European education and became, according to ethnopsychiatrists, significantly "detribalized" through their urbanization.

67. For a concise analysis of the plight of the "detribalized" African, see Tooth, *Studies in Mental Illness*.

68. Carothers, *African Mind in Health and Disease*, 132–33.

69. Medical Officer in charge of Yaba Lunatic Asylum to Senior Medical Officer, Lagos, 30 October 1954, NNAI MH 3420, 50.

70. Acting Permanent Secretary, Department of Internal Affairs, to Permanent Secretary, Ministry of Health, Eastern Region, Enugu, 20 December 1957, NNAI MH 3313, B.

71. Superintendent of Prisons, Port Harcourt, to Director of Prisons, Prisons Department, Lagos, 18 July 1955, NNAI MH 3313, 31.

CHAPTER 2: DECOLONIZING PSYCHIATRIC INSTITUTIONS AND NETWORKS

Epigraph: Quoted in Philip Singer, "Traditional Healing and the Medical/Psychiatric Mafia," in *Traditional Healing: New Science or New Colonialism?*, ed. Philip Singer (Owerri: Conch Magazine, 1977), 245–46.

1. For general background on the politics of decolonization in Nigeria, see, for example, Toyin Falola and Matthew M. Heaton, *A History of Nigeria* (Cambridge:

Cambridge University Press, 2008), 136–57; Michael Crowder, *The Story of Nigeria*, 4th ed. (London: Faber and Faber, 1978), 207–58; and James S. Coleman, *Nigeria: Background to Nationalism* (Berkeley: University of California Press, 1960).

2. Toyin Falola, *Development Planning and Decolonization in Nigeria* (Gainesville: University Press of Florida, 1996), 60.

3. R. Olufemi Ekundare, *An Economic History of Nigeria, 1860–1960* (London: Methuen, 1973), 356–60.

4. Ralph Schram, *A History of the Nigerian Health Services* (Ibadan: Ibadan University Press, 1971), 432.

5. Ibid., 298, 433.

6. Tolani Asuni, "Aro Hospital in Perspective," *American Journal of Psychiatry* 124, no. 6 (1967): 764.

7. *West African Pilot*, 21 November 1945, p. 2. The government denied all charges.

8. Dozens upon dozens of requests for release from Yaba asylum can be found in Nigerian National Archives, Ibadan [NNAI] COMCOL/1 735/S.1, vol. 2, 393.

9. Moses Ogede to Commissioner of the Colony, Lagos, 3 February 1951, NNAI COMCOL/1 735/S.1, vol. 2, 393.

10. For example, Mr. Wilson D. Agagah to Commissioner of the Colony, Lagos, 19 January 1948, NNAI COMCOL/1 735/S.1, vol. 1, 157; P. O. Ihezue to Commissioner of the Colony, Lagos, 27 April 1948, NNAI COMCOL/1 735/S.1, vol. 1, 163.

11. Asuni, "Aro Hospital," 764.

12. Jonathan H. Sadowsky, *Imperial Bedlam: Institutions of Madness in Colonial Southwest Nigeria* (Berkeley: University of California Press, 1999), 30.

13. Donald Cameron, Senior Specialist (Alienist), Lunatic Asylum, Lantoro, Abeokuta, to the Director of Medical Services, Northern Region, Kaduna, the Director of Medical Services, Eastern Region, Enugu, and Director of Medical Services, Western Region, Ibadan, 12 March 1952, Nigerian National Archives, Kaduna [NNAK] MH 2549, 44.

14. As seen in NNAK MH 312.

15. Cameron to Directors of Medical Services, NNAK MH 2549, 44.

16. Director of Medical Services, Northern Region, to the Inspector-General of Medical Services, Lagos, 10 May 1952, NNAK MH 312, 112.

17. Ibid.

18. Ibid.

19. Director of Medical Services, Enugu, to the Inspector-General of Medical Services, Lagos, 15 July 1952, NNAK MH 312, 113.

20. Donald Cameron, Senior Specialist (Alienist), Aro Hospital (Mental), Abeokuta, 20 November 1952, NNAK MH 312, 126.

21. Ibid.

22. Ibid.

23. Alexander Boroffka, *"Psychiatry in Nigeria": (A Partly Annotated Bibliography) with an Introductory Chapter on "The History of Psychiatry in Nigeria"* (Kiel: Brunswiker Universitätsbuchhandlung—Medizin, 2006), 22.

24. For a brief biography of Lambo, see Jonathan H. Sadowsky, "Thomas Adeoye Lambo," in *Doctors, Nurses, and Medical Practitioners: A Bio-Bibliographical Sourcebook*, ed. Lois N. Magner (Westport, CT: Greenwood Press, 1997), 172–76.

25. Asuni, "Aro Hospital," 764.

26. Edgar Jones, Shahina Rahman, and Robin Woolven, "The Maudsley Hosptial: Design and Strategic Direction, 1923–39," *Medical History* 51, no. 3 (2007): 357–78.

27. Sadowsky, *Imperial Bedlam*, 42n90.

28. As noted by al-Mahi in his introductory comments at the First Pan-African Psychiatric Conference; see T. Adeoye Lambo, ed., *First Pan-African Psychiatric Conference, Abeokuta, Nigeria* (Ibadan: Government Printer, 1961), 11.

29. Asuni, "Aro Hospital," 765.

30. Ibid., 765–66.

31. Tolani Asuni, "Therapeutic Communities of the Hospital and Villages in Aro Hospital Complex in Nigeria," *African Journal of Psychiatry* 1 (1979): 41.

32. Although he gives no figures for this. See T. Adeoye Lambo, "Further Neuropsychiatric Observations in Nigeria," *British Medical Journal* 2, no. 1060 (1956): 1697.

33. Asuni, "Aro Hospital," 769.

34. Tolani Asuni, "Social, Cultural and Economic Determinants of Psychiatric Services in Western Nigeria," *African Journal of Psychiatry* 1 (1975): 10.

35. Ben Park, *The Healers of Aro* (New York: United Nations, 1960), film.

36. T. Adeoye Lambo, "A Form of Social Psychiatry in Africa," *World Mental Health* 13 (1960): 198

37. Asuni, "Aro Hospital," 767.

38. Ibid., 766.

39. Ibid., 768.

40. J. D. A. Makanjuola, "The Aro Drug Addiction Research and Treatment Centre: A First Report," *British Journal of Addiction* 81 (1986): 809–14.

41. D. O. Utomi, "Clinical Psychology at Aro Psychiatric Hospital," in *Clinical Psychology in Africa: South of the Sahara, the Caribbean and Afro-Latin America*, ed. Karl Peltzer and Peter O. Ebigbo (Enugu: Working Group for African Psychology, 1989), 691.

42. Asuni, "Aro Hospital," 766.

43. Asuni, "Therapeutic Communities," 39.

44. Asuni, "Aro Hospital," 766.

45. T. Adeoye Lambo, "Socioeconomic Changes in Africa and Their Implications for Mental Health," in *Man in Africa*, ed. Gordon Wolstenholme and Maeve O'Connor (Boston: Little, Brown, 1965), 138.

46. Lambo, "Socioeconomic Changes," 134.

47. T. Adeoye Lambo, "Thomas Lambo," in *Psychiatrists on Psychiatry*, ed. Michael Shepherd (Cambridge: Cambridge University Press, 1982), 117.

48. Lambo, "Form of Social Psychiatry," 200–201.

49. Park, *Healers of Aro*.

50. Asuni, "Aro Hospital," 767.

51. Utomi, "Clinical Psychology," 691.

52. T. Adeoye Lambo, "The Role of Cultural Factors in Paranoid Psychosis among the Yoruba Tribe," *Journal of Mental Science* 101 (1955): 241.

53. Ibid.

54. Ibid.

55. Ibid., 245.

56. Ibid., 249.

57. Park, *Healers of Aro*.

58. Ibid.

59. Ibid.

60. Ayo Binitie, "Experiences in the Development and Planning of Psychiatric Services in Mid-Western State of Nigeria," *Psychopathologie africaine* 6 (1970): 201–8, describes the

Uselu Village Scheme in Benin City. See Charles R. Swift and Tolani Asuni, *Mental Health and Disease in Africa: With Special Reference to Africa South of the Sahara* (New York: Churchill Livingstone, 1975), 215, for a brief description of the psychiatric convalescent villages Swift helped to establish in Tanzania. Henri Collomb's efforts to integrate indigenous belief systems into Western psychiatric hospital care in Senegal, which became known as the "Fann School," is discussed in Alice Bullard, "The Critical Impact of Frantz Fanon and Henri Collomb: Race, Gender and Personality Testing of North and West Africans," *Journal of the History of Behavioral Sciences* 41, no. 3 (2005): 225–48.

61. Jatinder Bains, "Race, Culture and Psychiatry: A History of Transcultural Psychiatry," *History of Psychiatry* 16, no. 2 (2005): 141.

62. H. B. M. Murphy, "The Historical Development of Transcultural Psychiatry," in *Transcultural Psychiatry*, ed. John L. Cox (London: Croom Helm, 1986), 14–15.

63. Alexander H. Leighton, T. Adeoye Lambo, Charles C. Hughes, Dorothea C. Leighton, Jane M. Murphy, and David B. Macklin, *Psychiatric Disorder among the Yoruba: A Report from the Cornell-Aro Mental Health Research Project in the Western Region, Nigeria* (Ithaca, NY: Cornell University Press, 1963), 64 (hereafter cited in text as *PDY*).

64. T. Adeoye Lambo, "Important Areas of Ignorance and Doubt in the Psychology of the African," in *The Proceedings of the First International Congress of Africanists*, ed. Lalage Bown and Michael Crowder (Evanston, IL: Northwestern University Press, 1964).

65. Femi Oyebode, "Obituary: Thomas Adeoye Lambo, O.B.E.," *Psychiatric Bulletin* 28 (2004): 469.

66. World Health Organization Archives (WHOA), M4 136, 1–3.

67. World Health Organization, "The Promotion and Development of Traditional Medicine," *World Healh Organization Technical Report Series*, no. 622 (1978).

68. A large literature exists on this subject. See, for example, Toyin Falola, *Nationalism and African Intellectuals* (Rochester, NY: University of Rochester Press, 2001).

69. Lambo, "Role of Cultural Factors," 249.

70. Ibid., 245.

71. T. Adeyoe Lambo, "Schizophrenic and Borderline States," in *Transcultural Psychiatry*, ed. A. V. S. de Reuck and Ruth Porter (Boston: Little, Brown, 1965), 75.

72. T. Adeoye Lambo, "Early Childhood Experience and Adult Personality," in *Cultural Adaptation within Modern Africa*, ed. S. H. Irvine and J. T. Sanders (New York: Teachers College Press, 1972), 117.

73. T. Adeoye Lambo, "Changing Patterns of Mental Health Needs in Africa," *Contemporary Review* 222, no. 1286 (1973): 147.

74. Lambo, "Socioeconomic Changes," 144.

75. Lambo, "Changing Patterns," 146.

76. Lambo, "Thomas Lambo," 109.

77. Ibid., 111.

78. T. Adeoye Lambo, "Towards Justice in Health," *World Health* (July 1979): 2.

79. T. Adeoye Lambo, "A New World in the Making," *World Health* (April 1980): 2.

80. Lambo, "Changing Patterns," 147.

81. Boroffka, "*Psychiatry in Nigeria*," 26.

82. R. Olukayode Jegede, "Nigerian Psychiatry in Perspective," *Acta Psychiatrica Scandinavia* 63 (1981): 46–47, notes that as of 1981 the first batch of internally trained psychiatrists were currently completing their training at the University College Hospital, Ibadan, the University of Benin Teaching Hospital, and the Lagos University Teaching Hospital.

83. Ayodele Obembe, "Nigerian Psychiatry—Past, Present, Future," in *Psychiatry in Developing Countries*, ed. Stephen Brown (London: Gaskill, 1983), 5.

84. Boroffka, "*Psychiatry in Nigeria*," 5.

85. Ibid., 23, 26.

86. A. O. Odejide, "A Nigerian Psychiatric Outpatient Clinic: A Point Prevalence Study," *Journal of Clinical Psychiatry* 41, no. 4 (1980): 130.

87. For a full list of the various psychiatric institutions in Nigeria, see Boroffka, "*Psychiatry in Nigeria*," 537–55.

88. Jegede, "Nigerian Psychiatry in Perspective," 46.

89. Tolani Asuni, "Development of Psychiatry in Africa," in *Mental Health in Africa and the Americas Today*, ed. Samuel O. Okpaku (Nashville, TN: Chrisolith Books, 1991), 23.

90. Ibid., 17.

91. A. C. Raman, ed. *Proceedings of the Second Pan-African Psychiatric Workshop* (Port Louis: Association of Psychiatrists in Africa, 1972); Association of Psychiatrists in Africa, *Report of the 3rd Pan African Psychiatric Workshop* (Ibadan: Government Printer, 1971); and Association of Psychiatrists in Africa, *Proceedings of the 1974 Workshop of the Association of Psychiatrists in Africa* (Lausanne: ICAA, 1974).

92. See the bibliography of this book for copious examples of the high-level international publishing record of Nigerian psychiatrists in the 1960s, 1970s, and 1980s.

93. Asuni, "Development of Psychiatry," 21.

94. Boroffka, "*Psychiatry in Nigeria*," 25.

95. Ibid., 5.

96. David N. Livingstone, *Putting Science in Its Place: Geographies of Scientific Knowledge* (Chicago: University of Chicago Press, 2003), 135–78.

CHAPTER 3: MENTALLY ILL NIGERIAN IMMIGRANTS IN THE UNITED KINGDOM

1. Richard C. Keller has made a similar argument about the ways that theories about maladaptivity of racial "others" have circulated between France and North Africa in the postcolonial era, where concerns about the effect that North African immigrants are having on French "culture" have often taken on psychological-cum-racial connotations. See Keller, *Colonial Madness: Psychiatry in French North Africa* (Chicago: University of Chicago Press, 2007), 191–226.

2. John Solomos, *Race and Racism in Britain*, 3rd ed. (New York: Palgrave Macmillan, 2003), 40–47.

3. Oscar Gish, "Color and Skill: British Immigration, 1955–1968," *International Migration Review* 3, no. 1 (1968): 22.

4. This standard story of increasing racism leading up to the passage of the 1962 Commonwealth Immigrants Act has been contested somewhat by historians who argue that accusations of institutional racism should be balanced with narratives that account for the efforts that were being made to promote interracial harmony at the time. For example, Randall Hansen, *Citizenship and Immigration in Post-War Britain* (Oxford: Oxford University Press, 2000), argues that Commonwealth citizenship was a noble and unconventional idea and that, at least at the level of government, major strides were made in the postwar era to provide social services for colonial and Commonwealth immigrants and to promote cultural integration that became the basis for the development of a multicultural Britain.

5. Solomos, *Race and Racism*, 55.

6. Kathleen Paul, *Whitewashing Britain: Race and Citizenship in the Postwar Era* (Ithaca, NY: Cornell University Press, 1997), 124.

7. On the 1962 Commonwealth Immigrants Act and its successors, see, for example, Ian R. G. Spencer, *British Immigration Policy Since 1939: The Making of Multi-Racial Britain* (New York: Routledge, 1997), 129–52.

8. See, for example, L. K. Hemsi, "Psychiatric Morbidity of West Indian Immigrants," *Social Psychiatry* 2 (1967): 95–100. On psychiatric racism and the difficulties attendant to providing psychiatric care to ethnic minorities and immigrants in the United Kingdom, see, for example, Roland Littlewood and Maurice Lipsedge, *Aliens and Alienists: Ethnic Minorities and Psychiatry* (New York: Penguin, 1982); Julian P. Leff, *Psychiatry around the Globe: A Transcultural View* (London: Gaskell, 1988), 179–96; and Philip H. Rack, *Race, Culture, and Mental Disorder* (London: Tavistock, 1982).

9. On the conflation of race and class in postwar Britain, see Paul Gilroy, *"There Ain't No Black in the Union Jack": The Cultural Politics of Race and Nation* (Chicago: University of Chicago Press, 1987).

10. Margaret J. Field, *Search for Security: An Ethno-Psychiatric Study of Rural Ghana* (Evanston, IL: Northwestern University Press, 1960), 318–19.

11. Raymond H. Prince, "The 'Brain Fag' Syndrome in Nigerian Students," *Journal of Mental Science* 106 (1960): 559.

12. R. J. Still, "Mental Health in Overseas Students," *Proceedings of the British Student Health Association* (1961): 59–60.

13. Cecil B. Kidd, "Psychiatric Morbidity among Students," *British Journal of Preventive and Social Medicine* 19, no. 4 (1965): 148.

14. See Gerald N. Grob, ed., *Immigrants and Insanity: Dissenting Views, 1883–1914* (New York: Arno Press, 1980).

15. As described in Philip H. Rack, "Migration and Mental Illness," in *Transcultural Psychiatry*, ed. John L. Cox (London: Croom Helm, 1986), 60.

16. The popularization of this idea is typically linked to two articles by Roland Littlewood and Maurice Lipsedge: "Some Social and Phenomenological Characteristics of Psychotic Immigrants," *Psychological Medicine* 11 (1981): 289–302; and "Acute Psychotic Reactions in Caribbean-Born Patients," *Psychological Medicine* 11 (1981): 303–18.

17. See National Archives of the United Kingdom [NAUK] HO 45/1606; HO 45/7642; HO 45/9294/8452; HO 45/10289/110706; HO 45/10360/154554; HO 45/10560/169330; HO 45/10995/167955 for detailed correspondence between the United Kingdom and other European governments on the issue of reciprocal repatriation of foreign "lunatics."

18. Alex Fiddian to G. A. S. Northcote, esq., 20 September 1932, National Archives of Ghana, Accra (NAGA) CSO 11/8/16.

19. J. C. Carothers, "A Study of Mental Derangement in Africans, and an Attempt to Explain Its Peculiarities, More Especially in Relation to the African Attitude of Life," *Journal of Mental Science* 93 (1947): 560.

20. Secretary of State for the Colonies to Officer Administering the Government of the Federation of Nigeria, Lagos, 29 November 1955, Nigerian National Archives, Ibadan [NNAI] CSO 26 03028/S.1080, 17.

21. J. S. Knox, Medical Officer, H. M. Prison, Brixton, to Thames Magistrate Court, 28 February 1956, Nigerian National Archives, Ibadan NNAI CSO 26 03028/S.1080, 25.

22. Ibid.

23. Ibid.

24. Secretary of State for the Colonies to the Officer Administering the Government of Nigeria, 23 August 1950, NNAI CSO 03028/S.978, 1.

25. Secretary of State for the Colonies to the Officer Administering the Government of Nigeria, 12 August 1952, NNAI CSO 03028/S.1051, 1.

26. Chief Secretary of the Federation, Nigeria, to Permanent Secretary, Ministry of Social Services, 10 January 1956, NNAI MH 59/S.4/C.4, 2.

27. Extract from Letter from Consultant Psychiatrist at Long Grove Hospital, Epsom, Surrey, to Colonial Office, 7 October 1958, NNAI MH 59/S.4/C.27, 3.

28. Medical Report, 19 June 1956, NNAI MH 59/S.4/C.9, 3.

29. Inspector-General of Medical Services to Chief Secretary to the Government, Lagos, 10 November 1953, NNAI CSO 03028/S.1051, 18.

30. Secretary of State for the Colonies to Governor-General, Nigeria, 26 November 1954, NNAI CSO 03028/S.1088, 31.

31. J. Ernest Nicole, Medical Superintendent, Winwick Hospital, Winwick, Warrington, to W. Bate, Esq., Colonial Office, London, 18 November 1952, NNAI CSO 26 03028/S/977, 8.

32. Secretary of State for the Colonies to Officer Administering the Government of Nigeria, 10 December 1953, NNAI CSO 26 03028/S/977, 22.

33. Ibid., emphasis mine.

34. Secretary of State for the Colonies to Officer Administering the Government of Nigeria, 17 April 1954, NNAI CSO 26 03028/S/977, 26.

35. E. P. H. Charlton, Physician Superintendent, Banstead Hospital, Sutton, Surrey to E. B. Gumbrell, Esq., Colonial Office, London, 2 June 1958, NNAI MH 59/S.4/C.32, 3.

36. E. P. H. Charlton, Physician Superintendent, Banstead Hospital, Sutton, Surrey to E. B. Gumbrell, Esq., Colonial Office, London, 29 August 1958, NNAI MH 59/S.4/C.32, 4.

37. Secretary of State for the Colonies to the Officer Administering the Government of Nigeria, 2 September 1950, NNAI CSO 26 03028/S.988, 1.

38. Ibid.

39. Acting Governor, Nigeria, to Secretary of State for the Colonies, 11 October 1950, NNAI CSO 26 03028/S.988, 6.

40. Governor, Nigeria, to Secretary of State for the Colonies, 28 May 1951, NNAI CSO 26 03028/S.988, 10.

41. Physician Superintendent, Freirn Hospital, to Secretary, Board of Control, London, 9 June 1951, NNAI CSO 26 03028/S.988, 12.

42. Secretary of State for the Colonies to Officer Administering the Government of the Federation of Nigeria, 8 January 1957, NNAI CSO 26 03028/S.988, 27.

43. Ibid.

44. For details on this event, see the full file NNAI MH 59/S4/3.

45. Unknown to Acting Secretary Health, Nigeria, 4 July 1955, NNAI MH 59/S4, 3.

46. L. H. Thorpe, Board of Control, London to A. H. Jordan, Esq., Colonial Office, London, 12 March 1951, NNAI CSO 26 03028/S.976, 8.

47. Director of Medical Services, Nigeria, to Chief Secretary to the Government, Lagos, 29 May 1951, NNAI CSO 26 03028/S.976, 11.

48. K. Sagoe, Medical Officer in charge of Yaba Lunatic Asylum, to Senior Medical Officer, Lagos, 19 June 1952, NNAI CSO 26 03028/S.976, 39.

49. Medical Report, 19 June 1956, NNAI MH 59/S4/C9, 3.

50. Governor General, Nigeria, to Secretary of State for the Colonies, 28 September 1956, NNAI MH59/S4/C9, 6.

51. Hakim Adi, "West African Students in Britain, 1900–1960: The Politics of Exile," *Immigrants and Minorities* 12, no. 3 (1993): 108.

52. Political and Economic Planning, *Colonial Students in Britain: A Report* (London: PEP, 1955), 213.

53. T. Adeoye Lambo, *A Study of Social and Health Problems of Nigerian Students in Great Britain and Ireland* (Ibadan: Government Printer, 1958), 7 (hereafter cited in text as *SSH*). A copy of this report is available in the file "Mental Illness among Students," Nigerian National Archives, Kaduna [NNAK] AGNN 1031.

54. T. Adeoye Lambo, "Socioeconomic Changes in Africa and Their Implications for Mental Health," in *Man and Africa*, ed. Gordon Wolstenholme and Maeve O'Connor (Boston: Little, Brown, 1965), 133–34.

55. Ibid., 128.

56. T. Adeoye Lambo, "Patterns of Psychiatric Care in Developing African Countries," in *Magic, Faith, and Healing: Studies in Primitive Psychiatry Today*, ed. Ari Kiev (London: Free Press, 1964), 445–46.

57. Amechi Anumonye, *African Students in Alien Cultures* (Buffalo, NY: Black Academy Press, 1970), 101.

58. Ibid., 49.

59. Ibid., 77–80.

60. Ibid., 76.

61. Ibid., 16.

62. Tolani Asuni, "The Review of Nigerian Students Repatriated on Psychiatric Grounds," *West AfricanMedical Journal* 17 (1968): 7.

63. Amechi Anumonye, "Emotional Stresses among African Students in Britain," *Scottish Medical Journal* 12 (1967): 319.

64. Asuni, "Review of Nigerian Students," 7.

65. Ibid., 5–6.

66. A. W. Burke, "The Consequences of Unplanned Repatriation," *British Journal of Psychiatry* 123 (1973): 109–11.

67. Rack, *Race, Culture, and Mental Disorder*, 220.

68. This estimate is based on the cumulative total of case files I have acquired of Nigerians repatriated from the United Kingdom due to mental illness during this time period. It is therefore a conservative estimate, as the actual number could be higher, owing to the possible incompleteness of the records.

69. Rack, *Race, Culture, and Mental Disorder*, 213.

CHAPTER 4: SCHIZOPHRENIA, DEPRESSION, AND "BRAIN-FAG SYNDROME"

1. Edward Shorter, *A Historical Dictionary of Psychiatry* (Oxford: Oxford University Press, 2005), 267–75.

2. Edward Shorter, *A History of Psychiatry: From the Era of the Asylum to the Age of Prozac* (New York: John Wiley, 1997), 241–45.

3. See, for example, Irving I. Gottesman, *Schizophrenia Genesis: The Origins of Madness* (New York: W. H. Freeman, 1991), 104–32, for an in-depth history of twin studies of schizophrenia.

4. Sander L. Gilman, "Constructing Schizophrenia as a Category of Mental Illness," in *History of Psychiatry and Medical Psychology*, ed. Edwin R. Wallace IV and John Gach (New York: Springer, 2008), 461–83.

5. Horace Shelley and W. H. Watson, "An Investigation Concerning Mental Disorder in the Nyasaland Natives," *Journal of Mental Sciences*, 82 (1936): 704.

6. J. C. Carothers, "A Study of Mental Derangement in Africans, and an Attempt to Explain Its Peculiarities, More Especially in Relation to the African Attitude to Life," *Journal of Mental Science* 93 (1947): 570.

7. J. C. Carothers, *The African Mind in Health and Disease: A Study in Ethnopsychiatry* (Geneva: World Health Organization, 1953), 139.

8. R. Cunyngham Brown, *Report III on the Care and Treatment of Lunatics in British West African Colonies: Nigeria* (London: Garden City Press, 1937), 39.

9. Roland Littlewood and Maurice Lipsedge, *Aliens and Alienists: Ethnic Minorities and Psychiatry* (New York: Penguin, 1982), 117–20, makes this point. Although it should be noted that in some places colonial authorities consulted with indigenous leaders to determine whether the symptoms exhibited by individuals were consistent with "insane" behavior in their own cultural settings. This, of course, has its own social and political complications. See Megan Vaughan, "Idioms of Madness: Zomba Lunatic Asylum, Nyasaland, in the Colonial Period," *Journal of Southern African Studies* 9, no. 2 (1983): 218–38.

10. See Megan Vaughan, *Curing Their Ills: Colonial Power and African Illness* (Stanford, CA: Stanford University Press, 1991); Jock McCulloch, *Colonial Psychiatry and "The African Mind"* (Cambridge: Cambridge University Press, 1995).

11. McCulloch, *Colonial Psychiatry*, 51–52.

12. J. C. Carothers, "Some Speculations on Insanity in Africans in General," *East African Medical Journal* 17 (1940): 99.

13. Carothers, *African Mind in Health and Disease*, 140–42.

14. Eugen Bleuler, *Textbook of Psychiatry* (New York: Macmillan, 1976), 200–210, cited in Jonathan M. Metzl, *The Protest Psychosis: How Schizophrenia Became a Black Disease* (Boston: Beacon Press, 2009), 34.

15. B. J. F. Laubscher, *Sex, Custom and Psychopathology: A Study of South African Pagan Natives* (London: George Routledge, 1937). Carothers completely disagreed with Laubscher on this point, saying, "The present writer cannot agree with this; the structure is too altered," in Carothers, *African Mind in Health and Disease*, 142.

16. Carothers, *African Mind in Health and Disease*, 142.

17. T. Adeoye Lambo, "The Role of Cultural Factors in Paranoid Psychosis among the Yoruba Tribe," *Journal of Mental Science* 101 (1955): 239–66; T. Adeoye Lambo, "Some Unusual Features of Schizophrenia among Primitive Peoples," *West African Medical Journal* 6 (1957): 147–52.

18. Lambo, "Role of Cultural Factors," 246.

19. Ibid.

20. McCulloch, *Colonial Psychiatry*, 52.

21. Lambo, "Role of Cultural Factors," 240.

22. Ibid., 249.

23. Lambo, "Some Unusual Features," 148, 150.

24. Lambo, "Role of Cultural Factors," 253.
25. Ibid., 242.
26. T. Adeoye Lambo, "Further Neuropsychiatric Observations in Nigeria," *British Medical Journal* 2, no. 5214 (1960): 1696.
27. Ibid.
28. For a historical schematic of schizophrenia follow-up studies, see World Health Organization [WHO], *Schizophrenia: An International Follow-up Study* (Geneva: World Health Organization, 1979), 20–23.
29. Lambo, "Further Neuropsychiatric Observations," 1697.
30. Ibid.
31. The others were Aarhus, Denmark; Agra, India; Cali, Colombia; London; Moscow; Taipei; Prague; and Washington, DC. WHO, *International Pilot Study of Schizophrenia* (Geneva: WHO, 1973).
32. Ibid., 161.
33. For summaries of these studies, see ibid., 25–30.
34. Eric D. Wittkower, H. B. M. Murphy, J. Fried, and H. Ellenberger, "Crosscultural Inquiry into the Symptomatology of Schizophrenia," *Annals of the New York Academy of Science* 84 (1960): 855.
35. H. B. M. Murphy, Eric D. Wittkower, J. Fried, and H. Ellenberger, "A Cross-Cultural Survey of Schizophrenic Symptomatology," *International Journal of Social Psychiatry* 9 (1963): 247.
36. WHO, *International Pilot Study*, 168–75.
37. WHO, *Schizophrenia*, 113–64.
38. Ibid., 163.
39. Wittkower, Murphy, Fried, and Ellenberger, "Crosscultural Inquiry," 862.
40. For example, see H. B. M. Murphy, "The Historical Development of Transcultural Psychiatry," in *Transcultural Psychiatry*, ed. John L. Cox (London: Croom Helm, 1986), 19. For specific critique of the Ibadan data, see Robert B. Edgerton, "Traditional Treatment for Mental Illness in Africa: A Review," *Culture, Medicine and Psychiatry* 4 (1980): 167–89.
41. For a general history of melancholy and depression in the Western context, see Stanley W. Jackson, *Melancholia and Depression: From Hippocratic Times to Modern Times* (New Haven, CT: Yale University Press, 1986); and Clark Lawlor, *From Melancholia to Prozac: A History of Depression* (Oxford: Oxford University Press, 2012).
42. Arthur S. Reber, *Dictionary of Psychology*, 2nd ed. (New York: Penguin, 1995), 197–99.
43. For a background on the perceived lack of depressive illnesses in blacks, see Littlewood and Lipsedge, *Aliens and Alienists*, 68–86; and McCulloch, *Colonial Psychiatry*, 111–13.
44. Carothers, *African Mind in Health and Disease*, 142–48.
45. Brown, *Report III*, 39.
46. Carothers went so far as to say that the diagnosis of depression "depends" on a patient's admission of feelings of "misery." See Carothers, *African Mind in Health and Disease*, 146.
47. See, for example, Suman Fernando, "Depression and Ethnic Minorities," in Cox, *Transcultural Psychiatry*, 107–38.
48. Lawlor, *From Melancholia to Prozac*, throughout.
49. Littlewood and Lipsedge, *Aliens and Alienists*, 71–74.

50. T. Adeoye Lambo, "Neuropsychiatric Observations in the Western Region of Nigeria," *British Medical Journal* 2, no. 5006 (1956): 1390.

51. Lambo, "Further Neuropsychiatric Observations," 1698–99.

52. Ibid.

53. Ibid., 1696.

54. Henri Collomb and Jacques Zwingelstein, "Depressive States in an African Community," in *First Pan-African Psychiatric Conference, Abeokuta, Nigeria*, ed. T. Adeoye Lambo (Ibadan: Government Printer, 1961), 227–34; L. S. Gillis, "Observations from South Africa," in Lambo, *First Pan-African Psychiatric Conference*, 236–68; and E. F. B. Forster, "Treatment of the African Mental Patient," in Lambo, *First Pan-African Psychiatric Conference*, 276–79.

55. Alexander H. Leighton, T. Adeoye Lambo, Charles C. Hughes, Dorothea C. Leighton, Jane M. Murphy, and David B. Macklin, *Psychiatric Disorder among the Yoruba: A Report from the Cornell-Aro Mental Health Research Project in the Western Region, Nigeria* (Ithaca, NY: Cornell University Press, 1963), 112.

56. Ibid., 139–42.

57. H. B. M. Murphy, Eric D. Wittkower, N. A. Chance, "Crosscultural Inquiry into the Symptomatology of Depression: A Preliminary Report," *Transcultural Psychiatry* 1 (1964): 5–18.

58. Ibid., 6, 7.

59. Ibid., 16.

60. See Raymond H. Prince, "The Changing Picture of Depressive Syndromes in Africa: Is It Fact or Diagnostic Fashion?," *Canadian Journal of African Studies* 1 (1967): 177–92.

61. Michael O. Olatawura, "The Problem of Diagnosing Depression in Nigeria," *Psychopathologie africaine* 9 (1973): 389.

62. G. G. C. Rwegellera, "Cultural Aspects of Depressive Illness; Clinical Aspects and Psychopathology," *Psychopathologie africaine* 17 (1981): 49.

63. A. Kalunta, "Depressive Illness: Its Cultural Aspects," *Psychopathologie africaine* 17 (1981): 113.

64. John C. Ebie, "Some Observations on Depressive Illness in Nigerians Attending a Psychiatric Out-Patient Clinic," *African Journal of Medical Science* 3 (1972): 149–55.

65. Rwegellera, "Cultural Aspects," 51–54.

66. See P. M. Yap, "Mental Diseases Peculiar to Certain Cultures: A Survey of Comparative Psychiatry," *Journal of Mental Science* 97 (1951): 313–27.

67. See, for example, P. M. Yap, "*Koro*—A Culture-Bound Depersonalization Syndrome," *British Journal of Psychiatry* 111 (1965): 43–50; and P. M. Yap, "The Culture-bound Reactive Syndromes," in *Mental Health Research in Asia and the Pacific*, ed. William Caudill and Tsung-Yi Lin (Honolulu: East-West Center Press, 1969), 33–53.

68. For more on culture-bound syndromes, see Ari Kiev, *Transcultural Psychiatry* (New York: Free Press, 1972); and Ronald C. Simons and Charles C. Hughes, *The Culture-Bound Syndromes: Folk Illnesses of Psychiatric and Anthropological Interest* (Dordrecht: D. Reidel, 1985).

69. American Psychiatric Association, *Diagnostic and Statistical Manual of Mental Disorders*, 4th ed. (Washington, DC: American Psychiatric Association, 1994), 843 (hereafter cited as *DSMV-IV*).

70. Raymond H. Prince, "Transcultural Aspects of Affective Disorders in Adolescents: The Brain-Fag Syndrome in African Students," in *The Adolescent and Mood*

Disturbance, ed. Harvey Golombek and Barry D. Garfinkel (New York: International Universities Press, 1983), 54–55.

71. Raymond H. Prince, "The 'Brain Fag' Syndrome in Nigerian Students," *Journal of Mental Science* 106 (1960): 559–70; and Raymond H. Prince, "Functional Symptoms Associated with Study in Nigerian Students," *West African Medical Journal* 11 (1962): 198–206.

72. Prince, "Functional Symptoms," 198.

73. Prince, "'Brain Fag' Syndrome," 562.

74. Ibid., 559.

75. Prince, "Functional Symptoms," 199.

76. Alexander Boroffka and A. A. Marinho, "Psychoneurotic Syndromes in Urbanized Nigerians," *Transcultural Psychiatric Research Review* 15 (1963): 45.

77. Prince, "'Brain Fag' Syndrome," 560.

78. Ibid., 565.

79. Prince, "Functional Symptoms," 203.

80. Prince, "'Brain Fag' Syndrome," 565.

81. Prince, "Functional Symptoms," 205.

82. Prince, "'Brain Fag' Syndrome," 567, 568.

83. Ibid., 568–69.

84. Prince, "Transcultural Aspects," 55–56.

85. Raymond H. Prince, "Report from Nigeria: Psychotherapy with Herb Medicine and Magic: 'Curse' as a Possible Precipitating Factor for Neurosis and Psychosis," *Transcultural Psychiatric Research Review* 6 (1959): 42–44; and Raymond H. Prince, "Curse, Invocation and Mental Health among the Yoruba," *Canadian Psychiatric Association Journal* 5 (1960): 65–79.

86. Raymond H. Prince, "The Yoruba Image of the Witch," *Journal of Mental Science* 107 (1961): 795–805.

87. Raymond H. Prince, *Ifa: Yoruba Divination and Sacrifice* (Ibadan: University of Ibadan Press, 1963).

88. Raymond H. Prince, "Some Notes on Yoruba Native Doctors and Their Management of Mental Illness," in Lambo, *First Pan-African Psychiatric Conference*, 279–88; and Raymond H. Prince, "Indigenous Yoruba Psychiatry," in Kiev, *Magic, Faith, and Healing*, 84–120.

89. Allen German and O. P. Arya, "Psychiatric Morbidity amongst a Uganda Student Population," *British Journal of Psychiatry* 115 (1969): 1323–29; and R. M. Wintrob, "The Cultural Dynamics of Student Anxiety: A Report from Liberia," *Psychopathologie africaine* 9 (1973): 267–83.

90. Brian Harris, "A Case of Brain Fag in East Africa," *British Journal of Psychiatry* 138 (1981): 162–63.

91. Paul Parin, "A Case of 'Brain Fag' Syndrome: Psychotherapy of the Patient Adou A. in the Village of Yosso, Ivory Coast Republic," *Psychoanalytic Study of Society* 10 (1984): 1–52.

92. E. A. Guinness, "Profile and Prevalence of the Brain Fag Syndrome: Psychiatric Morbidity in School Populations in Africa," *British Journal of Psychiatry* 160, suppl. 16 (1992): 42–52.

93. Karl Peltzer, Varghese I. Cherian, and Lily Cherian, "Brain Fag Symptoms in Rural South African Secondary School Pupils," *Psychological Reports* 83 (1998): 1187–96.

94. R. Durst, S. Minuchin-Itzigsohn, and K. Jabotinsky-Rubin, "'Brain-Fag' Syndrome: Manifestation of Transculturation in an Ethiopian Jewish Immigrant," *Israel Journal of Psychiatry and Related Sciences* 30, no. 4 (1993): 223–32.

95. Amechi Anumonye, "Emotional Illness among Students of Developing Countries," *Papua New Guinea Medical Journal* 16 (1973): 187.

96. Olufemi Morakinyo, "Personality Variables in Psychiatric Illness Associated with Study among Africans," *African Journal of Psychiatry* 6 (1980): 2.

97. Ibid., 4.

98. Anumonye, "Emotional Illness," 187.

99. Amechi Anumonye, "Efficacy and Tolerance of Injectable Doxepin," *African Journal of Psychiatry* 2 (1975): 167.

100. Peter F. Omoluabi, "Psychophysiological Indicants of Brain-Fag Syndrome," in *Psychology and Society: Selected Readings*, ed. Eileen B. Wilson (Ile-Ife: Nigerian Psychological Association, 1986), 107–19.

101. Olufemi Morakinyo, "A Psychophysiological Theory of a Psychiatric Illness (the Brain Fag Syndrome) Associated with Study among Africans," *Journal of Nervous and Mental Disease* 168, no. 2 (1980): 86.

102. Omoluabi, "Psychophysiological Indicants."

103. R. Olukayode Jegede, "Psychiatric Illness in African Students: 'Brain Fag' Syndrome Revisited," *Canadian Journal of Psychiatry* 28 (1983): 190.

104. Ibid., 191.

105. Raymond H. Prince, "The Concept of Culture-Bound Syndromes: Anorexia Nervosa and Brain-Fag," *Social Science and Medicine* 21, no. 2 (1985): 201.

106. Omoluabi, "Psychophysiological Indicants," 119.

107. Jegede, "Psychiatric Illness," 191.

108. Ibid., 192.

109. Rwegellera, "Cultural Aspects," 48.

110. APA, *DSM-IV*, 846.

111. Olufemi Morakinyo and Karl Peltzer, "'Brain Fag' Symptoms in Apprentices in Nigeria," *Psychopathology* 35 (2002): 362–66; and O. Ayonrinde, "Brain Fag Syndrome: New Wine in Old Bottles or Old Wine in New Bottles?," *Nigerian Journal of Psychiatry* 6, no. 2 (2008): 47–50.

CHAPTER 5: GATEKEEPERS OF THE MIND

Epigraphs: C. Ramanohisoa, "The African Region," in *Traditional Medicine and Health Care Coverage: A Reader for Health Administrators and Practitioners*, ed. Robert H. Bannerman, John Burton, and Ch'en Wen-Chieh (Geneva: World Health Organization, 1983), 209; and Philip Singer, "Traditional Healing and the Medical/Psychiatric Mafia," in *Traditional Healing: New Science or New Colonialism?*, ed. Philip Singer (Owerri: Conch Magazine, 1977), 247.

1. For much more on this subject, see Steven Feierman and John M. Janzen, eds., *The Social Basis of Health and Healing in Africa* (Berkeley: University of California Press, 1992); and Karen E. Flint, *Healing Traditions: African Medicine, Cultural Exchange, and Competition in South Africa, 1820–1948* (Athens: Ohio University Press, 2008).

2. See, for example, Jacob K. Olupona, *City of 201 Gods: Ile-Ife in Time, Space, and the Imagination* (Berkeley: University of California Press, 2011), for a perspective on

how Yoruba religious beliefs have changed over time within Nigeria. A good deal of scholarship has also been conducted on the ways that Yoruba religious beliefs crossed the Atlantic Ocean in the context of the transatlantic slave trade. In the New World, Yoruba beliefs proved versatile and adaptable, but the core of the belief system remained intact in many places in the Americas, perhaps most notably in Cuba and Brazil. See, for example, Sandra T. Barnes, ed., *Africa's Ogun: Old World and New*, 2nd ed. (Bloomington: Indiana University Press, 1997); Joseph M. Murphy and Mei-Mei Sanford, eds., *Osun across the Waters: A Yoruba Goddess in Africa and the Americas* (Bloomington: Indiana University Press, 2001); and Toyin Falola and Matt D. Childs, eds., *The Yoruba Diaspora in the Atlantic World* (Bloomington: Indiana University Press, 2004).

3. On diversity of Yoruba beliefs, see, for example, Toyin Falola and Ann Genova, *Orisa: Yoruba Gods and Spiritual Identity in Africa and the Diaspora* (Trenton, NJ: Africa World Press, 2005).

4. Although, as in other areas, there is significant diversity in the origin tale of the Yoruba. Samuel Johnson's monumental *The History of the Yorubas* (Lagos: CCS, 2006), first published 1921, famously has Odudwa as a son of Lamuduru, one of the "kings of Mecca." The version of the tale presented here can be found in Olupona, *City of 201 Gods*, 29–30.

5. Anthony D. Buckley, *Yoruba Medicine* (Oxford: Clarendon, 1985).

6. W. R. Bascom, *Ifa Divination: Communication between Gods and Men in West Africa* (Bloomington: Indiana University Press, 1969).

7. Roger O. A. Makanjuola, "Yoruba Traditional Healers in Psychiatry, I: Healers' Concepts of the Nature and Aetiology of Mental Disorders," *African Journal of Medicine and Medical Sciences* 16 (1987): 53–59.

8. Roger O. A. Makanjuola and A. A. Jaiyeola, "Yoruba Traditional Healers in Psychiatry, II: Management of Psychiatric Disorders," *African Journal of Medicine and Medical Sciences* 16 (1987): 61–73. On Sọ̀npọ̀nnọ́, see Raymond H. Prince, "Indigenous Yoruba Psychiatry," in *Magic, Faith, and Healing: Studies in Primitive Psychiatry Today*, ed. Ari Kiev (London: Free Press, 1964), 84–120.

9. The best example of this in the Yoruba context being Buckley, *Yoruba Medicine*.

10. On such debates in medical anthropology, see Byron J. Good, *Medicine, Rationality, and Experience: An Anthropological Perspective* (Cambridge: Cambridge University Press, 1994).

11. A process that occurred in non-Western environments around the globe in the first half of the twentieth century. See Warwick P. Anderson, Deborah Jenson, and Richard C. Keller, eds., *Unconscious Dominions: Psychoanalysis, Colonial Trauma, and Global Sovereignties* (Durham, NC: Duke University Press, 2011).

12. For a general overview of psychoanalysis, see Joseph Schwartz, *Cassandra's Daughter: A History of Psychoanalysis* (New York: Viking, 1999).

13. Christiane Hartnack, *Psychoanalysis in Colonial India* (New Delhi: Oxford University Press, 2001).

14. Warwick P. Anderson, Deborah Jenson, and Richard C. Keller, "Introduction: Globalizing the Unconscious," in *Unconscious Dominions*, 9.

15. Frantz Fanon, *The Wretched of the Earth*, trans. Constance Farrington (New York: Monthly Review Press, 1978), first published 1961; and Octave Mannoni, *Prospero and Caliban: The Psychology of Colonization* (Ann Arbor: University of Michigan Press, 1990), first published 1950.

16. Ashis Nandy, "The Savage Freud: The First Non-Western Psychoanalyst and the Politics of Secret Selves in Colonial India," in *The Savage Freud and Other Essays on Possible and Retrievable Selves* (Princeton, NJ: Princeton University Press, 1995), 81–144; and Sudhir Kakar, *Culture and Psyche: Psychoanalysis and India* (New York: Psyche Press, 1996).

17. See, for example, Ranjana Khanna, *Dark Continents: Psychoanalysis and Colonialism* (Durham, NC: Duke University Press, 2003).

18. Anderson, Jenson, and Keller, "Introduction," 17.

19. Sigmund Freud, *Totem and Taboo: Some Points of Agreement between the Mental Lives of Savages and Neurotics*, trans. James Strachey (New York: Norton, 1950), 88, first published 1913.

20. J. J. Clarke, *Jung and Eastern Thought: A Dialogue with the Orient* (London: Routledge, 1994); and Blake W. Burleson, *Jung in Africa* (New York: Continuum, 2005).

21. See Jock McCulloch, *Colonial Psychiatry and "The African Mind"* (Cambridge: Cambridge University Press, 1995), 77–90.

22. Wulf Sachs, *Black Hamlet* (London: Geoffery Bles, 1937); Sachs, *Black Anger* (Boston: Little, Brown, 1947).

23. B. J. F. Laubscher, *Sex, Custom and Psychopathology* (New York: Humanities Press, 1952), xii, first published 1937.

24. Margaret J. Field, *Search for Security: An Ethno-Psychiatric Study of Rural Ghana* (Evanston, IL: Northwestern University Press, 1960).

25. Prince, "Indigenous Yoruba Psychiatry," 86–88.

26. Raymond H. Prince, "Curse, Invocation and Mental Health among the Yoruba," *Canadian Psychiatric Association Journal* 5, no. 2 (1960): 78.

27. Raymond H. Prince, "The Yoruba Image of the Witch," *Journal of Mental Science* 107 (1961): 796–97.

28. Ibid., 804.

29. Ibid.

30. Prince, "Curse, Invocation and Mental Health," 65–66.

31. T. Adeoye Lambo, *African Traditional Beliefs: Concepts of Health and Medical Practice* (Ibadan: Ibadan University Press, 1963), 4.

32. Ibid.

33. Ibid., 5.

34. Ibid.

35. T. Adeoye Lambo, "Traditional African Cultures and Western Medicine," in *Medicine and Culture*, ed. F. N. L. Poynter (London: Wellcome Institute of the History of Medicine, 1969), 206.

36. Lambo, *African Traditional Beliefs*, 8.

37. See, for example, Michael O. Olatawura, "Psychotherapy for the Nigerian Patient: Some Aspects of the Problems Involved," *Psychotherapy and Psychosomatics* 25 (1975): 259–66.

38. T. Adeoye Lambo, "Patterns of Psychiatric Care in Developing African Countries," in Kiev, *Magic, Faith, and Healing*, 443–44.

39. Ibid.

40. Lambo, *African Traditional Beliefs*, 8.

41. Lambo, "Traditional African Cultures," 202.

42. J. A. G. Johnson and J. B. Omopetu to Chief Secretary to the Government, Lagos, 15 January 1935, Nigerian National Archives, Ibadan [NNAI] CSO 26/1 01507/S.2, 68.

43. R. D. Ross, for Acting Chief Secretary to the Government, Lagos, to the Herbal Kingdom Society, Lagos, 21 January 1935, NNAI CSO 26/1 01507/S.2, 69.

44. R. Cunyngham Brown, *Report III on the Care and Treatment of Lunatics in the British West African Colonies: Nigeria* (Letchworth, UK: Garden City Press, 1938), 11.

45. Ibid.

46. J. C. Carothers, "A Report on the Psychiatric Services of Nigeria," (1955), NNAI MH 59/S.9, 10.

47. Ibid., 42–43.

48. See, for example, Kilton M. Stewart, *Pygmies and Dream Giants* (New York: Norton, 1954); Georges Devereux, *Reality and Dream: Psychotherapy of a Plains Indian* (New York: International Universities Press, 1951); and Marvin K. Opler, "Dream Analysis in Ute Indian Therapy," in *Culture and Mental Health: Cross-Cultural Studies*, ed. Marvin K. Opler (New York: Macmillan, 1959), 97–118. A good synthesis of this scholarship and its historical antecedents can be found in Ari Kiev, "The Study of Folk Psychiatry," in *Magic, Faith, and Healing*, 3–35, a book that, not coincidentally, contains chapters by Raymond H. Prince and T. Adeoye Lambo cited elsewhere in this chapter.

49. Prince, "Indigenous Yoruba Psychiatry," 110, 116.

50. Ibid., 110–11.

51. Ibid., 114.

52. The exact nature of Sọ̀npọ̀nnọ is variable across Yoruba communities. Buckley refers to Sọ̀npọ̀nnọ in the masculine singular and makes reference to the extent to which different cults "see Sopono in a significantly different manner" (*Yoruba Medicine*, 98–99). I provide the description of Sọ̀npọ̀nnọ as a family of spirits here because this particular interpretation formed the basis of Prince's analysis of the psychotherapeutic effects of the cult.

53. Raymond H. Prince, "The Problem of 'Spirit Possession' as a Treatment for Psychiatric Disorders," *Ethos* 2, no. 4 (1974): 318.

54. Prince, "Indigenous Yoruba Psychiatry," 114.

55. Raymond H. Prince, "Possession Cults and Social Cybernetics," in *Trance and Possession States*, ed. Raymond H. Prince (Montreal: R. M. Burke Memorial Society, 1968), 161.

56. Prince, "Indigenous Yoruba Psychiatry," 114.

57. A point he makes more explicitly in Raymond H. Prince, "Psychotherapy as the Manipulation of Endogenous Healing Mechanisms: A Transcultural Survey," *Transcultural Psychiatric Research Review* 13 (1976): 115–33.

58. Lambo, *African Traditional Beliefs*, 10.

59. Ibid.

60. Ibid.

61. T. Adeoye Lambo, "Neuropsychiatric Observations in the Western Region of Nigeria," *British Medical Journal*, 2, no. 5006 (1956): 10.

62. T. Adeoye Lambo, "Some Unusual Features of Schizophrenia among Primitive Peoples," *West African Medical Journal* 6 (1957): 150.

63. Lambo, "Neuropsychiatric Observations," 1389.

64. Lambo, *African Traditional Beliefs*, 10.

65. Lambo, "Neuropsychiatric Observations," 1389.
66. Prince, "Indigenous Yoruba Psychiatry," 116.
67. Ibid.
68. Raymond H. Prince, "Fundamental Differences of Psychoanalysis and Faith Healing," *International Journal of Psychiatry* 10 (1972): 125.
69. Ibid.
70. Ibid.
71. Ibid.
72. Raymond H. Prince, "Mental Health Workers Should be Trained at Home: Some Implications of Transcultural Psychiatric Research," *African Journal of Psychiatry* 2 (1972): 279.
73. Prince, "Indigenous Yoruba Psychiatry," 116.
74. Lambo, "Traditional African Cultures," 205.
75. Lambo, "Patterns of Psychiatric Care," 449–50.
76. Ibid., 443–44.
77. Prince, "Indigenous Yoruba Psychiatry," 116.
78. Tolani Asuni, "Aro Hospital in Perspective," *American Journal of Psychiatry* 124, no. 6 (1967): 767–68.
79. Ibid.
80. Tolani Asuni, "Existing Concepts of Mental Illness in Different Cultures and Traditional Forms of Treatment," in *Mental Health Services in Developing Countries: Papers Presented at a WHO Seminar on the Organization of Mental Health Services*, ed. Taha Ahmed Baasher, T. Adeoye Lambo, G. Morris Carstairs, Robert Giel, and F. R. Hassler (Addis Ababa: World Health Organization, 1975), 12.
81. Tolani Asuni, "Treatment of Depression," *Psychopathologie africaine* 17 (1981): 194–95.
82. Ibid.
83. Tolani Asuni, "Social, Cultural and Economic Determinants of Psychiatric Services in Western Nigeria," *African Journal of Psychiatry* 1 (1975): 12–13.
84. Asuni, "Existing Concepts," 12.
85. Ibid.
86. Asuni, "Treatment of Depression," 194–95.
87. Tolani Asuni, "Modern Medicine and Traditional Medicine," in *African Therapeutic Systems*, ed. Z. A. Ademuwagun, John A. A. Ayoade, Ira E. Harrison, and Dennis M. Warren (Waltham, MA: African Studies Association, 1979), 177.
88. Ibid.
89. Asuni, "Social, Cultural and Economic Determinants," 12–13.
90. Ibid.
91. Ibid.
92. See, for example, Lambo, *African Traditional Beliefs*, 4–5.
93. Prince, "Fundamental Differences," 125.
94. Prince, "Indigenous Yoruba Psychiatry," 113.
95. T. Adeoye Lambo, "The Village of Aro," in *Medical Care in Developing Countries: A Symposium from Makerere, Nairobi, Lusaka, Addis Ababa*, ed. M. King (London: Oxford University Press, 1966), 20:6.
96. Lambo, "Patterns of Psychiatric Care," 443–44.
97. Although it is beyond the scope of this work to discuss, it is important to note that traditional healers, for their part, engaged in the same gatekeeping processes as

they chose which elements of Western health systems to incorporate into their "traditional" practices.

98. Asuni, "Social, Cultural and Economic Determinants," 12–13.

99. R. Olukayode Jegede, "Aro Village System of Community Psychiatry in Perspective," *Canadian Journal of Psychiatry* 26 (1981): 174.

CHAPTER 6: THE PARADOXES OF PSYCHOACTIVE DRUGS

1. Edward Shorter, *A History of Psychiatry: From the Era of the Asylum to the Age of Prozac* (New York: John Wiley, 1997), 246–55.

2. For a background on the history of psychopharmacology and its detractors, see David Healy, "The Intersection of Psychopharmacology and Psychiatry in the Second Half of the Twentieth Century," in *History of Psychiatry and Medical Psychology*, ed. Edwin R. Wallace IV and John Gach (New York: Springer, 2008), 419–37; Charles Barber, *Comfortably Numb: How Psychiatry Is Medicating a Nation* (New York: Pantheon, 2003). A fascinating case study of the effects of the psychopharmaceutical revolution in twenty-first-century Argentina can be found in Andrew Lakoff, *Pharmaceutical Reason: Knowledge and Value in Global Psychiatry* (Cambridge: Cambridge University Press, 2005).

3. Andrew Sherratt, "Introduction: Peculiar Substances," in *Consuming Habits: Drugs in History and Anthropology*, ed. Jordan Goodman, Paul E. Lovejoy, and Andrew Sherratt (London: Routledge, 1995), 1.

4. Arthur S. Reber, *Dictionary of Psychology*, 2nd ed. (New York: Penguin, 1995), 612.

5. Healy, "Intersection of Psychopharmacology and Psychiatry," 431.

6. At least according to Asuni, Lambo and Boroffka: Tolani Asuni, "Socio-Psychiatric Problems of Cannabis in Nigeria," *UN Bulletin on Narcotics* 16 (1964): 17–28; T. Adeoye Lambo, "Medical and Social Problems of Drug Addiction in West-Africa with Special Emphasis on Psychiatric Aspects," *UN Bulletin on Narcotics* 17 (1965): 3–13; and Alexander Boroffka, "Mental Illness and Indian Hemp in Lagos," *East African Medical Journal* 43, no. 9 (1966): 377–84.

7. Key antipsychiatry texts include Ronald D. Laing, *The Divided Self: An Existential Study in Sanity and Madness* (London: Tavistock, 1960); Thomas Szasz, *The Myth of Mental Illness: Foundations of a Theory of Personal Conduct* (New York: Hober-Harper, 1961); and David Cooper, *Psychiatry and Anti-Psychiatry* (London: Tavistock, 1967).

8. David Healy, *The Creation of Psychopharmacology* (Cambridge, MA: Harvard University Press, 2002), provides an outstanding overview of the growth of the psychopharmaceutical industry and professional responses to it. Healy himself has been an active critic of the corporate promotion of antidepressants since the 1990s. See, for example, Healy, *The Antidepressant Era* (Cambridge, MA: Harvard University Press, 1997); and Healy, *Let Them Eat Prozac: The Unhealthy Relationship between the Pharmaceutical Industry and Depression* (New York: New York University Press, 2004).

9. David T. Courtwright, *Forces of Habit: Drugs and the Making of the Modern World* (Cambridge, MA: Harvard University Press, 2001), 168–73.

10. Asuni, "Socio-Psychiatric Problems," 17–28; Lambo, "Medical and Social Problems," 3–13; and Boroffka, "Mental Illness and Indian Hemp," 377–84.

11. Lambo, "Medical and Social Problems," 3.

12. Boroffka, "Mental Illness and Indian Hemp," 379.

13. See James H. Mills, *Cannabis Britannica: Empire, Trade, and Prohibition, 1800–1928* (Oxford: Oxford University Press, 2003).

14. See, for example, Paul E. Lovejoy, *Caravans of Kola: The Hausa Kola Trade, 1700–1900* (Oxford: Oxford University Press, 1980); and Edmund Abaka, *"Kola Is God's Gift": Agricultural Production, Export Initiatives, and the Kola Industry of Asante and the Gold Coast, c. 1820–1950* (Athens: Ohio University Press, 2005).

15. The literature on alcohol trade and consumption in Nigeria is large. See, for example, Charles Ambler, "Alcohol and the Slave Trade in West Africa, 1400–1850," in *Drugs, Labor, and Colonial Expansion*, ed. William Jankowiak and Daniel Bradburd (Tucson: University of Arizona Press, 2003), 73–88; Chima J. Korieh, "Alcohol and Empire: 'Illicit' Gin Prohibition and Control in Colonial Eastern Nigeria," *African Economic History* 31 (2003): 111–34; and A. Olorunfemi, "The Liquor Traffic Dilemma in British West Africa: The Southern Nigerian Example, 1895–1918," *International Journal of African Historical Studies* 17, no. 2 (1984): 229–41.

16. Asuni, "Socio-Psychiatric Problems," 20.

17. Ibid., 20, 21.

18. Lambo, "Medical and Social Problems," 7.

19. Asuni, "Socio-Psychiatric Problems," 21.

20. Lambo, "Medical and Social Problems," 7.

21. Asuni, "Socio-Psychiatric Problems," 29–30.

22. Traders and fishermen are listed specifically in this group. Boroffka, "Mental Illness and Indian Hemp," 380.

23. Lambo, "Medical and Social Problems," 6, emphasis in original.

24. Ibid., 6, 9.

25. Boroffka, "Mental Illness and Indian Hemp," 381.

26. Asuni, "Socio-Psychiatric Problems," 25–26.

27. Ibid., 30, 31.

28. Lambo, "Medical and Social Problems," 3; and Asuni, "Socio-Psychiatric problems," 21.

29. Asuni, "Socio-Psychiatric Problems," 31.

30. Ibid., 30.

31. Ibid.

32. Ibid., 29.

33. Lambo, "Medical and Social Problems," 6.

34. Ibid.,12.

35. Boroffka, "Mental Illness and Indian Hemp," 381.

36. Ibid., 383, emphasis in original.

37. Ibid.

38. Amechi Anumonye, "Alcohol and Drug Use in Youth," in *Proceedings of 6th International Institute on Prevention and Treatment of Drug Dependence*, ed. Eva Tongue and L. Graz (Hamburg: ICCA, 1976): 36–54.

39. Ibid., 42.

40. Moses O. Akindele, "Drugs and University Drop-Outs: Some Observations," in Association of Psychiatrists in Africa, *Proceedings of the 1974 Workshop of the Association of Psychiatrists in Africa: Alcohol and Drug Dependence* (Lausanne: ICCA, 1974), 77.

41. Ibid., 79.

42. Ibid., 78.

43. V. Olufemi Oviasu, "The Abuse of Cannabis in Nigeria," *Nigerian Medical Journal* 6 (1976): 359–66.

44. Ibid., 362.

45. Ibid.

46. John C. Ebie and Ona A. Pela, "Some Sociocultural Aspects of the Problem of Drug Abuse in Nigeria," *Drug and Alcohol Dependence* 8 (1981): 301–6; and M. H. Ahmed, "Drug Abuse, Women and Society: Some Demographic Characteristics of Female Cases in the University Department of Psychiatry, Kaduna, Nigeria, in 1980–1986," *West African Journal of Medicine* 8 (1989): 241–45.

47. A. O. Odejide and Michael O. Olatawura, "Alcohol Use in a Nigerian Rural Community," *African Journal of Psychiatry* 3 (1977): 69–74. See also A. O. Odejide, "Alcohol Use in a Sub-Group of Literate Nigerians," *African Journal of Psychiatry* 5 (1979): 15–20.

48. John C. Ebie and Ona A. Pela, "Substance Abuse in Nigeria: Review of Epidemiological Studies," in *Handbook of the Nigerian Training Course on Drug Dependence*, ed. John C. Ebie and Eve J. Tongue (Lausanne: ICCA, 1981), 5–10.

49. Ibid., 7, 8.

50. Ibid., 8, quoting J. Nevadomsky, "Patterns of Self-Reported Drug Use among Secondary School Students in Bendel State, Nigeria," *Narcotics Bulletin* 33, no. 1 (1981): 9–19.

51. M. H. Ahmed and Moses O. Akindele, "Drug Abuse as Seen in the Psychiatric Unit of Ahmadu Bello University Hospital, Kaduna," in *Proceedings of the 1974 Workshop of the Association of Psychiatrists in Africa*, 102.

52. A. O. Odejide, "Cross-Cultural Psychiatry: A Myth or Reality," *Comprehensive Psychiatry* 20, no. 2 (1979): 105–6.

53. T. Adeoye Lambo, "Further Neuropsychiatric Observations in Nigeria with Comments on the Need for Epidemiological Study in Africa," *British Medical Journal* 2 (1960): 1700.

54. Shorter, *History of Psychiatry*, 254; and Healy, *Creation of Psychopharmacology*, 130–36.

55. Raymond H. Prince, "The Use of Rauwolfia for the Treatment of Psychoses by Nigerian Native Doctors," *American Journal of Psychiatry* 117 (1960): 147–49.

56. A. O. Odejide, "Patterns of Psychotropic Drug Use in a Nigerian Psychiatric Outpatient Clinic," *International Pharmacopsychiatry* 15 (1980): 21.

57. Odejide, "Cross-Cultural Psychiatry," 106.

58. A. O. Odejide and Thomas A. Ban, "Psychotropic Drug Prescription Pattern in a Developing Country (Nigeria): The Need for an Essential Psychotherapeutic Drug List," *International Pharmacopsychiatry* 17 (1982): 163–69.

59. O. O. Famuyiwa, "Psychotropic Drug Prescription in Nigeria," *Acta Psychiatrica Scandinavia* 68 (1983): 73–81.

60. Ibid., 79.

61. A. O. Oejide and O. Ayinde, "Psychotropic and Antiparkinsonian Drug Use: An Examination of Prescription Practices," *African Journal of Psychiatry* 4 (1978): 31–36.

62. Ibid., 36.

63. Ibid., 35.

64. Odejide, "Patterns of Psychotropic Drug Use," 21–22.

65. See Healy, "Intersection of Psychopharmacology and Psychiatry."

66. Healy, *Creation of Psychopharmacology*, 245–51.

67. Ibid., 225–75.

68. Discussed in Christopher M. Callahan and German E. Berrios, *Reinventing Depression: A History of the Treatment of Depression in Primary Care, 1940–2004* (Oxford: Oxford University Press, 2005), 103–20.

69. Rick Mayes and Allan V. Horowitz, "DSM-III and the Revolution in the Classification of Mental Illness," *Journal of the History of the Behavioral Sciences* 41, no. 3 (2005): 266.

70. Michael O. Olatawura, "Effectiveness of Psychotropic Drugs in Patients in a Poor Nutritional State—A Review," *African Journal of Psychiatry* 2 (1976): 343–49.

71. Michael O. Olatawura, "The Effects of Psychotropic Drugs in Different Populations," *Bulletin of the World Health Organization* 56, no. 4 (1978): 519.

72. Olatawura, "Effectiveness of Psychotropic Drugs," 346.

73. Lambo, "Medical and Social Problems," 9.

74. Ibid., 8–9.

75. Anumonye, "Alcohol and Drug Use," 47.

76. A. O. Odejide, "Pattern of Psychotropic Drug Use: A Survey of Civil Service Workers in Ibadan, Nigeria" (paper presented at Thirty-Third International Congress on Alcoholism and Drug Dependence, Tangiers, Morocco, 10–15 October 1982), 34–43.

77. Ibid.

78. Olayiwola Erinosho, "Socio-Cultural Factors in Drug Use: The Case of Nigeria," in Ebie and Tongue, *Handbook*, 68.

79. Amechi Anumonye, "Drug Use among Young People in Lagos, Nigeria," *Bulletin on Narcotics* 32, no. 4 (1980): 39.

80. Erinosho, "Socio-Cultural Factors," 66.

81. Ibid.

82. Anumonye, "Alcohol and Drug Use," 40.

83. Erinosho, "Socio-Cultural Factors," 66.

CONCLUSION: NIGERIAN PSYCHIATRISTS AND THE GLOBALIZATION OF PSYCHIATRY

1. Raymond H. Prince, "The Changing Picture of Depressive Syndromes in Africa: Is It Fact or Diagnostic Fashion?," *Canadian Journal of African Studies* 1 (1967): 177–92.

2. Peter O. Ebigbo and U. H. Ihezue, "Uncertainty in the Use of Western Diagnostic Illness Categories for Labelling Mental illness in Nigeria," *Psychopathologie africaine* 18 (1982): 64.

3. Ibid., 66.

4. Roger O. A. Makanjuola, "'Ode Ori': A Culture-Bound Disorder with Prominent Somatic Features in Yoruba Nigerian Patients," *Acta Psychiatrica Scandinavia* 75 (1987): 231–36.

5. Ibid.

6. Raymond H. Prince, "Indigenous Yoruba Psychiatry," in *Magic, Faith, and Healing: Studies in Primitive Psychiatry Today*, ed. Ari Kiev (London: Free Press, 1964), 87.

7. Makanjuola, "Ode Ori," 234.

8. Ibid.

9. Sunny T. C. Ilechukwu, "Ogbanje/Abiku: A Culture-Bound Construct of Childhood and Family Psychopathology in West Africa," *Psychopathologie africaine* 23, no. 1 (1990–91): 54.

10. Ibid.

11. Ebigbo and Ihezue, "Uncertainty," 69.

12. Roger O. A. Makanjuola and A. A. Jaiyeola, "Yoruba Traditional Healers in Psychiatry, II: Management of Psychiatric Disorders," *African Journal of Medicine and Medical Science* 16 (1987): 69.

13. For a background on religious tensions in postindependence Nigeria, see, for example, Toyin Falola, *Violence in Nigeria: The Crisis of Religious Politics and Secular Ideologies* (Rochester, NY: University of Rochester Press, 1998); and Simeon O. Ilesanmi, *Religious Pluralism and the Nigerian State* (Athens: Ohio University Press, 1997).

14. A good overview of the Nigerian civil war of 1967–70 and the tensions that brought it about can be found in John de St. Jorre, *The Brothers' War: Biafra and Nigeria* (Boston: Houghton Mifflin, 1972).

15. On the political regimes of postindependence Nigeria, see Eghosa E. Osaghae, *Crippled Giant: Nigeria Since Independence* (Bloomington: Indiana University Press, 1998).

16. On the development of the petro-economy in the 1970s, see Tom G. Forrest, *Politics and Economic Development in Nigeria* (Boulder, CO: Westview Press, 1993).

17. On effects of structural adjustment on Nigeria, see Osaghae, *Crippled Giant*; Forrest, *Politics and Economic Development*; Adebayo O. Olukoshi, *The Politics of Structural Adjustment in Nigeria* (London: James Currey, 1993); Julius O. Ihonvbere, *Nigeria: The Politics of Adjustment and Democracy* (New Brunswick, NJ: Transaction, 1994); and Gary G. Moser, Scott Rogers, and Reinhold van Til, *Nigeria: Experience with Structural Adjustment* (Washington, DC: International Monetary Fund, 1997).

18. See, for example, Tolani Asuni, "Social, Cultural and Economic Determinants of Psychiatric Services in Western Nigeria," *African Journal of Psychiatry* 1 (1975): 3–15; and U. H. Ihezue, "Out Patient Psychiatric Clinic of a Nigerian University Teaching Hospital: Survey of Its Services," *Psychopathologie africaine* 18 (1982): 349–51.

19. R. Olukayode Jegede, "Aro Village System of Community Psychiatry in Perspective," *Canadian Journal of Psychiatry* 26 (1981): 174.

20. Alexander Boroffka, *"Psychiatry in Nigeria": (A Partly Annotated Bibliography) with an Introductory Chapter on "The History of Psychiatry in Nigeria"* (Kiel: Brunswiker Universitätsbuchhandlung—Medizin, 2006), 540.

21. Dr. Timothy Adebowale, Director of Clinical Services, Aro Neuropsychiatric Hospital, personal communication, 24 August 2012.

22. Although not always. Many psychiatrists also considered the difficulties of psychiatry to lie primarily in the discipline's inability to explain or treat mental illnesses in ways that would allow them to become more culturally relevant than traditional healers, whom psychiatrists well recognized continued to be the option of first resort for most of their patients. See A. Kalunta, "Depressive Illness: Its Cultural Aspects," *Psychopathologie africaine* 17 (1981): 122–26.

23. John C. Ebie and Ona A. Pela, "Some Sociocultural Aspects of the Problem of Drug Abuse in Nigeria," *Drug and Alcohol Dependence* 8 (1981): 301–6.

24. Benjamin O. Osuntokun and Alexander Boroffka, "Hysteria in Nigerians," *Nigerian Medical Journal* 5 (1975): 6–13.

25. S. Ejiofo Mbanefo, "The Effect of Crisis on the Mental Health of a Community," *Journal of the Royal College of General Practitioners* 21 (1971): 52.

26. Kalunta, "Depressive Illness," 121.

27. On dependency theory in Africa, see, in particular, Walter Rodney, *How Europe Underdeveloped Africa*, rev. ed. (Washington, DC: Howard University Press, 1982),

originally published in 1972; and Samir Amin, *Neo-Colonialism in West Africa*, trans. Francis McDonagh (New York: Monthly Review Press, 1973), originally published as *L'Afrique de L'Ouest Bloquée* (Paris: Les Editions de Minuit, 1971).

28. Key texts outlining the postcolonial critique include Edward W. Said, *Culture and Imperialism* (New York: Knopf, 1993); Homi K. Bhabha, *The Location of Culture* (New York: Routledge, 1994); Gayatri C. Spivak, *A Critique of Postcolonial Reasoning: Toward a History of the Vanishing Present* (Cambridge, MA: Harvard University Press, 1999); and Achille Mbembe, *On the Postcolony* (Berkeley: University of California Press, 2001).

29. For a literature review, see Byron J. Good, *Medicine, Rationality, and Experience: An Anthropological Perspective* (Cambridge: Cambridge University Press, 1994), 25–64.

30. Ibid., 53.

31. Roland Littlewood, "From Categories to Contexts: A Decade of the 'New Cross-Cultural Psychiatry,'" *British Journal of Psychiatry* 156 (1990): 308.

32. Arthur M. Kleinman, "Depression, Somatization, and the 'New Cross-Cultural Psychiatry," *Social Science and Medicine* 11 (1977): 3, 5.

33. Ibid., 5.

34. Ibid., 4, emphasis in original.

35. A distinction that was already being made in sociology by this time. Ibid., 9.

36. For an overview of research conducted using the methodology of the "new cross-cultural psychiatry" in the 1980s, see Littlewood, "From Categories to Contexts," 308–27.

37. Roland Littlewood, "How Universal Is Something We Can Call 'Therapy'? Some Implications of Non-Western Healing Systems for Intercultural Work," *Holistic Medicine* 5 (1990): 49–65.

38. As in Julian P. Leff, "The 'New Cross-Cultural Psychiatry': A Case of the Baby and the Bathwater," *British Journal of Psychiatry* 156 (1990): 305–7.

39. American Psychiatric Association, *Diagnostic and Statistical Manual of Mental Disorders*, 3rd ed. (Washington, DC: American Psychiatric Association, 1980).

40. For example, Benjamin R. Barber, *Jihad vs. McWorld* (New York: Ballantine, 1995).

41. Ethan Watters, *Crazy Like Us: The Globalization of the American Psyche* (New York: Free Press, 2010).

42. Frederick Cooper refers to this narrative style as a "leapfrogging legacy," which he defines as "claiming that something in time A caused something in time C without considering time B, which lies in between." See Cooper, *Colonialism in Question: Theory, Knowledge, History* (Berkeley: University of California Press, 2005), 17–18.

43. See, for example, A. G. Hopkins, "The History of Globalization—and the Globalization of History?," in *Globalization in World History*, ed. A. G. Hopkins (New York: Norton, 2001), 12–44.

44. A great example of this kind of scholarship linking Africa to processes of globalization and global history is Jeremy Prestholdt, *Domesticating the World: African Consumerism and the Genealogies of Globalization* (Berkeley: University of California Press, 2008).

45. As in, for example, Warwick P. Anderson, Deborah Jenson, and Richard C. Keller, eds., *Unconscious Dominions: Psychoanalysis, Colonial Trauma, and Global Sovereignties* (Durham, NC: Duke University Press, 2011).

Bibliography

ARCHIVES CONSULTED

National Archives of the United Kingdom, Public Record Office, Kew
Nigerian National Archives, Ibadan
Nigerian National Archives, Kaduna
World Health Organization Archives, Geneva

NEWSPAPERS

West African Pilot

BOOKS AND ARTICLES

Abaka, Edmund. *"Kola Is God's Gift": Agricultural Production, Export Initiatives and the Kola Industry of Asante and the Gold Coast, c. 1820–1950*. Athens: Ohio University Press, 2005.

Adas, Michael. *Machines as the Measure of Men: Science, Technology, and Ideologies of Western Dominance.* Ithaca, NY: Cornell University Press, 1989.

Adi, Hakim. "West African Students in Britain, 1900–1960: The Politics of Exile." *Immigrants and Minorities* 12, no. 3 (1993): 107–28.

Afigbo, Adiele E. "Sir Ralph Moor and the Economic Development of Southern Nigeria: 1896–1903." In *Nigerian History, Politics and Affairs: The Collected Essays of Adiele Afigbo*, edited by Toyin Falola, 185–212. Trenton, NJ: Africa World Press, 2005.

———. *The Warrant Chiefs: Indirect Rule in Southeastern Nigeria, 1891–1929*. London: Longman, 1972.

Ahmed, M. H. "Drug Abuse, Women and Society, Some Demographic Characteristics of Female Cases in the University Department of Psychiatry, Kaduna, Nigeria, in 1980–1986." *West African Journal of Medicine* 8 (1989): 241–45.

Ahmed, M. H., and Moses O. Akindele. "Drug Abuse as Seen in the Psychiatric Unit of Ahmadu Bello University Hospital, Kaduna." In Association of Psychiatrists in Africa, *Proceedings of the 1974 Workshop of the Association of Psychiatrists in Africa: Alcohol and Drug Dependence*, 102–4.

Akindele, Moses O.. "Drugs and University Drop-Outs: Some Observations." In Association of Psychiatrists in Africa, *Proceedings of the 1974 Workshop of the Association of Psychiatrists in Africa: Alcohol and Drug Dependence*, 77–79.

Ambler, Charles. "Alcohol and the Slave Trade in West Africa, 1400–1850." In *Drugs, Labor, and Colonial Expansion*, edited by William Jankowiak and Daniel Bradburd, 73–88. Tucson: University of Arizona Press, 2003.
American Psychiatric Association. *Diagnostic and Statistical Manual of Mental Disorders*. 3rd ed. Washington, DC: American Psychiatric Association, 1980.
——. *Diagnostic and Statistical Manual of Mental Disorders*. 4th ed. Washington, DC: American Psychiatric Association, 1994.
Amin, Samir. *Neo-Colonialism in West Africa*. Translated by Francis McDonagh. New York: Monthly Review Press, 1973. Originally published as *L'Afrique de L'Ouest Bloquée* (Paris: Les Editions de Minuit, 1971).
Anderson, Warwick P. "Where Is the Postcolonial History of Medicine?," *Bulletin of the History of Medicine* 72 (1998): 522–30.
Anderson, Warwick P., Deborah Jenson, and Richard C. Keller, eds. *Unconscious Dominions: Psychoanalysis, Colonial Trauma, and Global Sovereignties*. Durham, NC: Duke University Press, 2011.
Anumonye, Amechi. *African Students in Alien Cultures*. Buffalo, NY: Black Academy Press, 1970.
——. "Alcohol and Drug Use in Youth." In *Proceedings of 6th International Institute on Prevention and Treatment of Drug Dependence*, edited by Eva Tongue and L. Graz, 36–54. Hamburg: ICCA, 1976.
——. "Drug Use among Young People in Lagos, Nigeria." *Bulletin on Narcotics* 32, no. 4 (1980): 39–45.
——. "Efficacy and Tolerance of Injectable Doxepin." *African Journal of Psychiatry* 2 (1975): 165–67.
——. "Emotional Illness among Students of Developing Countries." *Papua New Guinea Medical Journal* 16 (1973): 183–88.
——. "Emotional Stresses among African Students in Britain." *Scottish Medical Journal* 12 (1967): 314–19.
Arnold, David, ed. *Colonizing the Body: State Medicine and Epidemic Disease in Nineteenth-Century India*. Berkeley: University of California Press, 1993.
——. *Imperial Medicine and Indigenous Societies*. Manchester: Manchester University Press, 1992.
Association of Psychiatrists in Africa. *Proceedings of the 1974 Workshop of the Association of Psychiatrists in Africa: Alcohol and Drug Dependence*. Lausanne: ICCA, 1974.
——. *Report of the Third Pan-African Psychiatric Workshop*. Ibadan: Government Printer, 1971.
Asuni, Tolani. "Aro Hospital in Perspective." *American Journal of Psychiatry* 124, no. 6 (1967): 763–70.
——. "Development of Psychiatry in Africa." In *Mental Health in Africa and the Americas Today*, edited by Samuel O. Okpaku, 17–32. Nashville, TN: Chrisolith Books, 1991.
——. "Existing Concepts of Mental Illness in Different Cultures and Traditional Forms of Treatment." In *Mental Health Services in Developing Countries: Papers Presented at a WHO Seminar on the Organization of Mental Health Services*, edited by Taha Ahmed Baasher, T. Adeoye Lambo, G. Morris Carstairs, Robert Giel, and F. R. Hassler, 12–17. Addis Ababa: World Health Organization, 1975.
——. "Modern Medicine and Traditional Medicine." In *African Therapeutic Systems*, edited by Z. A. Ademuwagun, John A. A. Ayoade, Ira E. Harrison, and Dennis M. Warren, 176–81. Waltham, MA: African Studies Association, 1979.

———. "The Review of Nigerian Students Repatriated on Psychiatric Grounds." *West African Medical Journal* 17 (1968): 3–7.
———. "Social, Cultural and Economic Determinants of Psychiatric Services in Western Nigeria." *African Journal of Psychiatry* 1 (1975): 3–15.
———. "Socio-Psychiatric Problems of Cannabis in Nigeria." *UN Bulletin on Narcotics* 16 (1964): 17–28.
———. "Therapeutic Communities of the Hospital and Villages in Aro Hospital Complex in Nigeria." *African Journal of Psychiatry* 1 (1979): 35–42.
———. "Treatment of Depression." *Psychopathologie africaine* 17 (1981): 190–96.
Ayonrinde, O. "Brain Fag Syndrome: New Wine in Old Bottles or Old Wine in New Bottles?" *Nigerian Journal of Psychiatry* 6, no. 2 (2008): 47–50.
Bains, Jatinder. "Race, Culture and Psychiatry: A History of Transcultural Psychiatry." *History of Psychiatry* 16, no. 2 (2005): 139–54.
Barber, Benjamin R. *Jihad vs. McWorld.* New York: Ballantine, 1995.
Barber, Charles. *Comfortably Numb: How Psychiatry Is Medicating a Nation.* New York: Pantheon, 2003.
Barnes, Sandra T., ed. *Africa's Ogun: Old World and New.* 2nd ed. Bloomington: Indiana University Press, 1997.
Bascom, W. R. *Ifa Divination: Communication between Gods and Men in West Africa.* Bloomington: Indiana University Press, 1969.
Basalla, George. "The Spread of Western Science." *Science* 156 (1967): 611–22.
Bégué, Jean-Michel. "French Psychiatry in Algeria (1830–1962): From Colonial to Transcultural." *History of Psychiatry* 7 (1996): 533–48.
Bell, Leland V. *Mental and Social Disorder in Sub-Saharan Africa: The Case of Sierra Leone, 1787–1990.* Westport, CT: Greenwood Press, 1991.
Bhabha, Homi K. *The Location of Culture.* New York: Routledge, 1994.
Biehl, João, Byron J. Good, and Arthur M. Kleinman, eds. *Subjectivity: Ethnographic Investigations.* Berkeley: University of California Press, 2007.
Binitie, Ayo. "Experiences in the Development and Planning of Psychiatric Services in Mid-Western State of Nigeria." *Psychopathologie africaine* 6 (1970): 201–8.
Bleuler, Eugen. *Textbook of Psychiatry.* New York: Macmillan, 1976.
Boroffka, Alexander. "The History of Mental Hospitals in Nigeria." *Psychiatry* 8 (1985): 37–43.
———. "A History of Psychiatry in Nigeria." *Psychiatry* 8 (1985): 709–14.
———. "Mental Illness and Indian Hemp in Lagos." *East African Medical Journal* 43, no. 9 (1966): 377–84.
———. *"Psychiatry in Nigeria": (A Partly Annotated Bibliography) with an Introductory Chapter on "The History of Psychiatry in Nigeria."* Kiel: Brunswiker Universitätsbuchhandlung—Medizin, 2006.
Boroffka, Alexander, and A. A. Marinho. "Psychoneurotic Syndromes in Urbanized Nigerians." *Transcultural Psychiatric Research Review* 15 (1963): 44–46.
Borstelmann, Thomas. *The Cold War and the Color Line: American Race Relations in the Global Arena.* Cambridge, MA: Harvard University Press, 2001.
Brown, R. Cunyngham. *Report III on the Care and Treatment of Lunatics in the British West African Colonies: Nigeria.* Letchworth, UK: Garden City Press, 1938.
Buckley, Anthony D. *Yoruba Medicine.* Oxford: Clarendon, 1985.
Bullard, Alice. "The Critical Impact of Frantz Fanon and Henri Collomb: Race, Gender and Personality Testing of North and West Africans." *Journal of the History of Behavioral Sciences* 41, no. 3 (2005): 225–48.

——. "Imperial Networks and Postcolonial Independence: The Transition from Colonial to Transcultural Psychiatry." In Mahone and Vaughan, *Psychiatry and Empire*, 197–219.
Burke, A. W. "The Consequences of Unplanned Repatriation." *British Journal of Psychiatry* 123 (1973): 109–11.
Burleson, Blake W. *Jung in Africa*. New York: Continuum, 2005.
Callahan, Christopher M., and German E. Berrios. *Reinventing Depression: A History of the Treatment of Depression in Primary Care, 1940–2004*. Oxford: Oxford University Press, 2005.
Carothers, J. C. *The African Mind in Health and Disease: A Study in Ethnopsychiatry*. Geneva: World Health Organization, 1953.
——. "Some Speculations on Insanity in Africans in General." *East African Medical Journal* 17 (1940): 90–105.
——. "A Study of Mental Derangement in Africans, and an Attempt to Explain Its Peculiarities, More Especially in Relation to the African Attitude to Life." *Journal of Mental Science* 93 (1947): 548–97.
Chakrabarty, Dipesh. "The Legacies of Bandung: Decolonization and the Politics of Culture." In *Making a World After Empire: The Bandung Moment and Its Political Afterlives*, edited by Christopher J. Lee, 45–68. Athens: Ohio University Press, 2010.
——. *Provincializing Europe: Postcolonial Thought and Historical Difference*. Princeton, NJ: Princeton University Press, 2000.
Chambers, David W., and Richard Gillespie. "Locality in the History of Science: Colonial Science, Technoscience, and Indigenous Knowledge." *Osiris* 15 (2000): 221–40.
Clarke, J. J. *Jung and Eastern Thought: A Dialogue with the Orient*. London: Routledge, 1994.
Coleman, James S. *Nigeria: Background to Nationalism*. Berkeley: University of California Press, 1960.
Collomb, Henri, and Jacques Zwingelstein. "Depressive States in an African Community." In Lambo, *First Pan-African Psychiatric Conference*, 227–34.
Comaroff, Jean, and John L. Comaroff. "The Madman and the Migrant: Work and Labor in the Historical Consciousness of a South African People." *American Ethnologist* 14, no. 2 (1987): 191–209.
Cooper, David. *Psychiatry and Anti-Psychiatry*. London: Tavistock, 1967.
Cooper, Frederick. *Colonialism in Question: Theory, Knowledge, History*. Berkeley: University of California Press, 2005.
——. "Conflict and Connection: Rethinking Colonial African History." *American Historical Review* 99, no. 5 (1994): 1516–45.
Courtwright, David T. *Forces of Habit: Drugs and the Making of the Modern World*. Cambridge, MA: Harvard University Press, 2001.
Cox, John L., ed. *Transcultural Psychiatry*. London: Croom Helm, 1986.
Crowder, Michael. *The Story of Nigeria*. 4th ed. London: Faber and Faber, 1978.
Curtin, Philip D. "Medical Knowledge and Urban Planning in Tropical Africa." *American Historical Review* 90, no. 3 (1985): 594–613.
Davidson, S. "Psychiatric Work among the Bemba." *Rhodes-Livingstone Journal* 7 (1949): 75–86.
Deacon, Harriet J. "Madness, Race and Moral Treatment: Robben Island Lunatic Asylum, Cape Colony, 1846–1890." *History of Psychiatry* 7 (1996): 287–97.

Devereux, Georges. *Reality and Dream: Psychotherapy of a Plains Indian.* New York: International Universities Press, 1951.
Drayton, Richard H. *Nature's Government: Science, Imperial Britain, and the "Improvement" of the World.* New Haven, CT: Yale University Press, 2000.
Durst, R., S. Minuchin-Itzigsohn, and K. Jabotinsky-Rubin. "'Brain-Fag' Syndrome: Manifestation of Transculturation in an Ethiopian Jewish Immigrant." *Israel Journal of Psychiatry and Related Sciences* 30, no. 4 (1993): 223–32.
Ebie, John C. "Some Observations on Depressive Illness in Nigerians Attending a Psychiatric Out-Patient Clinic." *African Journal of Medical Science* 3 (1972): 149–55.
Ebie, John C., and Ona A. Pela. "Some Sociocultural Aspects of the Problem of Drug Abuse in Nigeria." *Drug and Alcohol Dependence* 8 (1981): 301–6.
——. "Substance Abuse in Nigeria: Review of Epidemiological Studies." In Ebie and Tongue, *Handbook of the Nigerian Training Course on Drug Dependence*, 5–10.
Ebie, John C., and Eve J. Tongue, eds. *Handbook of the Nigerian Training Course on Drug Dependence.* Lausanne: ICCA, 1981.
Ebigbo, Peter O., and U. H. Ihezue. "Uncertainty in the Use of Western Diagnostic Illness Categories for Labelling Mental Illness in Nigeria." *Psychopathologie africaine* 18 (1982): 59–74.
Echenberg, Myron J. *Black Death, White Medicine: Bubonic Plague and the Politics of Public Health in Colonial Senegal, 1914–1945.* Portsmouth, NH: Heinemann, 2002.
Edgerton, Robert B. "Traditional Treatment for Mental Illness in Africa: A Review." *Culture, Medicine and Psychiatry* 4 (1980): 167–89.
Ekundare, R. Olufemi. *An Economic History of Nigeria, 1860–1960.* London: Methuen, 1973.
Erinosho, Olayiwola. "Socio-Cultural Factors in Drug Use: The Case of Nigeria." In Ebie and Tongue, *Handbook of the Nigerian Training Course on Drug Dependence*, 65–69.
Falola, Toyin. *Development Planning and Decolonization in Nigeria.* Gainesville: University Press of Florida, 1996.
——. *Nationalism and African Intellectuals.* Rochester, NY: University of Rochester Press, 2001.
——. *Violence in Nigeria: The Crisis of Religious Politics and Secular Ideologies.* Rochester, NY: University of Rochester Press, 1998.
Falola, Toyin, and Matt D. Childs, eds. *The Yoruba Diaspora in the Atlantic World.* Bloomington: Indiana University Press, 2004.
Falola ,Toyin, and Ann Genova. *Orisa: Yoruba Gods and Spiritual Identity in Africa and the Diaspora.* Trenton, NJ: Africa World Press, 2005.
Falola, Toyin, and Matthew M. Heaton. *A History of Nigeria.* Cambridge: Cambridge University Press, 2008.
Famuyiwa, O. O. "Psychotropic Drug Prescription in Nigeria." *Acta Psychiatrica Scandinavia* 68 (1983): 73–81.
Fanon, Frantz. *Black Skin, White Masks.* Translated by Charles Lam Markmann. New York: Grove Press, 1967. First published 1952.
——. *A Dying Colonialism.* Translated by Haakon Chevalier. New York: Grove Press, 1965. First published 1959.
——. *The Wretched of the Earth.* Translated by Constance Farrington. New York: Monthly Review Press, 1978. First published 1961.

Fassin, Didier. "Ethnopsychiatry and the Postcolonial Encounter: A French Psychopolitics of Otherness." In Anderson, Jenson, and Keller, *Unconscious Dominions*, 223–46.

Feierman, Steven. "Struggles for Control: The Social Roots of Health and Healing in Modern Africa." *African Studies Review* 28, nos. 2–3 (1985): 73–147.

Feierman, Steven, and John M. Janzen, eds. *The Social Basis of Health and Healing in Africa*. Berkeley: University of California Press, 1992.

Fernando, Suman. "Depression and Ethnic Minorities." In Cox, *Transcultural Psychiatry*, 107–38.

Field, Margaret J. *Search for Security: An Ethno-Psychiatric Study of Rural Ghana*. Evanston, IL: Northwestern University Press, 1960.

Flint, Karen E. *Healing Traditions: African Medicine, Cultural Exchange, and Competition in South Africa, 1820–1948*. Athens: Ohio University Press, 2008.

Forrest, Tom G. *Politics and Economic Development in Nigeria*. Boulder, CO: Westview Press, 1993.

Forster, E. F. B. "Treatment of the African Mental Patient." In Lambo, *First Pan-African Psychiatric Conference*, 276–79.

Foucault, Michel. *Madness and Civilization: A History of Insanity in the Age of Reason*. Translated by Richard Howard. New York: Vintage, 1965.

Freud, Sigmund. *Totem and Taboo: Some Points of Agreement between the Mental Lives of Savages and Neurotics*. Translated by James Strachey. New York: Norton, 1950. First published 1913.

Gailey, Harry A. *The Road to Aba: A Study of British Administrative Policy in Eastern Nigeria*. New York: New York University Press, 1970.

Gaines, Kevin K. *American Africans in Ghana: Black Expatriates and the Civil Rights Era*. Chapel Hill: University of North Carolina Press, 2006.

Gallais, P., and L. Planques. "Etudes sur la deficiences mentale dans les terretoires d'outre mer: Perspectives ethnopsychiatriques dans l'Union francaise." *Medicine tropicale* 11 (1951): 5–30.

German, Allen, and O. P. Arya. "Psychiatric Morbidity amongst a Uganda Student Population." *British Journal of Psychiatry* 115 (1969): 1323–29.

Gillis, L.S. "Observations from South Africa." In Lambo, *First Pan-African Psychiatric Conference*, 236–38.

Gilman, Sander L. "Constructing Schizophrenia as a Category of Mental Illness." In Wallace and Gach, *History of Psychiatry and Medical Psychology*, 461–83.

Gilroy, Paul. *"There Ain't No Black in the Union Jack": The Cultural Politics of Race and Nation*. Chicago: University of Chicago Press, 1987.

Gish, Oscar. "Color and Skill: British Immigration, 1955–1968." *International Migration Review* 3, no. 1 (1968): 19–37.

Good, Byron J. *Medicine, Rationality, and Experience: An Anthropological Perspective*. Cambridge: Cambridge University Press, 1994.

Good, Mary-Jo DelVecchio, Sandra T. Hyde, Sarah Pinto, and Byron J. Good, eds. *Postcolonial Disorders*. Berkeley: University of California Press, 2008.

Gottesman, Irving I. *Schizophrenia Genesis: The Origins of Madness*. New York: W. H. Freeman, 1991.

Grob, Gerald N., ed. *Immigrants and Insanity: Dissenting Views, 1883–1914*. New York: Arno Press, 1980.

Grove, Richard. *Green Imperialism: Colonial Expansion, Tropical Island Edens and the Origins of Environmentalism, 1600–1860*. Cambridge: Cambridge University Press, 1995.
Guinness, E. A. "Profile and Prevalence of the Brain Fag Syndrome: Psychiatric Morbidity in School Populations in Africa." *British Journal of Psychiatry* 160, suppl. 16 (1992): 42–52.
Hansen, Randall. *Citizenship and Immigration in Post-War Britain*. Oxford: Oxford University Press, 2000.
Harris, Brian. "A Case of Brain Fag in East Africa." *British Journal of Psychiatry* 138 (1981): 162–63.
Hartnack, Christiane. *Psychoanalysis in Colonial India*. New Delhi: Oxford University Press, 2001.
——. "Vishnu on Freud's Desk: Psychoanalysis in Colonial India." *Social Research* 57, no. 4 (1990): 921–49.
Headrick, Daniel R. *The Tools of Empire: Technology and European Imperialism in the Nineteenth Century*. Oxford: Oxford University Press, 1991.
Healy, David. *The Antidepressant Era*. Cambridge, MA: Harvard University Press, 1997.
——. *The Creation of Psychopharmacology*. Cambridge, MA: Harvard University Press, 2002.
——. "The Intersection of Psychopharmacology and Psychiatry in the Second Half of the Twentieth Century." In Wallace and Gach, *History of Psychiatry and Medical Psychology*, 419–37.
——. *Let Them Eat Prozac: The Unhealthy Relationship between the Pharmaceutical Industry and Depression*. New York: New York University Press, 2004.
Hemsi, L. K. "Psychiatric Morbidity of West Indian Immigrants." *Social Psychiatry* 2 (1967): 95–100.
Heussler, Robert. *The British in Northern Nigeria*. London: Oxford University Press, 1968.
Hobsbawm, Eric J., and Terence Ranger. *The Invention of Tradition*. Cambridge: Cambridge University Press, 1983.
Hodge, Joseph M. *Triumph of the Expert: Agrarian Doctrines of Development and the Legacies of British Colonialism*. Athens: Ohio University Press, 2007.
Hopkins, A. G. "The History of Globalization—and the Globalization of History?" In *Globalization in World History*, edited by A. G. Hopkins, 12–44. New York: Norton, 2001.
Howells, John G., ed. *World History of Psychiatry*. New York: Brunner/Mazel, 1975.
Ihezue, U. H. "Out Patient Psychiatric Clinic of a Nigerian University Teaching Hospital: Survey of Its Services," *Psychopathologie africaine* 18 (1982): 349–51.
Ihonvbere, Julius O. *Nigeria: The Politics of Adjustment and Democracy*. New Brunswick, NJ: Transaction, 1994.
Ilechukwu, Sunny T. C. "Ogbanje/Abiku: A Culture-Bound Construct of Childhood and Family Psychopathology in West Africa." *Psychopathologie africaine* 23, no. 1 (1990–91): 19–60.
Ilesanmi, Simeon O. *Religious Pluralism and the Nigerian State*. Athens: Ohio University Press, 1997.
Iliffe, John. *East African Doctors: A History of the Modern Profession*. Cambridge: Cambridge University Press, 1998.

Isichei, Elizabeth. *A History of the Igbo People.* London: Macmillan, 1976.
Jackson, Lynette A. *Surfacing Up: Psychiatry and Social Order in Colonial Zimbabwe, 1908–1968.* Ithaca, NY: Cornell University Press, 2005.
Jackson, Stanley W. *Melancholia and Depression: From Hippocratic Times to Modern Times.* New Haven, CT: Yale University Press, 1986.
Janzen, John M. *The Quest for Therapy: Medical Pluralism in Lower Zaire.* Berkeley: University of California Press, 1978.
Jegede, R. Olukayode. "Aro Village System of Community Psychiatry in Perspective." *Canadian Journal of Psychiatry* 26 (1981): 173–77.
——. "Nigerian Psychiatry in Perspective." *Acta Psychiatrica Scandinavia* 63 (1981): 45–56.
——. "Psychiatric Illness in African Students: 'Brain Fag' Syndrome Revisited." *Canadian Journal of Psychiatry* 28 (1983): 188–92.
Johnson, Samuel. *The History of the Yorubas.* Lagos: CCS, 2006. First Published 1921.
Jones, Edgar, Shahina Rahman, and Robin Woolven. "The Maudsley Hosptial: Design and Strategic Direction, 1923–39." *Medical History* 51, no. 3 (2007): 357–78.
Kakar, Sudhir. *Culture and Psyche: Psychoanalysis and India.* New York: Psyche Press, 1996.
Kalunta, A. "Depressive Illness: Its Cultural Aspects." *Psychopathologie africaine* 17 (1981): 113–26.
Keller, Richard C. *Colonial Madness: Psychiatry in French North Africa.* Chicago: University of Chicago Press, 2007.
Khanna, Ranjana. *Dark Continents: Psychoanalysis and Colonialism.* Durham, NC: Duke University Press, 2003.
Kidd, Cecil B. "Psychiatric Morbidity among Students." *British Journal of Preventive and Social Medicine* 19, no. 4 (1965): 143–50.
Kiev, Ari, ed. *Magic, Faith, and Healing: Studies in Primitive Psychiatry Today.* London: Free Press, 1964.
——. *Transcultural Psychiatry.* New York: Free Press, 1972.
Kleinman, Arthur M. "Depression, Somatization, and the 'New Cross-Cultural Psychiatry.'" *Social Science and Medicine* 11 (1977): 3–10.
——. *Patients and Healers in the Context of Culture: An Exploration of the Borderland between Anthropology, Medicine, and Psychiatry.* Berkeley: University of California Press, 1980.
Korieh, Chima J. "Alcohol and Empire: 'Illicit' Gin Prohibition and Control in Colonial Eastern Nigeria." *African Economic History* 31 (2003): 111–34.
Laing, Ronald D. *The Divided Self: An Existential Study in Sanity and Madness.* London: Tavistock, 1960.
Lakoff, Andrew. *Pharmaceutical Reason: Knowledge and Value in Global Psychiatry.* Cambridge: Cambridge University Press, 2005.
Lambo, T. Adeoye. *African Traditional Beliefs: Concepts of Health and Medical Practice.* Ibadan: Ibadan University Press, 1963.
——. "Changing Patterns of Mental Health Needs in Africa." *Contemporary Review* 222, no. 1286 (1973): 146–54.
——. "Early Childhood Experience and Adult Personality." In *Cultural Adaptation within Modern Africa*, edited by S. H. Irvine and J. T. Sanders, 117–27. New York: Teachers College Press, 1972.

——, ed. *First Pan-African Psychiatric Conference, Abeokuta, Nigeria.* Ibadan: Government Printer, 1961.

——. "A Form of Social Psychiatry in Africa." *World Mental Health* 13 (1960): 190–203.

——. "Further Neuropsychiatric Observations in Nigeria: With Comments on the Need for Epidemiological Study in Africa." *British Medical Journal* 2, no. 5214 (1960): 1696–1704.

——. "Important Areas of Ignorance and Doubt in the Psychology of the African." In *The Proceedings of the First International Congress of Africanists,* edited by Lalage Bown and Michael Crowder, 337–44. Evanston, IL: Northwestern University Press, 1964.

——. "Medical and Social Problems of Drug Addiction in West-Africa: With Special Emphasis on Psychiatric Aspects." *UN Bulletin on Narcotics* 17 (1965): 3–13.

——. "Neuropsychiatric Observations in the Western Region of Nigeria." *British Medical Journal* 2, no. 5006 (1956): 1388–94.

——. "A New World in the Making." *World Health* (April 1980): 2–5.

——. "Patterns of Psychiatric Care in Developing African Countries." In Kiev, *Magic, Faith, and Healing,* 443–53.

——. "The Role of Cultural Factors in Paranoid Psychosis among the Yoruba Tribe." *Journal of Mental Science* 101 (1955): 239–66.

——. "Schizophrenic and Borderline States." In *Transcultural Psychiatry,* edited by Anthony V. S. de Reuck and Ruth Porter, 62–75. Boston: Little, Brown, 1965.

——. "Socioeconomic Changes in Africa and Their Implications for Mental Health." In *Man and Africa,* edited by Gordon Wolstenholme and Maeve O'Connor, 121–45. Boston: Little, Brown, 1965.

——. "Some Unusual Features of Schizophrenia among Primitive Peoples." *West African Medical Journal* 6 (1957): 147–52.

——. *A Study of Social and Health Problems of Nigerian Students in Great Britain and Ireland.* Ibadan: Government Printer, 1958.

——. "Thomas Lambo." In *Psychiatrists on Psychiatry,* edited by Michael Shepherd, 98–123. Cambridge: Cambridge University Press, 1982.

——. "Towards Justice in Health." *World Health* (July 1979): 2–5.

——. "Traditional African Cultures and Western Medicine." In *Medicine and Culture,* edited by F. N. L. Poynter, 201–10. London: Wellcome Institute of the History of Medicine, 1969.

——. "The Village of Aro." In *Medical Care in Developing Countries: A Symposium from Makerere, Nairobi, Lusaka, Addis Ababa,* edited by M. King, 20:6. London: Oxford University Press, 1966.

Last, Murray. "Introduction: The Professionalisation of African Medicine: Ambiguities and Definitions." In *The Professionalisation of African Medicine,* edited by Murray Last and G. L. Chavunduka, 1–19. Manchester: Manchester University Press, 1986.

Laubscher, B. J. F. *Sex, Custom and Psychopathology: A Study of South African Pagan Natives.* New York: Humanities Press, 1952. First published 1937.

Lawlor, Clark. *From Melancholia to Prozac: A History of Depression.* Oxford: Oxford University Press, 2012.

Leff, Julian P. "The 'New Cross-Cultural Psychiatry': A Case of the Baby and the Bathwater." *British Journal of Psychiatry* 156 (1990): 305–7.

——. *Psychiatry around the Globe: A Transcultural View.* London: Gaskell, 1988.

Leighton, Alexander H., T. Adeoye Lambo, Charles C. Hughes, Dorothea C. Leighton, Jane M. Murphy, and David B. Macklin. *Psychiatric Disorder among the Yoruba: A Report from the Cornell-Aro Mental Health Research Project in the Western Region, Nigeria.* Ithaca, NY: Cornell University Press, 1963.
Lester, Alan. "Imperial Circuits and Networks: Geographies of the British Empire." *History Compass* 4, no. 1 (2006): 124–41.
Levine, Philippa. *Prostitution, Race, and Politics: Policing Venereal Disease in the British Empire.* New York: Routledge, 2003.
Leys, Colin. *The Rise and Fall of Development Theory.* Bloomington: Indiana University Press, 1996.
Littlewood, Roland. "From Categories to Contexts: A Decade of the 'New Cross-Cultural Psychiatry.'" *British Journal of Psychiatry* 156 (1990): 308–27.
——. "How Universal Is Something We Can Call 'Therapy'? Some Implications of Non-Western Healing Systems for Intercultural Work." *Holistic Medicine* 5 (1990): 49–65.
Littlewood, Roland, and Maurice Lipsedge. "Acute Psychotic Reactions in Caribbean-Born Patients." *Psychological Medicine* 11 (1981): 303–18.
——. *Aliens and Alienists: Ethnic Minorities and Psychiatry.* New York: Penguin, 1982.
——. "Some Social and Phenomenological Characteristics of Psychotic Immigrants." *Psychological Medicine* 11 (1981): 289–302.
Livingstone, David N. *Putting Science in Its Place: Geographies of Scientific Knowledge.* Chicago: University of Chicago Press, 2003.
Lovejoy, Paul E. *Caravans of Kola: The Hausa Kola Trade, 1700–1900.* Oxford: Oxford University Press, 1980.
Luedke, Tracy J., and Harry G. West, eds. *Borders and Healers: Brokering Therapeutic Resources in Southeast Africa.* Bloomington: Indiana University Press, 2006.
Lugard, Frederick. *The Dual Mandate in British Tropical Africa.* 5th ed. London: Archon, 1965.
Lyons, Maryinez. *The Colonial Disease: A Social History of Sleeping Sickness in Northern Zaire, 1900–1940.* Cambridge: Cambridge University Press, 1992.
Mahone, Sloan, and Megan Vaughan, eds. *Psychiatry and Empire.* New York: Palgrave Macmillan, 2007.
Makanjuola, J. D. A. "The Aro Drug Addiction Research and Treatment Centre: A First Report." *British Journal of Addiction* 81 (1986): 809–14.
Makanjuola, Roger O. A. "'Ode Ori': A Culture-Bound Disorder with Prominent Somatic Features in Yoruba Nigerian Patients." *Acta Psychiatrica Scandinavia* 75 (1987): 231–36.
——. "Yoruba Traditional Healers in Psychiatry, I: Healers' Concepts of the Nature and Aetiology of Mental Disorders." *African Journal of Medicine and Medical Sciences* 16 (1987): 53–59.
Makanjuola, Roger O. A., and A. A. Jaiyeola. "Yoruba Traditional Healers in Psychiatry, II: Management of Psychiatric Disorders." *African Journal of Medicine and Medical Science* 16 (1987): 67–73.
Mannoni, Octave. *Prospero and Caliban: The Psychology of Colonization.* Ann Arbor: University of Michigan Press, 1990. First published 1950.
Marks, Shula. "What Is Colonial about Colonial Medicine? And What Has Happened to Imperialism and Health?" *Social History of Medicine* 10, no. 2 (1997): 205–19.

Mayes, Rick, and Allan V. Horowitz. "DSM-III and the Revolution in the Classification of Mental Illness." *Journal of the History of the Behavioral Sciences* 41, no. 3 (2005): 249–67.
Mbanefo, S. Ejiofo. "The Effect of Crisis on the Mental Health of a Community." *Journal of the Royal College of General Practitioners* 21 (1971): 44–52.
Mbembe, Achille. *On the Postcolony.* Berkeley: University of California Press, 2001.
McCulloch, Jock. *Colonial Psychiatry and "The African Mind."* Cambridge: Cambridge University Press, 1995.
Meriwether, James H. *Proudly We Can Be Africans: Black Americans and Africa, 1935–1961.* Chapel Hill: University of North Carolina Press, 2002.
Metzl, Jonathan M. *The Protest Psychosis: How Schizophrenia Became a Black Disease.* Boston: Beacon Press, 2009.
Mills, James H. *Cannabis Britannica: Empire, Trade, and Prohibition, 1800–1928.* Oxford: Oxford University Press, 2003.
Morakinyo, Olufemi. "Personality Variables in Psychiatric Illness Associated with Study among Africans." *African Journal of Psychiatry* 6 (1980): 1–5.
———. "A Psychophysiological Theory of a Psychiatric Illness (the Brain Fag Syndrome) Associated with Study among Africans." *Journal of Nervous and Mental Disease* 168, no. 2 (1980): 84–89.
Morakinyo, Olufemi, and Karl Peltzer. " 'Brain Fag' Symptoms in Apprentices in Nigeria." *Psychopathology* 35 (2002): 362–66.
Moser, Gary G., Scott Rogers, and Reinhold van Til. *Nigeria: Experience with Structural Adjustment.* Washington, DC: International Monetary Fund, 1997.
Murphy, H. B. M. "The Historical Development of Transcultural Psychiatry," in Cox, *Transcultural Psychiatry*, 7–22.
Murphy, H. B. M., Eric D. Wittkower, and N. A. Chance. "Crosscultural Inquiry into the Symptomatology of Depression: A Preliminary Report." *Transcultural Psychiatry* 1 (1964): 5–18.
Murphy, H. B. M., Eric D. Wittkower, J. Fried, and H. Ellenberger. "A Cross-Cultural Survey of Schizophrenic Symptomatology." *International Journal of Social Psychiatry* 9 (1963): 237–49.
Murphy, Joseph M., and Mei-Mei Sanford, eds. *Osun across the Waters: A Yoruba Goddess in Africa and the Americas.* Bloomington: Indiana University Press, 2001.
Nandy, Ashis."The Savage Freud: The First Non-Western Psychoanalyst and the Politics of Secret Selves in Colonial India." In *The Savage Freud and Other Essays on Possible and Retrievable Selves*, 81–144. Princeton, NJ: Princeton University Press, 1995.
Nevadomsky, J. "Patterns of Self-Reported Drug Use among Secondary School Students in Bendel State, Nigera." *Narcotics Bulletin* 33, no. 1 (1981): 9–19.
Nicholson, I. F. *The Administration of Nigeria, 1900–1960: Men, Methods, and Myths.* Oxford: Clarendon Press, 1969.
Obembe, Ayodele. "Nigerian Psychiatry—Past, Present, Future." In *Psychiatry in Developing Countries*, edited by Stephen Brown, 4–6. London: Gaskill, 1983.
Odejide, A. O. "Alcohol Use in a Sub-Group of Literate Nigerians." *African Journal of Psychiatry* 5 (1979): 15–20.
———. "Cross-Cultural Psychiatry: A Myth or Reality?" *Comprehensive Psychiatry* 20, no. 2 (1979): 103–9.

———. "A Nigerian Psychiatric Outpatient Clinic: A Point Prevalence Study." *Journal of Clinical Psychiatry* 41, no. 4 (1980): 130–33.
———. "Pattern of Psychotropic Drug Use: A Survey of Civil Service Workers in Ibadan, Nigeria." Paper presented at the Thirty-Third International Congress on Alcoholism and Drug Dependence, Tangiers, Morocco, 10–15 October 1982..
———. "Patterns of Psychotropic Drug Use in a Nigerian Psychiatric Outpatient Clinic." *International Pharmacopsychiatry* 15 (1980): 14–23.
Odejide, A. O., and O. Ayinde. "Psychotropic and Antiparkinsonian Drug Use: An Examination of Prescription Practices." *African Journal of Psychiatry* 4 (1978): 31–36.
Odejide, A. O., and Thomas A. Ban. "Psychotropic Drug Prescription Pattern in a Developing Country (Nigeria): The Need for an Essential Psychotherapeutic Drug List." *International Pharmacopsychiatry* 17 (1982): 163–69.
Odejide, A. O., and Michael O. Olatawura. "Alcohol Use in a Nigerian Rural Community." *African Journal of Psychiatry* 3 (1977): 69–74.
Olatawura, Michael O. "Effectiveness of Psychotropic Drugs in Patients in a Poor Nutritional State—A Review." *African Journal of Psychiatry* 2 (1976): 343–49.
———. "The Effects of Psychotropic Drugs in Different Populations." *Bulletin of the World Health Organization* 56, no. 4 (1978): 519–23.
———. "The Problem of Diagnosing Depression in Nigeria." *Psychopathologie africaine* 9 (1973): 389–403.
———. "Psychotherapy for the Nigerian Patient: Some Aspects of the Problems Involved." *Psychotherapy and Psychosomatics* 25 (1975): 259–66.
Olorunfemi, A. "The Liquor Traffic Dilemma in British West Africa: The Southern Nigerian Example, 1895–1918." *International Journal of African Historical Studies* 17, no. 2 (1984): 229–41.
Olukoshi, Adebayo O. *The Politics of Structural Adjustment in Nigeria*. London: James Currey, 1993.
Olupona, Jacob K. *City of 201 Gods: Ile-Ife in Time, Space, and the Imagination*. Berkeley: University of California Press, 2011.
Omoluabi, Peter F. "Psychophysiological Indicants of Brain-Fag Syndrome." In *Psychology and Society: Selected Readings*, edited by Eileen B. Wilson, 107–19. Ile-Ife: Nigerian Psychological Association, 1986.
Opler, Marvin K. "Dream Analysis in Ute Indian Therapy." In *Culture and Mental Health: Cross-Cultural Studies*, edited by Marvin K. Opler, 97–118. New York: Macmillan, 1959.
Osaghae, Eghosa E. *Crippled Giant: Nigeria Since Independence*. Bloomington: Indiana University Press, 1998.
Osuntokun, Benjamin O., and Alexander Boroffka. "Hysteria in Nigerians." *Nigerian Medical Journal* 5 (1975): 6–13.
Oviasu, V. Olufemi. "The Abuse of Cannabis in Nigeria." *Nigerian Medical Journal* 6 (1976): 359–66.
Oyebode, Femi. "Obituary: Thomas Adeoye Lambo, O.B.E." *Psychiatric Bulletin* 28 (2004): 469.
Packard, Randall M. *White Plague, Black Labor: Tuberculosis and the Political Economy of Health and Disease in South Africa*. Berkeley: University of California Press, 1989.
Parin, Paul. "A Case of 'Brain Fag' Syndrome: Psychotherapy of the Patient Adou A. in the Village of Yosso, Ivory Coast Republic." *Psychoanalytic Study of Society* 10 (1984): 1–52.
Park, Ben. *The Healers of Aro*. New York: United Nations, 1960. Film.

Parle, Julie. "The Fools on the Hill: The Natal Government Asylum and the Institutionalisation of Insanity in Colonial Natal." *Journal of Natal and Zulu History* 19 (2001): 1–40.
Patton, Adell, Jr. *Physicians, Colonial Racism, and Diaspora in West Africa.* Gainesville: University of Florida Press, 1996.
Paul, Kathleen. *Whitewashing Britain: Race and Citizenship in the Postwar Era.* Ithaca, NY: Cornell University Press, 1997.
Peltzer, Karl, Varghese I. Cherian, and Lily Cherian. "Brain Fag Symptoms in Rural South African Secondary School Pupils." *Psychological Reports* 83 (1998): 1187–96.
Perham, Margery. *Native Administration in Nigeria.* London: Oxford University Press, 1937.
Political and Economic Planning. *Colonial Students in Britain: A Report.* London: PEP, 1955.
Porter, Roy. *Mind Forg'd Manacles: A History of Madness in England from the Restoration to the Regency.* Cambridge, MA: Harvard University Press, 1987.
Prestholdt, Jeremy. *Domesticating the World: African Consumerism and the Genealogies of Globalization.* Berkeley: University of California Press, 2008.
Prince, Raymond H. "The 'Brain Fag' Syndrome in Nigerian Students." *Journal of Mental Science* 106 (1960): 559–70.
———. "The Changing Picture of Depressive Syndromes in Africa: Is It Fact or Diagnostic Fashion?" *Canadian Journal of African Studies* 1 (1967): 177–92.
———. "The Concept of Culture-Bound Syndromes: Anorexia Nervosa and Brain-Fag." *Social Science and Medicine* 21, no. 2 (1985): 197–203.
———. "Curse, Invocation and Mental Health among the Yoruba." *Canadian Psychiatric Association Journal* 5 (1960): 65–79.
———. "Functional Symptoms Associated with Study in Nigerian Students." *West African Medical Journal* 11 (1962): 198–206.
———. "Fundamental Differences of Psychoanalysis and Faith Healing." *International Journal of Psychiatry* 10 (1972): 125–28.
———. *Ifa: Yoruba Divination and Sacrifice.* Ibadan: University of Ibadan Press, 1963.
———. "Indigenous Yoruba Psychiatry." In Kiev, *Magic, Faith, and Healing*, 84–120.
———. "Mental Health Workers Should Be Trained at Home: Some Implications of Transcultural Psychiatric Research." *African Journal of Psychiatry* 2 (1972): 277–82.
———. "Possession Cults and Social Cybernetics." In *Trance and Possession States*, edited by Raymond Prince, 157–65. Montreal: R. M. Burke Memorial Society, 1968.
———. "The Problem of 'Spirit Possession' as a Treatment for Psychiatric Disorders." *Ethos* 2, no. 4 (1974): 315–33.
———. "Psychotherapy as the Manipulation of Endogenous Healing Mechanisms: A Transcultural Survey." *Transcultural Psychiatric Research Review* 13 (1976): 115–33.
———. "Report from Nigeria: Psychotherapy with Herb Medicine and Magic: 'Curse' as a Possible Precipitating Factor for Neurosis and Psychosis." *Transcultural Psychiatric Research Review* 6 (1959): 42–44.
———. "Some Notes on Yoruba Native Doctors and Their Management of Mental Illness." In Lambo, *First Pan-African Psychiatric Conference*, 279–88.
———. "Transcultural Aspects of Affective Disorders in Adolescents: The Brain-Fag Syndrome in African Students." In *The Adolescent and Mood Disturbance*, edited by Harvey Golombek and Barry D. Garfinkel, 53–71. New York: International Universities Press, 1983.

——. "The Use of Rauwolfia for the Treatment of Psychoses by Nigerian Native Doctors." *American Journal of Psychiatry* 117 (1960): 147–49.
——. "The Yoruba Image of the Witch." *Journal of Mental Science* 107 (1961): 795–805.
Rack, Philip H. "Migration and Mental Illness." In Cox, *Transcultural Psychiatry*, 59–75.
——. *Race, Culture, and Mental Disorder.* London: Tavistock, 1982.
Raj, Kapil. *Relocating Modern Science: Circulation and the Construction of Knowledge in South Asia and Europe, 1650–1900.* New York: Palgrave Macmillan, 2007.
Raman, A. C., ed. *Proceedings of the Second Pan-African Psychiatric Workshop.* Port Louis: Association of Psychiatrists in Africa, 1972.
Ramanohisoa, C. "The African Region." In *Traditional Medicine and Health Care Coverage: A Reader for Health Administrators and Practitioners*, edited by Robert H. Bannerman, John Burton, and Ch'en Wen-Chieh, 209–21. Geneva: World Health Organization, 1983.
Ranger, Terence, and Paul Slack, eds. *Epidemics and Ideas: Essays on the Historical Perception of Pestilence.* Cambridge: Cambridge University Press, 1992.
Reber, Arthur S. *Dictionary of Psychology.* 2nd ed. New York: Penguin, 1995.
Rodney, Walter. *How Europe Underdeveloped Africa.* Rev. ed. Washington, DC: Howard University Press, 1982.
Rwegellera, G. G. C. "Cultural Aspects of Depressive Illness: Clinical Aspects and Psychopathology." *Psychopathologie africaine* 17 (1981): 41–63.
Sachs, Wulf. *Black Anger.* Boston: Little, Brown, 1947.
——. *Black Hamlet.* London: Geoffery Bles, 1937.
Sadowsky, Jonathan H. "The Confinements of Isaac O.: A Case of 'Acute Mania' in Colonial Nigeria." *History of Psychiatry* 7 (1996): 91–112.
——. *Imperial Bedlam: Institutions of Madness in Colonial Southwest Nigeria.* Berkeley: University of California Press, 1999.
——. "Thomas Adeoye Lambo." In *Doctors, Nurses, and Medical Practitioners: A Bio-Bibliographical Sourcebook*, edited by Lois N. Magner, 172–76. Westport, CT: Greenwood Press, 1997.
Said, Edward W. *Culture and Imperialism.* New York: Knopf, 1993.
Scheff, Thomas J. *Being Mentally Ill: A Sociological Theory.* 2nd ed. Chicago: Aldine de Gruyter, 1982.
Schram, Ralph. *A History of the Nigerian Health Services.* Ibadan: Ibadan University Press, 1971.
Schwartz, Joseph. *Cassandra's Daughter: A History of Psychoanalysis.* New York: Viking, 1999.
Scull, Andrew. *Social Order/Mental Disorder: Anglo-American Psychiatry in Historical Perspective.* London: Routledge, 1989.
Shelley, Horace, and W. H. Watson. "An Investigation Concerning Mental Disorder in the Nyasaland Natives." *Journal of Mental Sciences* 82 (1936): 701–30.
Sherratt, Andrew. "Introduction: Peculiar Substances." In *Consuming Habits: Drugs in History and Anthropology*, edited by Jordan Goodman, Paul E. Lovejoy, and Andrew Sherratt, 1–10. London: Routledge, 1995.
Shorter, Edward. *A Historical Dictionary of Psychiatry.* Oxford: Oxford University Press, 2005.
——. *A History of Psychiatry: From the Era of the Asylum to the Age of Prozac.* New York: John Wiley, 1997.

Simons, Ronald C., and Charles C. Hughes. *The Culture-Bound Syndromes: Folk Illnesses of Psychiatric and Anthropological Interest.* Dordrecht: D. Reidel, 1985.

Singer, Philip. "Traditional Healing and the Medical/Psychiatric Mafia." In *Traditional Healing: New Science or New Colonialism?*, edited by Philip Singer, 242–52. Owerri, Nigeria: Conch Magazine, 1977.

Smith, Robert S. *The Lagos Consulate, 1851–1861.* London: Macmillan, 1978.

Solomos, John. *Race and Racism in Britain.* 3rd ed. New York: Palgrave Macmillan, 2003.

Spencer, Ian R. G. *British Immigration Policy Since 1939: The Making of Multi-Racial Britain.* New York: Routledge, 1997.

Spivak, Gayatri C. *A Critique of Postcolonial Reasoning: Toward a History of the Vanishing Present.* Cambridge, MA: Harvard University Press, 1999.

Stewart, Kilton M. *Pygmies and Dream Giants.* New York: Norton, 1954.

Still, R. J. "Mental Health in Overseas Students." *Proceedings of the British Student Health Association* (1961): 59–61.

St. Jorre, John de. *The Brothers' War: Biafra and Nigeria.* Boston: Houghton Mifflin, 1972.

Swartz, Sally. "Colonizing the Insane: Causes of Insanity in the Cape, 1891–1920." *History of the Human Sciences* 8, no. 4 (1995): 39–57.

Swift, Charles R., and Tolani Asuni. *Mental Health and Disease in Africa: With Special Reference to Africa South of the Sahara.* New York: Churchill Livingstone, 1975.

Szasz, Thomas S. *The Manufacture of Madness: A Comparative Study of the Inquisition and the Mental Health Movement.* New York: Dell, 1970.

———. *The Myth of Mental Illness: Foundations of a Theory of Personal Conduct.* New York: Hoeber-Harper, 1961.

Tamuno, Tekena N. *The Evolution of the Nigerian State: The Southern Phase, 1898–1914.* London: Longman, 1972.

Tassin, Kristen S. "'Lift Up Your Head, My Brother': Nationalism and the Genesis of the Non-Aligned Movement." *Journal of Third World Studies* 23, no. 1 (2006): 147–68.

Tooth, Geoffrey C. *Studies in Mental Illness in the Gold Coast.* London: His Majesty's Stationery Office, 1950.

Union of South Africa. *Annual Report of the Commissioner of Mental Hygiene.* Pretoria: Government Printer, 1950.

Utomi, D. O. "Clinical Psychology at Aro Psychiatric Hospital." In *Clinical Psychology in Africa: South of the Sahara, the Caribbean and Afro-Latin America*, edited by Karl Peltzer and Peter O. Ebigbo, 691–95. Enugu: Working Group for African Psychology, 1989.

Vaughan, Megan. *Curing Their Ills: Colonial Power and African Illness.* Stanford, CA: Stanford University Press, 1991.

———. "Idioms of Madness: Zomba Lunatic Asylum, Nyasaland, in the Colonial Period." *Journal of Southern African Studies* 9, no. 2 (1983): 218–38.

Von Eschen, Penny M. *Race against Empire: Black Americans and Anticolonialism, 1937–1957.* Ithaca, NY: Cornell University Press, 1997.

Wallace, Edwin R., IV, and John Gach, eds. *History of Psychiatry and Medical Psychology.* New York: Springer, 2008.

Watters, Ethan. *Crazy Like Us: The Globalization of the American Psyche.* New York: Free Press, 2010.

Wintrob, R. M. "The Cultural Dynamics of Student Anxiety: A Report from Liberia." *Psychopathologie africaine* 9 (1973): 267–83.

Wittkower, Erik D., H. B. M. Murphy, J. Fried, and H. Ellenberger. "Crosscultural Inquiry into the Symptomatology of Schizophrenia." *Annals of the New York Academy of Science* 84 (1960): 854–63.

World Health Organization. *International Pilot Study of Schizophrenia*. Geneva: World Health Organization, 1973.

——. "The Promotion and Development of Traditional Medicine." *World Health Organization Technical Report Series*, no. 622 (1978).

——. *Schizophrenia: An International Follow-up Study*. Geneva: World Health Organization, 1979.

Yap, P. M. "The Culture-bound Reactive Syndromes." In *Mental Health Research in Asia and the Pacific*, edited by William Caudill and Tsung-Yi Lin, 33–53. Honolulu: East-West Center Press, 1969.

——. "*Koro*—A Culture-Bound Depersonalization Syndrome." *British Journal of Psychiatry* 111 (1965): 43–50.

——. "Mental Diseases Peculiar to Certain Cultures: A Survey of Comparative Psychiatry." *Journal of Mental Science* 97 (1951): 313–27.

Index